THE PSYCHOLOGY OF THE
INFANT

Founded by C. K. Ogden

The International Library of Psychology

DEVELOPMENTAL PSYCHOLOGY
In 32 Volumes

I	The Child's Discovery of Death	*Anthony*
II	The Psychology of the Infant	*Bernfeld*
III	The Psychology of Special Abilities and Disabilities	*Bronner*
IV	The Child and His Family	*Bühler*
V	From Birth to Maturity	*Bühler*
VI	The Mental Development of the Child	*Bühler*
VII	The Psychology of Children's Drawings	*Eng*
VIII	Educational Psychology	*Fox*
IX	A Study of Imagination in Early Childhood	*Griffiths*
X	Understanding Children's Play	*Hartley et al*
XI	Intellectual Growth in Young Children	*Isaacs*
XII	Conversations with Children	*Katz*
XIII	The Growth of the Mind	*Koffka*
XIV	The Child's Unconscious Mind	*Lay*
XV	Infant Speech	*Lewis*
XVI	The Growth of Reason	*Lorimer*
XVII	The Growing Child and its Problems	*Miller*
XVIII	The Child's Conception of Physical Causality	*Piaget*
XIX	The Child's Conception of Geometry	*Piaget et al*
XX	The Construction of Reality in the Child	*Piaget*
XXI	The Early Growth of Logic in the Child	*Inhelder et al*
XXII	The Growth of Logical Thinking from Childhood to Adolescence	*Inhelder et al*
XXIII	Judgement and Reasoning in the Child	*Piaget*
XXIV	The Moral Judgment of the Child	*Piaget*
XXV	Play, Dreams and Imitation in Childhood	*Piaget*
XXVI	The Psychology of Intelligence	*Piaget*
XXVII	Mental Health and Infant Development, V1	*Soddy*
XXVIII	Mental Health and Infant Development, V2	*Soddy*
XXIX	Modern Psychology and Education	*Sturt*
XXX	The Dynamics of Education	*Taba*
XXXI	Education Psychology	*Thorndike*
XXXII	The Principles of Teaching	*Thorndike*

THE PSYCHOLOGY OF THE INFANT

SIEGFRIED BERNFELD

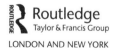

Taylor & Francis Group

LONDON AND NEW YORK

First published in 1929 by
Routledge

Reprinted in 1999, 2000, 2002 by
Routledge
2 Park Square, Milton Park, Abingdon, Oxfordshire OX14 4RN
711 Third Avenue, New York, NY 10017
Transferred to Digital Printing 2007

Routledge is an imprint of the Taylor & Francis Group, an informa business

First issued in paperback 2013

© 1929 Siegfried Bernfeld, Translated by Rosetta Hurwitz

The publishers have made every effort to contact authors/copyright holders
of the works reprinted in the *International Library of Psychology*.
This has not been possible in every case, however, and we would
welcome correspondence from those individuals/companies
we have been unable to trace.

These reprints are taken from original copies of each book. In many cases
the condition of these originals is not perfect. The publisher has gone to
great lengths to ensure the quality of these reprints, but wishes to point
out that certain characteristics of the original copies will, of necessity, be
apparent in reprints thereof.

British Library Cataloguing in Publication Data
A CIP catalogue record for this book
is available from the British Library

The Psychology of the Infant
ISBN13: 978-0-415-20982-3 (hbk)
ISBN13: 978-0-415-86882-2 (pbk)
Developmental Psychology: 32 Volumes
ISBN13: 978-0-415-21128-4
The International Library of Psychology: 204 Volumes
ISBN13: 978-0-415-19132-7

TRANSLATOR'S NOTE

THE substance of this book, which I had the good fortune several years ago to cover in general outline under Dr. Bernfeld's private guidance before it appeared in book form, is uniquely interesting. On the one hand, Dr. Bernfeld confines himself to an intensive study of the brief period in infancy from birth to weaning. On the other hand, he undertakes a broad synthesizing task of twofold character. First, he has sought to extend his researches in this period of infancy back even to primitive beliefs and practices. Second, he has endeavoured to build a Freudian arch over the whole period of modern interest in child psychology—from 1865, through the Gestalt and Eidetic researches of the present day. In the course of his study, Dr. Bernfeld shows how the Freudian psychology and the other schools of psychology often supplement each other, and are not so greatly at variance as they are popularly conceived to be. Finally, he indicates possible lines for further research into the obscurity that veils the first year of human existence.

The range of Dr. Bernfeld's study naturally created terminological difficulties. My aim throughout the translation has been to follow the usage of the school discussed. Thus, *instinctive* is used in its general application, whereas *instinctual* is used in the specifically psychoanalytical passages. All other psycho-analytical terms were translated in accordance with the *Glossary* (Supplement No. 1 to the *International Journal of Psycho-Analysis*). Attention has been called to some of these in the translator's footnotes. In conclusion, I wish to express my grateful appreciation to Dr. Ruth Mack Brunswick for reading portions of the translation in proof, and for her valuable suggestions.

ROSETTA HURWITZ.

CONTENTS

PAGE

PREFACE ix

A. THE NEW-BORN 1

    BIRTH AND PSYCHO-PHYSICAL RETARDATION . 1
    THE FUNCTION OF INFANT REARING . . . 2
    SLEEP 11
    CRYING 19
    NURSING 24
    CONCERNING THE CONSCIOUSNESS OF THE NEW-
        BORN 29
    PSYCHOLOGY OF THE SENSES 35
    DISCHARGE MOVEMENTS 48
    REFLEXES 55
    ACTIONS 56
    THE STRUCTURE OF THE NEW-BORN . . . 58

B. FIRST PROGRESS 63

    SEEING 63
    THE ORAL ZONE 72
    HEARING 83
    INSTINCT GROUPS 93
    LAUGHING, WEEPING, AND FRIGHT . . . 102
    PERCEPTIONS 121
    STRUCTURE OF THE THREE-MONTHS-OLD CHILD . 138

C. THE INSTINCT OF MASTERY 149

    DEVELOPMENT OF THE HAND 149
    SITTING, CRAWLING, CLIMBING 154
    STANDING, WALKING 159
    MATURATION AND LEARNING 163
    FORMS OF MASTERY 178
    THE INSTINCTUAL COMPONENTS OF MASTERY . 186
    LIBIDO DEVELOPMENT OF THE INFANT AT THE
        GRASPING AGE 193

PAGE

D. TRAUMA AND FRUSTRATIONS 210

GENERALITIES 210
BIRTH AS A TRAUMA 214
THE WEANING PERIOD 226

1. DENTITION 228
2. BITING AND CHEWING 240
3. TAKING THE CHILD FROM THE BREAST . 245

E. THE INFANT AND ITS WORLD 261

THE BODY-EGO AND THE OUTER-WORLD . . 261
THE AFFECTIVE ATTITUDES 274
PERCEPTION AND INSTINCT 283
THE SIGNIFICANCE OF WEANING . . . 293

BIBLIOGRAPHY 303

INDEX 307

PREFACE

A MONOGRAPH which aims at being an independent comprehensive presentation of the mental phenomena of the infant during the nursing period has not yet, to my knowledge, been attempted. The fact that there are so many who are interested, both theoretically and practically, in this phase of infancy is sufficient justification for a book on this theme. But since it is not my intention to give merely a compilation, it is perhaps fitting to offer a few words, by way of orientation, concerning the purpose and the point of view of this publication.

I have endeavoured to attain a fairly complete acquaintance with all the recorded facts—that is to say, I have striven to take into consideration all that is to be found in literature on child-psychology, whether it was in works of broad scope or in works dealing with special experiments recording observations made of the period from birth to weaning. I regret that foreign works were not always available. It is not, however, necessarily to be supposed that essential gaps have therefore resulted. More serious was another unavoidable limitation, for I had to decide to omit from this volume certain mental phenomena of the suckling period. First, I was obliged to omit speech, and further to treat perception and intelligence-phenomena more briefly and incompletely than is suitable for the outline of a detailed monograph. This limitation was necessary because these phenomena which appear during the first year of life cannot be understood at their origin, but they can be explained retrospectively from the study of a more developed phase. If we are to remain within the bounds of the nursing period, we must accept this deficiency. Later works on the psychology of early childhood will have to elaborate on the speech, perception, and intelligence-phenomena of the infant. There are occasional references to this in a later connection.

On the other hand, by means of the data offered by history and ethnography, I have elaborated, copiously in some

ix

chapters and in others cursorily, the factual materials offered by psychology. The reader will probably be pleased with this attempt to use historical and ethnographic data, if not with the interpretation placed upon them, even if he should not be in agreement with the systematic reflections which are simultaneously introduced and stated with the data in their appropriate places. It is not my purpose to present new facts in this book. Consequently, where instances were necessary, I have cited not my own observations, but examples already published. Nevertheless, I of course interpreted and chose the material at hand, guided by impressions from my own experience, and this experience, when necessary, was the decisive factor in choosing between contradictory data.

In spite of my attempt at completeness, I do not intend this as a reference book. But I have developed a chain of thought which will make possible a systematic organization and interpretation of the facts found. The later chapters, therefore, presuppose the previous ones, and the discussions in the opening chapters are taken up again later and developed. This manner of presentation is designed to put the emphasis upon the " theory " contained in the book. I attempt to show the mental factors of the period treated from the viewpoint of the psychology of the development of instinct (*Trieb*). Since the theory of instincts has not yet been recognized in psychology to the extent that it deserves, a great many difficulties have arisen from which an equally great number of shortcomings derive. The author perceives these very clearly. But since child-psychology, if it is to be organized into principles, cannot permanently dispense with the explanation of the facts established by it, even a somewhat inadequate attempt is useful. It will perhaps act as a stimulus towards new observations and experiments.

It is not necessary here to forestall the assumptions and interpretations which will be stated in the following pages. The ideas advanced are substantiated in the book itself, in so far as they are not already established by other authors, which is true of most of them. In these instances, reference to the authors must suffice. Only in one case, that of the author most often referred to, does this natural proceeding call for justification. I have assumed that the reader's knowledge of Freudian literature is not less than his knowledge of other developmental psychologies, and I have therefore introduced no more of the Freudian texts than was absolutely essential to the immediate train of thought. This proposed psychology of the infant has its foundation in Freudian psychology. The detailed proofs of some of the general theoretical attitudes are, therefore, not contained in this book, but are contained in the works of the Freudian school included in the bibliographical appendix. This is undoubtedly a fault of this book, for which, however, the author is not be blamed. The deficiency, however, is the more grievous, since child-psychologists are less familiar with Freud's most important works on developmental psychology than they are with minor dissertations of experimental psycho-analytical content. An introduction to psycho-analysis along with the psychology of the infant could not be accomplished, for this is a separate task which would perhaps surpass Infant Psychology in scope and difficulty. I expect that to some readers the presentation of certain terms and ideas will not be intelligible in their full significance. I have tried conscientiously to avoid the criticism of being "uncritically biassed." It appears more likely that these other methods and psycho-analysis, both properly understood, do not exclude one another, but, as I hope to demonstrate, supplement one another, in that the Freudian psychology especially undertook an intensive study of the psychology of the instincts which the other schools have too much neglected. In this field, no one else has contributed anything of value. To omit Freud would be impossible, if only for this reason. Moreover, since we here set ourselves the task of establishing instinctual life as the foundation of a theoretical condensation, the Freudian psychology must become the foundation for this, since there exists at present in psychology no other all-embracing theory of instincts. Perhaps this book will help to enrich child-psychology through the findings of psychoanalysis and Freud's theories, since it demonstrates their fruitfulness for the understanding of facts established from other sources, and for the development of the fundamental ideas of other schools.

SIEGFRIED BERNFELD.

VIENNA,
July, 1925.

THE
PSYCHOLOGY OF THE INFANT

A. THE NEW-BORN

BIRTH AND PSYCHO-PHYSICAL RETARDATION

BIRTH is the greatest sudden alteration which the fundamental phenomena of life impose upon mankind. Irrespective of the physiological changes in circulation, nourishment, and temperature, etc., the environment of the child is basically altered within a few hours. He is transplanted out of the uniformly liquid contents of the womb undisturbed by stimuli into an adult world of limitless stimuli, diversified, intense, and continuously changing, where the most elementary physiological needs are no longer automatically gratified. Metabolism no longer takes place within the limits of the united organism, the mother-fœtus, but requires to be started from outside for the newly-developed independent organism—the child. Exchange of gases stops for a few minutes and must be set into operation by a new act of lung breathing, which thenceforth usually functions automatically, although under muscular control.

It must, of course, be observed that certain devices minimize to some extent the abruptness of this transition. The organism, to be sure, is thrust by birth into the adult world of stimuli, but the mental apparatus does not respond completely to the stimuli. One sense organ, the ear, is incapable of functioning immediately after birth. The middle ear contains liquid, not air, and several hours of breathing are undoubtedly needed before it contains air as well as liquid (Preyer). When hearing starts is still a matter for investigation. It is still, in spite of all research, uncertain whether auditory stimuli are perceived before the fourth day (Dix). It is also doubtful whether the olfactory sense is capable of functioning during the " first hours of life "—as we shall, for the sake of brevity, call it henceforth, instead of using the more exact expression, post-fœtal life. One is inclined to decide affirmatively in accordance with many investigations. The

I

senses of sight, touch, and taste undoubtedly function a few minutes after birth. In fact, they function partially during birth, so that the complete omission of whole categories of stimuli, which would greatly weaken the effect of the change of environment at birth, is true only of the auditory, and perhaps of the olfactory, stimuli.

But it is to be noted that even the functioning sense organs are considerably limited. The entire neurological apparatus is considerably reduced in the capacity for excitation of its sense paths as well as of its motor paths (Solltmann). The legs, feet, back, breast, and belly, the greatest portion of the bodily surface, are presumably less sensitive than they are a few weeks after birth. Sight is limited to the differentiation between light and darkness. In fact, the vernix caseosa can perhaps be considered as one form of protection against stimuli.

THE FUNCTION OF INFANT REARING

The new-born is, indeed, anatomically and physiologically an independent organism, but only in this respect: the manifestations of its being cannot be described, certainly not understood, unless everything that its environment—the mother first of all—does for it and with it is observed. The new-born is not capable of maintaining. life for itself. The inherent instincts and impulses are not sufficiently extensive, the motor apparatus at their disposal not sufficiently developed for the maintenance of the new life. On the other hand, the instinctual and impulse activities (as at present we shall call them, without having as yet given the justifying explanation, although the term is doubtless comprehensible) need the supplementary activities either of the mother or of substitutes. The determining factor is a physiological process in the mother such as the secretion of the milk glands, but among no people and at no time does this service of the mother for the new-born exhaust her tasks, at least so far as I can learn from Ethnography and History. The baby is not only nursed, but in some degree and manner reared and tended by the mother. And the great majority of all activities which belong to the whole of this complicated process are impulse and instinctual activities on the part of the mother. A part surely originates in religious and social outlook and conditions, and, finally— among people of definite culture—in empirically tested thinking, science. A combination of both series of impulsive or instinctual activities, the behaviour of the child and rearing ritual of the mother together, make possible the maintenance and development of the new-born. They are as indivisible a unit as the blood circulation of the fœtus and mother.

The manifold prescriptions which science gives the mother for the care of the new-born can be summarized in one phrase: warmth and protection from stimuli. This means that our care of the infant attempts to reconstruct and strengthen the psycho-physical condition in which we found the fœtus. The abruptness of the alteration in the environment—that is, in the biosphere—must be minimized. The demand for punctilious cleanliness is common to scientific hygiene and medicine, and, of course, pertains to the care of the nursling, but it is not specifically intended for it.

The traditional methods of rearing the child, as they were used for many centuries, and certainly since the thirteenth century in Western and Central Europe, are consistent with science (Müllerheim). Immediately after birth the child is bathed for the first time, and during the first few weeks it is often bathed in warm water: It is enveloped in warm clothes that protect it as much as possible from stimuli, and it is placed in a cradle or in a contrivance similar in principle, which protects it from cold, strong light, and sudden changes. On awakening it is suckled. It is kept sleeping as much as possible, not in the least disturbed by the rhythmic movement of the swinging cradle. Superstition, custom, and changing medical opinion modify now one and now another of the details, but in essentials the process remains constant. Instead of the cradle the bassinet is used, or the mother's bed is often shared by the child, and the swaddling varies up to the most confining wrapping.

These two are the most important variations in this scheme. The first is reconcilable with our notions of child rearing; the second, perhaps, not so well, but we shall have more to say about this later. The sleeping new-born in the traditional rocking cradle, closed by curtains, packed in coverings, and enveloped by a moist atmosphere, recalls the fœtus and its biosphere even more clearly than the infant who sleeps, lying according to the rules of present-day scientific hygiene. Both methods are identical in principle; nevertheless, science has taught us to discriminate against the use of one group of customary methods: the cradle, its enclosed warm, damp atmosphere, for example, being condemned as harmful or unnecessary.

This pre-scientific popular and customary method of caring for the new-born infant during the first few days is by no means limited to Western and Central Europe. The same customs or the most important elements of them are found in all climates and latitudes. They are primal, for they are found among people of every form of culture and every stage of primitiveness. They are independent of geographic, social, and economic factors, as Ploss (2) frequently emphasizes, and it seems to me that his theory is very plausible.

The following detailed summary can be made:

Warm baths and *ablutions* are reported among the Malabar of East India, the Persians, the Armenians, and the Southern Arabians; also among the African Hoer and Ewe, the negroes in Old Calabar, and the Lower Congo, the Dravidian-Nair (India proper), Kirghiz, Samoyeds, Esthonians, Sume Indians in Nicaragua. To these may be added the Australians and, of course, the Japanese and Chinese. (This paragraph in Ploss is slightly ambiguous.) The practice of hot baths can well be included in this enumeration, and is reported of the Armenians, Russians, African Meroë, Taukluhs in Manipur, the Tartars, and of aristocratic Turkish groups. The Jews can be added, at least since the days of the Talmud (Feldman).

Warm and protective coverings are used by many peoples. To enumerate these would be tedious. I will therefore quote from Ploss (2) the list of peoples who on principle keep their new-born naked: the Arabians, Negroes, Malays, Polynesian tribes, Dravidian Maldivian Islanders, Caribs, Tupis (South America), the people of the Fire Islands, and the Eskimos; furthermore, the poor classes of the ancient Germans and the Japanese, and, it may be supposed, of many other peoples.

The *cradle* is commonly used. If we include the sack, basket, hammock, and all other similar portable apparatus, the list of peoples who recreate more or less the fœtus situation for the new-born becomes very inclusive, and embraces representatives of all racial groups: the Indo-Europeans, Caucasian tribes, Semites, Hamites, Sudanese, Bantu-Negroes, Hottentots and Bushmen, Malay-Polynesian tribes, Australians,

Japanese, Koreans, Chinese, Siamese, Ural-Altains, Hyperboreans and Indians.

The peoples who carry their infants on their backs in coverings or portable apparatus of this kind recreate the fœtus situation more exactly. Wernich writes (Ploss, 2) of the Japanese: "The continuous carrying of the child on the back in the garments of the mother . . . so that it lives like a parasite on its mother's back . . . appears to be a prolongation of the intra-uterine life of the child." This analogy has occasionally been touched upon by other authors, but in my opinion it has nowhere been considered as seriously as it deserves. The cradle and carrying the child about in arms have called forth intense discussion among physicians, and will occupy us later, but I shall here quote from this discussion the opinion of Ploss (2), since it has immediate bearing.

He considers passive movements, such as carrying the child in the arms or gentle rocking, to be useful, " because Nature maintains for the child in the womb quite similar passive movements, in that the mother transfers all her movements to the child who is lightly buoyed up in the embryonic water."

,In accordance with these facts one might easily feel inclined to propose a very simple, obvious, indisputable, and also affectively satisfying formula, namely, that the function of infant care is, generally speaking, to recreate the fœtus situation. In fact, however, the described form of caring for the new-born child is by no means the only one. It is not possible to make a statistical or a more or less exact numerical statement in the present state of ethnographic knowledge of adolescence, but it is certain that the customs, principally of other kinds, which we encounter are likewise in common use among people of all cultural stages, climates, and social conditions.

For these other customs a unifying characteristic cannot so easily be found. The forms appear to be more varied. It is easy to distinguish straight away one very frequent type, whose chief characteristic lies in the fact that it is, item for item, the exact opposite of those described. We have already mentioned peoples who do not swaddle their new-born and infants in warm and protective coverings, but allow them to go naked. Similar contrasts can be established for the other customs.

Cold baths are used for the new-born, according to Ploss-Renz, among the following peoples: the ancient and modern Indians, the ancient Persians, Medes, Bactrians, the Hungarian

Gypsies, the original inhabitants of Italy, Germany, and England; in ancient Rome and Greece, among the African Senegalese, the Congo Negroes, Yumas, Bubastis, the Kaffirs, the Hottentots; on the Damon Islands, the Philippines, the Carolina Islands, the Sandwich Islands, New Guinea, Samoa, and in Australia; by the Scythians, in Asiatic Turkey; by the Ostyaks, Samoyeds, Yuroks, Laplanders; by the Aleutian and Koluschan Indians, the Indians of New Scotland on the Hudson, in Virginia, the Mohave in California de Santa Marta, in old Peru, in Chili, in Caingang, Tapuya, Caraja, and Patagonia.

The *cradle* or other resting place, which is partially or completely closed, is not used by the Indians of Dekkan, the Icelanders, some tribes descended from Negroes of Guinea, some of the Kalmuks, the Finns, the Transylvanian Gypsies (Zelt), the Arabians, the extinct Comanche, the Hawaiians, the Naim-Naim, Wahamba. Among those tribes the child lies unwrapped on the bare floor or upon a flat padding, chosen for a certain degree of softness. To these can be added the numerous tribes who carry their naked new-born or the infant on their backs, hips, or shoulders, using at most a narrow strap, but no envelope, bag, or dress-folds covering most of the child's body.

The physicians of today are not alone in their opposition to rocking and swinging, for some races behave as if they were anxious to prevent every passive movement of the child, as if the child should rest, wherever possible, unmoved on a pad or in a fixed position as long as possible. The child is not even lifted for nursing, but the mother lies with it, or kneels over it. I merely mention this in passing, for more will be said of it in another connection.

Finally, the tight covering, the binding of the new-born child and suckling, which is used so widely, must be mentioned here, though it is, in any case, as far removed from the fœtus situation as the loose coverings in which the child has to some extent free play of arms and legs, and is not forced into a straitened, cramped position.

If we combine these details into a composite description, we gain a conception of child rearing which represents the exact opposite of the fœtus situation. The child immediately after birth—and from this time on with varying frequency—is bathed or washed in cold water; it is placed on a flat pad without coverings, or is swaddled and left to lie motionless. It seldom happens, indeed, that all the customs relating to infant-care are drawn from this type, just as a pure practice of the other type seldom occurs, but ideally two diametrically opposite poles result: the *fœtusphile* and the *fœtusphobia* care (if these words are permissible) between which the occasionally encountered concrete instances are to be found.

It is difficult to believe in the existence of the fœtus-phobia guardianship. It seems homicidal to us. We are so accustomed to the fœtusphile tendency, and so supported in our habits by science, though with some limitations, that we are forced to ask: Do not children so treated die? In fact, the answer is: Of course, some die, but not all. Exact and reliable reports on infant mortality were not accessible to me, but Ploss (2), in agreement with other authors, speaks of the high mortality figures, up to 80 per cent. of those born alive. One can hardly expect anything different from the fœtusphobia guardianship, especially when we consider the peculiar methods of feeding, of which we shall speak later. And the second question arises: "Why do these particular tribes employ this·irrational method?"

Before this question can be answered, the first must be thoroughly investigated. Actually we have no basis for the assumption that the high infant mortality is caused by fœtus-phobia rearing, for first, as already mentioned, this method is rarely ever found in purity, and secondly, we have no reliable statements which permit us to judge the ratio of these two tendencies and to know their respective influence on the mortality figures. We must remember that, in a large percentage of cases, rearing of children by any method does not suffice to combat the innumerable dangers to the new-born and suckling; but, on the other hand, all practised methods suffice to guarantee the preservation of the race.

We must realize that our present attitude toward the child, the present value we ascribe to life, is the result of a long psychological development. Not all races and civilizations feel that birth guarantees a child the privilege of living, not all regard the death of the child as disaster or the killing of it as a crime. The number of tribes who on principle kill a percentage of their children, a category (perhaps the first-born) or group (perhaps the weaklings), is very large and the motives very various. It is very probable that in earlier stages of development this was a custom among many peoples who today think and act differently. Reik has plausibly shown that the peculiar rites of Couvade (the custom of the man's taking to his bed during his wife's childbirth) and the initiation rites of puberty are distorted and stereotyped expressions of the once actual practice of killing the new-born, or a definite group or class of them. Ethnographers have often pointed this out.

Many traces of this ancient tendency, repressed for ages, can be found in contemporary cultured nations. If we take this into consideration we shall be inclined to suppose that the high child mortality of the races in question does not alarm them: it appears as a necessary evil. We shall have to take into consideration that some even desire this result, others put up with it as a gratification of unconscious wishes, although they view it as a (necessary) evil.

Here the reader will perhaps deplore the absence of condemnation, but it seems to me that we are not justified in condemning this custom. It is detrimental to the scientific understanding of the relationships we are here studying to postulate too great a hiatus between the actions and feelings of primitive peoples and the peoples of our day. I therefore wish, instead of expressing natural indignation, to show that the sudden growth of the protection of the infant in this century is not to be attributed to the absence of hostile tendencies, but primarily to the economic-political interest of the nations in large populations. (The psychological presupposition for this is probably, as Reik remarks, the reaction-formation for the repression of that hostile tendency.) And in spite of the advance in care and hygiene, the mortality figures for specific groups of European population are not as low as would be expected in view of the increase in medical knowledge and the indignation against the primitive custom of child-killing. Official statistics for Berlin show the proportionately low figure of 18·1 per cent. for infant mortality, but this Rühle proves to be an average figure, in which are included the rich Tiergarten section with 5·3 per cent. and the proletarian district, Wedding, with 42 per cent.

Wherever child mortality becomes a problem attempts are made to minimize it by the aid of magic or exorcism, by means of the rituals of animistic philosophies, by prayers, and by religious sacrifices according to religious philosophies. For

example, it is believed that the use of salt or other holy substances strengthens the child and makes it immune. Charms
are said to protect the infant against evil spirits, and offerings
propitiate the offended deity. Many remnants of these
customs exist even today as superstitions along with scientific
knowledge of child rearing. There is hardly any doubt that
those demons that threaten the child originate, like all evil
spirits, as projections of the evil impulses of the superstitious
themselves (Freud, 12). The tender devoted conscientious-
ness and concern with which the primitives from time to time
care for their children, and the cruel absurdities—indeed, the
murderous effects—of some of their customs, or of a whole group
of these customs, must be understood as manifestations of
an ambivalence of tender and at the same time hostile attitudes
which dominate them.

We cannot undertake in this book to explain the whole of
this problem, which will be attempted in a later work. Consequently all the necessary matter is merely summarized,
even if it is not convincing. A large proportion of those rearing
customs which belong neither to the fœtusphile nor fœtusphobia type can be shown to be distorted and modified expressions of repressed hostility or reactions to such. Some
positive hostility is altruistically justified, because its purpose
is supposed to be to accustom the child to the real difficulties
of life. The same is true for the fœtusphobia mode of action.
The duty which in Mexico the midwife has to perform after
the first bath of the child is nicely expressed in the prayer:
" Child precious above all! Ometecuhtli and Omecihuatl
have created you in the twelfth heaven, in order that you
should be born into this world. Know, then, that this world
is sorrowful, full of pain, troublesome and solitary; it is a
vale of tears; and that you, when an adult, must eat your
bread with pain, and earn it by your hands " (Ploss, 2).

The bearer of this hostile tendency seems to be the father,
or perhaps more correctly the men of the tribe, or of the race.
In support of this contention I quote: (1) Among mammalia,
the young are in danger of being eaten by the male (Mitchell,
Brehm). (2) Freud's *Totem and Taboo* and the work of Reik
already mentioned have disclosed motives in the life of peoples
which explain much of this hostility and which in this general
scheme apply only or almost exclusively to men.

To avoid misunderstanding I emphasize the fact that this

says nothing concerning the individual mental attitude of a particular man or woman.

Fœtusphobia rearing is therefore not an instinct. It is understood as a restraint (according to the Freudian assumption of the killing of the father in the Primal Horde and the resulting fear of retaliation) which the fear of retaliation progressively experiences, or as an outbreak of this fear—to name this one factor as a simplification in place of the countless operative factors. Perhaps a fragment of hostility remains as the instinctive behaviour of the man toward the helpless youngster; then we should have to a certain extent a small instinct kernel around which the complicated social-psychic structure is built. We can venture to assume an opposite development for the fœtusphile rearing form. Breeding, the function of the mother among mammalia and among marsupials, presents an extra-uterine fœtal life, and shows clearly, as in the case of the monkey, a fœtusphile tendency. For example, Brehm gives this description: " The baby monkey immediately after birth suspends itself by both forearms about the mother's neck, but with its legs on the mother's belly in a most convenient position, so as not to molest the mother and to nurse undisturbed." The mother, for her part, " immediately licks it (the monkey infant), she delouses it again, she presses it to her . . . she nurses it and rocks it to and fro. . . ." Essential manifestations of child rearing are here described, and the most involved form of pure fœtusphile infant care can be interpreted as an adaptation of these instincts to a complicated social condition, or as a dovetailing of discoveries which are repeatedly made in the instincts. Nevertheless we may perhaps desire to attribute a greater importance to the discoveries of mankind, including those in this field. In that case certain points may be noted. The primitive mother has no correct knowledge of the fœtus condition, nevertheless she can divine some characteristics of the fœtal biosphere, and, when confronted with the situation, provide for the helpless, weak child in some way; she will readily know how to imitate the prototype, which is herself when pregnant.

We perhaps come near the truth if we do not conceive this as a rational process. For we see that the mother is supported by the instinctual expressions of love in her devices for infant care, which the new-born receives as part and parcel of the mother's body: to be pressed to her, to be held close to her body, etc. And in conclusion one must mention what psycho-analysis regards as the " primal phantasy " of mankind, active perhaps in every person—namely, the longing, as a result of the sorrows and privations of life's path, to return to the prenatal world of sensationless quiet, into Nirvana or into the womb. In the devices for infant care, likewise, this phantasy may effect a satisfactory fulfilment towards that part of the body called child.

These should therefore be, to a certain extent, the social psychological correlatives of the conservative tendency which we found in the psychophysical condition of the new-born and in the expressions of its impulses, and which we shall still more clearly prove.

Krauss's observation that among the primitives the child is taboo because it is a part of the pregnant mother, the " bearer and nurser of a creation mysterious in its origin," is very probable and must be inserted in order to make some child-rearing customs understood (not, however, those customs belonging to the fœtusphile and fœtusphobia types) and will be evaluated and criticized in another connection.

'In the following sentences of Dr. T. Ischikawa, a Japanese ear specialist, I see a slight illustration of this conception: " I am inclined to the opinion that the natural development of the child could be perfected, if we, during certain periodic traumas, transplanted it into a new medium, an ' artificial womb,' so to speak, which should have relatively the same or nearly the same conditions with respect to light, sound, and temperature as the actual womb. . . ."

SLEEP

The infant's chief occupation, its principal activity, is sleep. When it is not hindered by hunger or some harsh disturbance, it sleeps about twenty hours a day (Vierordt). This long sleeping period only gradually diminishes, so that a year old child's sleeping period is still much longer than its waking period, and not until the fourth year is this ratio reversed. This fact has attracted general attention. Scarcely a single paper on the psychology of the infant omits to mention it, and yet it seems to have been studied insufficiently. The details, which appear to be well established, can be briefly stated.

If the sleeping period is considered as a whole, then the duration of a single unbroken sleeping period is short, seldom longer than two hours (Preyer). According to Preyer the length increases rapidly: in the second month often to a three-hour sleeping period, and sometimes from five to six hours; in the sixth month from six to eight-hour sleeping periods are frequent. The sleep of the infant therefore differs from that of the adult and child; it has a much faster rhythm. It should be mentioned here that the infant falls asleep more quickly, sleeps more lightly, and can be awakened easily. Yet this obviously is not true for all rousing stimuli; for in contradistinction to the easily observed fact that the child is sensitive and can be easily roused, we can just as easily prove that it reacts to a great many stimuli indeed (perhaps somewhat pantomimically) but does not wake. Dix gives a good example of this: " Bubi lies on his back, the little arms raised to his head as in the fœtus position. The electric car passing on the street frightens him slightly. The eyes quiver, draw together, the corners of the mouth are dropped as if to cry. But he sleeps on. Suddenly he forms his mouth for nursing. The fingers close from time to time; he clenches and unclenches his fists. His eyes roll upward and to the side under the closed eyelids. Suddenly he utters a slight groan. Immediately after he begins. to smile. He appears to be dreaming. Thereupon calm sleep again follows, which continues for ten minutes without any interruption. . . ."

This observation was made on the sixty-fifth day. It is valid also for the first days of life. Dix's son slept so soundly on the seventeenth day that not even screaming woke him. When he fell asleep at his mother's breast during nursing and was gently moved, he became frightened, sucked, growled, and fell asleep again. This much can be observed in every case: the infant spontaneously awakes for a short time after about two hours' sleep; the sleep periods can be shortened at discretion, by various stimuli; on the other hand, not all stimuli to which the sleeper reacts will wake it, and these stimuli are not always effective. In conclusion, it is often impossible to determine whether a sleep-disturbing stimulus will call forth any reaction. The stimuli which are found to cause awakening are: skin irritations, bright light, cold (see Ischikawa particularly); and noises of all kinds after the first few days. The changing of an uncomfortable position of the limbs during sleep shows, in addition to what has been said above, that not every stimulus which causes a re-action wakes the child. Caramaussel's researches concerning children about four weeks old show clearly how stimuli produce changes in breathing without waking the child. Regarding sleep in the first weeks, Caramaussel has further established that the breathing curve is entirely different from that of the later period; it is unusually irregular and expiration often does not immediately follow inspiration or *vice versa*, but there is a hiatus of breathing for about one second, as if the child had not yet learned how to breathe correctly. This registers a curve of plateaux characteristic of breathlessness. Of course, the graph soon approaches the curve of the unusual regularity of the adult. The month-old child no longer shows this remarkable hesitation between expiration and inspiration unless a disturbance to sleep occurs. If the infant is waked, it experiences a true " anxiety state "; the younger it is, the stronger the anxiety (Preyer): contracting of the body, quiver-ing of the limbs, at times resembling a kind of light cramp.

A theoretical classification of these facts results from repre-sentative views of sleep in general. Claparède (1) has under-taken a clear and impressive sifting of these views. Here we can only consider their application to the child's sleep. (i.) The oldest explanation merges with the conception that sleep is the result of intoxication due to fatigue products. The younger the organism, the more vigorous is metabolism. It follows therefore that, in relation to the meagre accomplish-ments of the organism, the infant becomes tired more quickly than the older child, and therefore it sleeps longer and after shorter waking periods (crying, nursing, or using the sense organs). Besides this, Preyer further assumes that the milk has a fatiguing (sleep-inducing) effect. (ii.) The second ex-planation includes the investigations of Solltmann which, in so far as they are here the subject of discussion, have proved that the capacity for fatigue of the nervous system of the new-born is large in the case of the young of animals; irrita-bility is minimal, a fact which helps to explain the quantity of sleep—that is, falling asleep quickly and sleeping lightly (Bühler-Koffka). Disturbances have no power of producing a waking state: as Dekker so well expressed it, the new-born sleeps because there is no reason for its being awake. (iii.) The third hypothesis is built on the recuperative effects of sleep;

during sleep not only are fatigue toxins removed and no new ones created in any great quantity, but also sleep is favourable to the development of growth, in that the organs are thereby rebuilt; the increase of fat amounts to 24 per cent. (Key). We find accordingly an increasing need for sleep during growing periods (Trömmer), and during the first weeks of life especially. This is Claparède's opinion, which, of course, is not substantiated without the further conceptions which he presents in the works mentioned in the appendix. According to him, sleep is not an automatic (reflex) result of a definite quantity of accumulated fatigue products, but an instinct whose function it is to prevent exhaustion (and, as we must add, to promote growth and recuperation); the means of which are perhaps to be considered under these physiological processes upon which the other conceptions are based, but which make sleep an active biological function.

It is not for us now to examine the accuracy of these theories, for the problem of sleep is obviously very complicated and the extensive literature—including the most recent—which de Sanctis surveys has not brought solution but contradictory facts and viewpoints. As formerly in such cases in science, so here, too, the different opinions present partial truths, but they lack classification. We shall often find ourselves in a similar predicament in this book; a question relating to child-psychology or to general knowledge of adolescence will be tied up with the solution of general psychological problems which have not yet been satisfactorily followed up. We certainly can never formulate a decision for which we, as author and reader of books on child-psychology, are not competent. But we shall attempt to work further with that hypothesis which, for our particular child psychological problem, or for our general standpoint, appears most fertile, which naturally can only be the case when the facts of our field are explained by it, or at least not contradicted.[1]

From this point of view, Claparède's opinion is the first to claim attention; he regards sleep phenomena as expressions of an impulse (*Trieb*),[2] (Claparède says instinct). Since we have set out to study the development of the

---

[1] More closely expounded: Bernfeld, *Die Psychoanalyse in der Jugendforschung.*

[2] I here translate *Trieb* as *impulse*, because the author intends to differentiate it from Claparède's use of *instinct*. Otherwise I reserve the word impulse for *Drang* or *Impulse.—Translator.*

child from the instincts as the centre, we should have to invent this view if it did not exist already. Observation and the available literature offer more facts to support this theory than the other views. These have several difficulties. The second hypothesis (ii.), which offers a plausible explanation for the quick sleep of the infant, makes it difficult to understand its awakening, especially the immediate awaking and the awaking after relatively weak stimuli, which is surely an established fact for the second week of life and perhaps for the first. Hypothesis (i.), which explains the short rhythm of sleep, is too inaccessible to proof to be accepted. The assumption that the new-born is easily habituated to longer sleep periods I find only briefly mentioned in the literature (Dyroff, Bühler), but it must not be overlooked. The diary which was kept for my oldest child from the eighth to the hundred-and-fiftieth day shows consistently that at the beginning of the third week six feedings at intervals of $3\frac{1}{2}$ hours and a continuous night of $6\frac{1}{2}$ hours were given, to which the child became accustomed. Sometimes, however, though not always, she awakened after $5\frac{1}{2}$ hours, cried for a few minutes, and then fell asleep again. Similar instances were confirmed by many mothers, and I remember that it was so of my second child, but I have kept no record of it. In Claparède's view, both difficulties unite. The latter is rather suited to confirm them.

Having once established the sleep instinct or impulse, it becomes very difficult to escape the obligation to add a few remarks as to the conception of its hypothetical origin. Claparède tries to explain the sleep instinct by starting from the phenomena of feigning death, regarding this as part of a general protection and defence instinct, the purpose of sleep being protection from exhaustion.

This idea will not be discussed here. But it is a useful principle of method that one should only have recourse to suppositions carrying us far back into our animal ancestry, when one is convinced that the explanation and resources within mankind are of no avail.

It appears that Claparède has not sufficiently deliberated upon this. For a group of sleep theories point out more or less convincingly that the almost uninterrupted sleep of the new-born approximating to sustained uninterrupted sleep is a continuation of the embryonic state. Among child psychologists this view is advocated, though, to be sure, only in a passing sentence; Stern and Perez write of the sleeping new-born: " It seems to return again to the secluded existence which was its normal state in the womb, and the organism seeks to retain that mode of life." Claparède mentions this reference and disposes of it quickly: the fœtus situation has nothing to do with sleep, which is relative, and does not exist where there are no waking states.   This point of view presents a considerable difficulty.   It is usually difficult to ascertain whether the new-born is asleep or awake.   The criteria for sleep of adults, children or older infants, are completely or partially absent in the first weeks of life.   Immobility may also be characteristic of a waking state, and is, on the other hand, only relative in sleep.   The same is valid for the closed eyes; sometimes they are half-open in sleep (Dix). Occasionally the child lies with one eye open and one blinking eye, and may be asleep or awake.   Closed eyes do not neces-sarily indicate sleep.   Generally speaking, the infant's reaction capacity is narrowly limited.   We have no basis for assuming positive sleep because there is no response and we find that reactions occur without awaking the infant (Caramaussel, Canestrini).   Bacalo has shown that the difference between the sleeping and the waking heart-beat and pulse is very small (de Sanctis).   Canestrini stresses the fact that the fontanel pulsation curve from rest to a waking condition generally shows no sharp line of demarcation in the infant.

Knowledge of the waking and the sleeping consciousness would be the deciding criterion.   We have no way of determin-ing these.   Shall we therefore say that the new-born does not sleep ?   Or shall we call sleep those culminating points of deep sleep which, according to Canestrini, are reached about one hour after falling asleep and immediately are lost again ? It seems to me preferable to retain the word sleep.   All the life-phenomena are much less differentiated in the new-born than they are later; they are more significant, the result of more numerous processes than later.   The same is valid for sleep; it, too, differentiates itself in the course of life.   The complete waking state, the somnolent state, the quiet state " without thought," the hypnagogic state, the deep " luxury " sleep, the after nap, etc., in the course of time, gradually differentiate themselves from the general state of being of the infant, in whom we can distinguish very short periods of undeniable complete awakeness and not much longer periods of positive deep sleep, while the greater part of the day passes in an undifferentiated condition, which has more similarity to later sleeping states than to later waking states. This corresponds throughout to the rule of scientific nomenclature, which is to attach to the indifferent state the name of that phenomenon which clearly develops from it, and has definite characteristics. We are right in speaking of the sleep of the new-born.

This is obviously less valid for the embryonic state. It may be even less differentiated than the sleep of the new-born; it may be even more significant; for it is, indeed, the beginning of the development of the later sleep phenomena and contains the most important characteristics of them. To a certain degree sleep reproduces regularly, normally, or very frequently the fœtus situation: increased and warm protection, darkness (both physiologically beneficial), and very frequently position. One can almost, in the case of the new-born, speak of a retention of the fœtus situation instead of a return to it, for the interruptions are so short that the time factor is negligible. Furthermore, these interruptions are of such fundamental significance for the development of the new-born, that we would do better to accept them and say: the sleep of the new-born is the return to the fœtus situation, to which the new-born tends to revert as soon as possible after interruption. The first interruption of this nature is birth. The extensive category of later sleep disturbances in the first few weeks of life is principally of the same kind: sudden skin irritation of all sorts, light, sensitivity to motion, sudden elevation. All other factors, such as fatigue, torpidity of the nervous system, may be added from the beginning and are organized with this tendency: to preserve the previous life-state. And all of this is certainly not the individual discovery of a single new-born, but deserves the designation, *instinct* (*Instinkt*), *impulse* (*Trieb*).

This conception has two advantages over Claparède's view (in-so-far as it is a development beyond it): it evades the difficulty of separating the sleep of the new-born from that of the older infant, which would result in establishing the relativity of sleep; it need not refer to the lower strata of the animal sequence. This enables us, as I see it, to classify sleep without any contradiction among those phenomena which

appear to us to be dominated by that conservative tendency ˈ
which we mentioned: to retain the fœtus situation, to return
to it after interruption.   Just as we find that there is a racial
psychic correlative to the psychophysical state of the new-
born, so, it seems to me, this conservative tendency works as
a residue in the life of the adult, who, according to Freud's (11)
profound observation, is perhaps impelled regularly every
night to give up a large portion of the gains of waking life
and to return to the starting-point of his life.   De Sanctis
observes that he has the feeling, after being suddenly awakened
from a deep sleep, of coming from some far-off place.   If this
òbservation is a general experience, it can be easily interpreted
as a consciousness of that regression; for one really returns
from afar, out of the fœtus condition.   Kempf cites a list·of
examples which illustrate this explanation of sleep in racial
customs and in the racial psyche as revealed in funeral
rites.

Sleep of the new-born (and especially of the infant) seems
almost holy because of naïve racial beliefs.   The wish, not
to be disturbed by the child, joins forces with the idea of
the importance of sleep which is based upon their own experience and experience with children.   Perhaps, too, something like unconscious understanding here plays a part, such
as remembering the psycho-economic value of the conservative
tendency of the infant's sleep, which is frequently expressed
in cradle songs.   Nevertheless it is often customary to wake
the infant (even in the first days) to cleanse or nurse it.
Physicians have often favoured this practice.   Today, to be
sure, they are unanimously opposed to waking the child,
partly because they consider sleep an incomparably important
activity, and partly because they wish to prevent the over-
frequent, unnecessarily frequent, frightening of the new-born
with its tendencies to tetanus.   An example of the combination of both conceptions, the recognition of the value of sleep
and the rationally founded recommendation of waking as it is
so often found in old authors, is seen in the following sentences
used in the careful and painstaking Medicus of the physicist,
John Helferecht Jungkens, M.D.:

"Concerning sleep, it is very good for children to sleep a
great deal, be it by day or by night, and the more they sleep
the healthier it is for them: if, however, they should sleep
excessively, they may be picked up and roused to be cleansed

and tidied when they have soiled themselves. For this purpose the child may be picked up two and three times daily."

Another reason besides the hygienic justification for waking small infants I know only from one instance, the Jews, of whom Feldman reports: " In some places the smiling of a child during sleep indicates . . . playing with Lilith (especially during the night of the Sabbath or new moon), and the child should be wakened."

CRYING

Proceeding from our conception of sleep, we must raise the question which has on occasion been asked—namely, why are we awake ? In particular, why does the new-born awake; why cannot the conservative tendency, which we believe we have recognized, enforce itself; what hinders it so constantly that the human being, when adult, considers the waking state to be the self-evident, actual life, and sleep to be the problem, very pleasant indeed, but nevertheless an interruption ? It is easy to perceive that this is the basic question bearing on the reason for the new-born's development in general. And no one will believe that scientific knowledge can answer the question adequately; on the contrary, it answers so inadequately that the contributions, which will be cited, can be disposed of in a few pages.

Obviously a whole series of factors are here operative, of which we shall recognize some. One is easily stated—namely, waking occurs for the purpose of making possible further sleep. This is not as odd as it might appear to some. Normally the new-born awakes crying, which produces the attending person, the mother. She supposes that her child is hungry or feels some discomfort and removes the disturbing irritation, and the child falls asleep again. Sleep is restored. Crying was, accordingly, a signal for help, and waking occurred to make possible this call.

Many psychologists, therefore, consider the crying of the new-born as an expressive gesture (*Ausdrucksbewegung*) (*e.g.*, Darwin, Preyer, Bühler, Koffka). Perhaps this is not quite exact, for the expressive gestures of the adult are fundamentally unintentional gestures which accompany the affect; it was assumed that they were either motor abreactions to strong affects or remnants of once useful (perhaps instinctual) activities. Neither of these applies to the crying of the new-born;

its crying is certainly much more "purposive," the only "purposive" thing, that, so to speak, the new-born can do in this case. But we understand what is meant by the term expressive gesture, and certainly the expressive gestures of the adult in great part develop out of the crying of the infant.

This call for help of the few-hours-old human being is so surprisingly purposeful and, since it composes a good part of the total waking period of the new-born, it is of such indubitable developmental importance that one would like to learn more of its details and origin.

Crying is a special form of breathing: it is spasmodic, exaggerated expiration (sometimes also inspiration) with a contracted glottis, wide opened mouth, and tightly closed eyes. Closing the eyes seems to occur automatically (as a reflex) at every strong exertion, presumably to prevent, by contracting the eyeballs and its vessels, the rush of blood to the eyes. Crying is accordingly always a repetition of those movements which the first breathing after birth produced. It almost seems that each awaking in the first days is associated with the "waking" out of the fœtus condition, and that the child repeats those motor reactions of birth. This alone—namely, the gestures and physiology of drawing the first breath, which in general is also the first cry—is not adequately explained. Nevertheless, the basis seems to be established; they arise from the need for air and serve to relieve it. Its reflexive release seems to be closely connected with the strong skin excitation, to which the child at birth is exposed for the first time. They are repeated at each crying, though without breathlessness in advance. There are, of course, a number of instances, such as the one mentioned above in reference to Caramaussel, in which breathlessness, too, is reproduced. If one wishes, one can say that, in the last analysis, crying—this strong and prolonged expiration, even if only for a fraction of a second—is induced breathlessness. All these physiological and gestural reactions remain for life the motor accompaniments, the expressive gestures of certain affects, and from these develops the expression of a whole series of other very important emotions (Darwin) about which much will be said later.

The excitations to which the new-born responds by crying are manifold. According to Preyer, they are hunger, thirst, wrappings, discomfort during nursing. Several similar kinds could be named. But for us it is important only to classify them, and this may be attempted somewhat in this manner: (1) Stimuli which are components of the birth situation: coldness, sudden light, pressure, sudden unusual changes of posture.[1] (2) Stimuli which have some relation to the birth situation: every sudden excitation of the sense organs. (3) Stimuli without any relation to the birth situation: in the first days of life, of course, only hunger and thirst. We must realize that internal bodily stimuli, which we do not know, and which we accept as a cause for spontaneous crying, cannot be classified, but there is nothing to prevent us from conceiving them as classifiable under (1) or (2).

Some of these stimuli are obviously of such a kind that awakening with a cry for help appears, when related to them, to be a " purposeful " manner of behaviour—*e.g.*, hunger, cold, which imperil life. And to save life, it is indeed purposive to sacrifice sleep for a short while. For other stimuli this is in nowise valid. They are of a harmless nature. It does not pay, so to speak, to trouble ourselves about them. It does not always happen, for waking does not necessarily follow, but often it does. The investigations referred to give no information here; they only contradict each other; sometimes, at the slamming of a door or casting light on the child's face, waking and crying are reported, at other times not. The more minute studies indicate reactions to definite stimuli regularly, but not always by waking and crying. We must assume that the stimulus must fulfil definite conditions, the most important of which is perhaps that it did not commence during the short period of true deep sleep. However that may be, it is certain it will respond with crying and, moreover, in a " purposeless " manner. In this case one can say with descriptive accuracy, but interpreting by analogy, that the stimulus recalls the already experienced co-existence of stimuli and reactions which we call birth, and calls forth the missing part through the motor reactions; or that one portion of the birth process is repeated. It is difficult to say why. If we accept an impression which forces itself on us, we would say with

[1] Research on this question was, I regret to say, not brought to my attention, although it might yield very interesting results: of course, the new-born reacts to posture changes, and, indeed, it appears to me, to any sudden strong changes, by crying, whereas to placid continuous, rhythmic changes it reacts by falling asleep.

Freud (11) that the new-born behaves as if birth were a traumatic experience, which—at a given excitation—it must repeat, particularly that part which it is capable of reproducing.

I must, of course, grant that I cannot expect this impression, at least for the present, to be taken as a serious proposal, because crying functions, even in these instances, as a sign of calling for help, or can function as such; it is, therefore, no meaningless repetition; rather a purposive attitude exists, co-exists, or at least could exist. Nevertheless, from the very beginning, it is probable that the crying of the new-born is a very ambiguous phenomenon, which will later differentiate itself, in which therefore the repetitive and expressive functions are intimately united.

Because of this, crying can also succeed stimuli which were not in the birth situation, in which stimuli we included hunger and thirst, because the more subtle, finer processes of both birth and hunger are unknown. The hunger-cry is not the repetition of the birth-cry. It is from the very beginning distinguishable from every other form of crying of the new-born; it first occurs, however, after crying for other reasons has frequently occurred. One does not assume that the new-born is hungry before twelve hours have passed, and certainly the processes are not sufficiently differentiated for one to have the right to assume that the child cries at one time because it is hungry, and at another time solely because it is reminded of birth. But one is tempted to separate, theoretically, these two forms from each other; I shall later show that their further development is completely different.

It is obvious that the hunger-cry is purposeful, and it fulfils a function of expression. To classify it under expressive movements is therefore not incorrect, but it benefits us little. The expressive movements in child-psychology would make up a small chapter by themselves; here they are isolated and are nothing more than an embarrassment. I should like to suggest that the hunger-cry be interpreted differently and more simply.

When the adult feels hungry, he makes a number of bodily movements such as will bring him to the dining-room, and others, which we call eating. If we wish to be exact we have to include all those which brought him into possession of food, such as occupation, marketing, preparation. All these movements issue from the hunger impulse (*Trieb*). They are activities which are necessary for the satisfaction of this impulse, activities which are necessary because the impulse is only gratified when a partial alteration in the environment is undertaken, even if it is as slight as a single outstretching and bending of the arm. The new-born is in just the same situation as the adult—*i.e.*, in fundamental contrast to the fœtus situation; in its case, too, a portion of the environment must experience change, if it is to be satisfied. Only in the case of the infant the necessary activities for this are divided between two persons, between it and its mother (foster-mother). It is not customary to designate the movements of the mother as activities for the gratification of hunger; we rather call them physiological activities (*e.g.*, milk-secretion) and activities of mother love. Speaking from the point of view of the child, we must not forget that these are the correlatives to the instinctual activities of the infant, a composite part of them. The infant depends upon the activities of the mother; there therefore remain, as the infant's share in these instinctual activities, sucking when the nipple is in its mouth, and crying until it is there. ˙

Crying is, therefore, an activity of the new-born and, in fact, an instinctual activity. Of course, it is part of a complex of activities, that part which the new-born's motor apparatus and its social situation (so to speak) make possible. From the standpoint of the adult, crying is an expressive gesture of the infant. Considered from the child's standpoint, it is an instinctual activity, and it is therefore capable of regulation and adjustment; it is subject to habit and experience. Nurses know this, and, as I have already mentioned, it is manifested in the fact that the new-born very soon learns to wake at feeding time, but sleeps between feedings if it is not otherwise disturbed. Although it is not fully dealt with, we cannot overlook the fact that not only hunger and the hunger-cry but also many others can be called instinctual activities, the removal (gratification) of which requires a change in the environment.

To return to the initial question of this chapter, we answer: waking results when a disturbance occurs which is fatal to life or which can become so if sustained, and it serves to bring about those changes in the environment which remove the disturbance. If that happens, sleep ensues. This we see clearly. Another factor appears, not quite so obvious, but nevertheless impressive and comprehensible enough to be mentioned: it seems as if birth were a process which can best be designated as a trauma, so that stimuli which belong to the syndrome of the birth situation compel the repetition of the reactions of the new-born to birth—at least under specific conditions—similar to the way in which Freud (9) assumes it for the dreams of the epileptic neurotic.

SUCKING

Crying and sucking are complementary processes in the new-born when awake, and to a certain degree in older infants too. Crying ceases as soon as the lips close round something capable of being sucked; crying continues until something which can be sucked appears. Strictly speaking, this is valid only for the hunger-cry, but all other crying can for a time be removed by sucking. The hunger-cry is nothing more than a preliminary step to sucking. The new-born is incapable of making an intentional movement to put something into its mouth. If it does not attain this by the mother's help or by accident (its own hands or a finger succeeding by random movements in getting into the mouth), then it resorts to the universal-instinctual activity, crying. Sucking dominates the infant from the very beginning with marvellous precision. If sometimes awkwardness is noticed at the first or second feeding, it is so insignificant and so quickly overcome that it is not of great importance at all,[1] as opposed to the well-supported facts, that in other instances the sucking movements have functioned even before the completion of birth (Preyer). It is by no means an ordinary reflex; on the contrary, sucking is a very complicated act, which is not altogether understood in all details. In any case, the child does not suck with the lips, but these serve only to make airtight the contact with the mammilla (aided by the Magitot membrane, which disappears as the child becomes older) (Vierordt).

The act of sucking, proper, is performed within the mouth, in which the tongue, gums, cheeks, and lower jaw act as a suction pump. Swallowing is closely associated with sucking,

[1] Tracy's expression, " far from perfect in the beginning," is greatly exaggerated.

but only when the fluid has reached the mouth. Sucking is actively ended even before the mammilla is withdrawn from the mouth, before the new-born expels it. This complicated process is undoubtedly innate; it is the only example of an instinct so complete and unlearned which is present from the beginning. It has attracted so much attention that some authors assume that sucking has, in fact, already come into play in the uterus (Tracy, Friedjung). The existence of this capacity cannot be explained more satisfactorily, nor, for that matter, less accurately than can the marvellous complete functioning of all physical and biological processes. But this is not the task of psychology, at least not of present-day psychology. Reference to the embryonic activity does not help us much in this case, because the problem would then be, to show from what rudiments and in what phases these sucking capacities develop; this is not possible, and therefore the problem must be put aside.

There is no choice but to assume that a highly synthesized process exists from the beginning and, as soon as it finds an adequate stimulus, functions perfectly. That this act is in the service of the hunger instinct is unquestionable, and it seems almost tautological to say so. And yet it must be emphasized that the relation between sucking and hunger is not very simple. Indeed, it contains many really serious problems. In a discussion of these, which we can only begin here, we must proceed from two facts. (1) At the beginning the child also sucks objects which are inadequate for the satisfaction of hunger. (2) Sucking also occurs when the child is satiated. This is as well established for the first weeks of the child's life as it is for many years in numerous instances, but strict proof of it from the first days of life cannot be produced. The difficulty consists in our ignorance of the emotions of the new-born; but we must make them accessible. The new-born falls asleep immediately after feeding; but we can surely assume, when it sucks its finger, that it is hungry. Of course, the existence of finger-sucking in the first hours of life during which hunger, at least insistent hunger, is hardly probable, is an indication that from the very beginning sucking is to a certain extent independent of hunger, and no facts contradict this assumption. Dix comments similarly on the first days: his son began to suck as soon as his tongue or lips were touched after his three-hour feeding interval; otherwise one had to tickle his tongue several times before he began to suck. The decision as to whether this independence dates back to the first sucking movement, or is acquired in the first day, is as unimportant as it is immaterial for our further reflections. The latter fact is absolutely indubitable, and is confirmed by every observer. The new-born sucks its own finger most frequently; but almost any object may serve as a releasing stimulus, if it is not too big, too rough, too hot, too cold, too bitter, salty or sour (Preyer).[1]

The new-born sucks even without any object—*in vacuo*, so to speak—in sleep and after nursing (perhaps after insufficient feeding), but in any case only until it has made the discovery of sucking objects.

The instinct of the new-born accordingly pertains to sucking in general, irrespective of whether satiation is thereby attained. Of course, sucking is finally replaced by crying if it continues to be ineffective, for this inborn activity is not in itself capable of quieting hunger, but only under the condition that an object containing milk will eventually reach the lips, a condition which the instinct takes into account. The instinct says, so to speak, " I want to suck," and not " I want to drink "; and this occurs to the new-born only when something capable of being sucked reaches its mouth.

It is not easy to propose this interpretation without attempting a slight correction of the concept of the instinct of self-preservation. For to establish the sucking activity is considered a matter of course (Kirkpatrick), if one is at all concerned with the instincts of the child; but this certainly seems to be remote from the purpose of almost all authors on child-psychology. The establishment of this instinct will stand the test, but it is not so simple and is problematical. Normally, eating in the case of the adult is only an indirect instinctual activity, which is released by hunger; it is a habit activity, whose time, quantity, and nature serve to prevent hunger. If a physiological condition of hunger were reached, it would be harmful indeed simply to gratify it by eating. The self-preservative instinct has experienced a change in its expres-

[1] My observation in the diary quoted where sucking is brought about in the twenty-five-hour-old child through stroking the cheeks is the only observation, as far as I know, in the literature of child psychological observations, if one does not consider Darwin's (2) remark: " It seemed clear to me that a warm soft hand, applied to his face, excited a wish to suck." Referred to by Popper in another connection.

sions—a change which is fitted for its purpose in every respect and adjusts to it prophylactically. Analogously with sleep:[1] we become sleepy before we are exhausted. We become hungry before we are hungry. Then, too, the acquisition of nourishment is not a direct effect of the instinct of self-preservation with adults—regardless of the level of civilization; we work and earn, not merely because of the instinct of self-preservation, but indeed in a manner very far removed from pure instinctive activity. The " desperate deeds " due to hunger are more qualified to give us a picture of the direct expressions of the self-preservative instinct. The difficulty of studying this instinct is considerable because all community life begins obviously to check it. But by analogy from animals and children one can perhaps reconstruct the instinct of self-preservation, in so far as it interests us here, as follows: if the individual is not completely satisfied and satiation is not frequent during waking—for if the individual is completely satiated it falls asleep—every article of food excites, as soon as it is apperceived, the impulsion to obtain possession of it, to take it into the mouth and eat it, to destroy it by mastication, without any other consideration except its own bodily capacities.[2] The name self-preservative instinct obscures the real fact in that it attributes to the instinct an aim which it does not contain.

The instinct is capable of adaptation within the bounds of its aim: this gorging one's self—as we rightly name the described act, *Fresstrieb* — occurs individually according to the conditions of the food-supply; if there is no food, then the individual inevitably starves. His aim is to eat, and only indirectly is it self-preservation. If this explanation seems natural and self-evident to some, it may appear subtle to others. I consider it necessary because it is not stated sufficiently clearly anywhere, and because it introduces a conception which was started in another field through similar reflections when it was decided to revise the theory of the reproductive instinct[3] by similar arguments. Likewise, the reproductive instinct has not reproduction as its aim, but a concrete act. Nevertheless, the sexual instincts do serve propagation, just as the nutritional instinct (one might say) serves self-preserva-

---

[1] It is alluded to repeatedly—*e.g.*, by de Sanctis.
[2] Numerous examples, of course, not interpreted in this way, in Köhler's *The Mentality of Apes*.
[3] Repeatedly and most energetically by Freud.

tion, but by a route very important psychologically. We have made similar observations about sleep. Sleep is instinctual and serves the waking state, assimilation in general.

This organic need has a mental representative which Freud conceives as the wish for sleep, which, however, in so far as it is psychical, avails itself of the psychic mechanisms, as we explained with reference to Claparède and Freud: the reproduction of the fœtus situation. The organic need for nourishment (self-preservation) has, as its mental representative, the nutritional instinct. The mental representative does not know, so to speak, the organic aims and needs, and it functions according to its own mechanisms, and is intelligible through them. Since we do not yet understand the relationship between the mental and the organic, we must assume it, without deeming it necessary to establish definite ideas concerning the organic in this psychological connection.

In the new-born the nutritional instinct is modified. It begins to function when the oral grasp is completed. As we have seen above, it is not entirely undifferentiated. Certain tactual perceptions—we shall try to learn more about this—hinder its function. Swallowing is linked with eating; it commences automatically when food reaches the mouth, obviously at the back of the tongue. It is gratified when a certain capacity of the stomach is reached. How the cessation of sucking occurs, we do not know. The simplest assumption would be that the instinct had attained its aim, satiation. This, however, would make the completion of the instinctual activity (satiation) more dependent upon hunger than the beginning of it, which leads to some difficulties. We are always prepared for being suddenly confronted with the ambiguousness of the phenomena studied in the new-born, and we are prepared to trace these varied relationships to the undifferentiated effects of two or even more factors. But in the state of our very limited knowledge of the details of the sucking act this is not necessary.

The observations which I find in literature permit of no definite statement as to whether the expulsion of the mammilla is an act of the frequent process of vomiting which occurs in the infant so naturally and for a long time without reaction of discomfort, and which starts when the stomach is filled to capacity. To this it may be added that the infant generally, after a short time, falls asleep for reasons which will be explained later.

The continuous sucking of the finger after satiation discloses a very important aspect of these processes in general, which cannot be discussed, however, without assuming pleasure in sucking. But before we use this term, we must insert a short interpolation. In any case, the important consequence of this fact will be better treated during the discussion of the actual infant period, because, as was observed, it is not established beyond doubt for the first days of life, and perhaps cannot be established at all.

CONCERNING THE CONSCIOUSNESS OF THE NEW-BORN

This interpolation, which has become more and more unavoidable, should give us a simplified terminology. In many places it has been very difficult to avoid the use of words which are only fully justified when it is assumed that the new-born has the same kind of consciousness as the adult. This assumption must be justified and exactly defined so that the abbreviation which we use shall be unmistakable when we speak of *pleasure* and *pain*, etc. In addition to the terminological interest, the question of the consciousness of the new-born is of theoretical interest, but it seems to me neither so profound nor so important as it occasionally is felt to be. Consciousness in the new-born has been as emphatically affirmed by some as it has been firmly denied by others, but at present child psychologists appear to affect discreet indecision. Bühler thinks that in order to assert anything final about the consciousness of the new-born one must have knowledge of the biological working of consciousness in general. It seems to me that he is right; and because we have no more than speculative ideas for a future outline, this question must remain open. Nevertheless, it is advisable to discuss it, at least for our terminological purpose.

There is no coercive reason for denying on principle *consciousness* in the new-born. The new-born is not merely a reflex being; to say the least, the reflexes are so complicated that nothing forbids us to think of them as accompanied by *consciousness*. The neurologic state of the cerebrum is not so undeveloped that the possibility of consciousness must be strictly excluded, even if a definite stage of development of

the cerebrum should be an essential prerequisite for consciousness. We know nothing about consciousness, its origin
and its functions, so that we cannot draw a conclusion from
these sources as to the absence of consciousness in the new-
born. On the other hand, consciousness must appear in the
infant sometime in the first weeks, for no one can reject the
impression that the three-months-old child has consciousness,
and to exclude it creates, it seems to me, insurmountable
difficulties for our understanding. But one cannot specify
the moment of the psychical development in the first few
weeks of life in which an essential change occurs, which gives
one the right, the opportunity, to speak of it as the hour of
the birth of consciousness. And therefore one is quite naturally justified in assuming its existence in some degree at the
beginning. Where this is not done, good reasons are necessary.
These are lacking, and one, therefore, receives the impression
that the view which assumes on principle the absence of
consciousness in the new-born is biassed, and that the
conjecture of consciousness, which is after all permissible
in an undecided scientific question, is denied because its
admission has unwished-for consequences for the new-born—
e.g., there is no reason against employing the same considerations for the fœtus of more mature stages of development, and
for certain groups of animals. This impression, that the child
in the first days makes upon us—namely, that it is indeed more
animal than human, but that it is by no means a machine—
is of as little value for scientific results as if it had been refuted
by reason. For one can understand the new-born life quite
well even without consciousness. And if one attempts to
assume consciousness as indubitable, even in this the non-
scientific attitude seems to bear out the facts. First of all
there is the fear of denying the psychical in the new-born.
This is only necessary as long as one continues to create un-
surmountable limitations to our understanding through the
systematic equation of mental and conscious, not only in this
instance but in general. This fear does not concern us
because we have established ourselves on the foundation of
Freudian psychology. There is no doubt that the new-born
reacts mentally; whether or not it happens consciously,
how far, and in what manner, is a question apart, which is
not of decisive significance if one is convinced of the existence of unconscious mental life or feels impelled toward

this assumption. We shall hereafter speak of pleasure and 'pain,'[1] perception, etc., as abbreviations for the more exact mode of terminology, without intending to imply anything concerning the quality, conscious or unconscious. If this process has the quality, consciousness, then the individual experiences it as pleasure, etc., presupposing that the relation of consciousness to the process is the same in this case as in those which we have experienced ourselves and have positively inferred in other people—on the basis of their verbal utterances; a prerequisite upon which are based the possibilities of all psychology of conscious phenomena.

I should like to add several remarks, although they can be better substantiated later, because they may create an apperceptive attitude in the reader, which will be useful further on. In all questions pertaining to the uncertainty of the problem of *consciousness* some investigators who have affirmed consciousness have made conjectures about the nature of primitive childish consciousness. As far as I can see, these suppositions incline to attribute to the new-born and young infant " dull, emotional states of consciousness," "the first traces " (Stern). These are, of course, conceivable, and I have neither the intention nor the means to contest these statements. But the possibility of thinking of this matter in a different way has been indicated. Freud (10) makes the important comment that it is not advisable to spoil the most certain and most direct knowledge we have, consciousness, through the assumption of its continuous transition through stages of progressively weakened consciousness until unconsciousness is reached. Psycho-Analysis, which recognizes an unconscious, makes possible to a certain degree the retention of consciousness in its precise meaning even in those states which, lacking the familiar clear unambiguous quality of consciousness, are ascribed by everyone to the *unconscious*. If it were necessary, these nuances would be tolerated. If one supports this idea of consciousness it is hardly impossible, but rather difficult, to imagine a progression through gradual stages from a vague consciousness; just as we can not trace a sense-quality to anything but a more simple state, one which contains this quality. This means, we should like to be able to say: when consciousness makes its appearance for the first time, it appears with the quality of consciousness—

[1] Unlust.

a definite clarity of experience which we cannot describe, but which without any intermediate stages we understand directly.[1] We can easily imagine that in the beginning mental processes seldom (perhaps in quite a limited degree) possess the quality of consciousness; though it is immaterial whether it was received while in the uterus or after birth, immediately after birth, or several weeks later, we should, however, like to think of having received this quality unclouded. Although we know little concerning the biological value of consciousness, still it is difficult to imagine what use a hazy, stupefied, dazed consciousness can be to the organism. Of course we are familiar with such states, but in them we are incapable of doing what consciousness requires of us; in this state especially consciousness does not function and everything blends imperceptibly as if we had been unconscious. In those states, which appear to give us our understanding of the function of consciousness, consciousness is a very perceptible quality— e.g., pleasure and 'pain.' One can imagine that distinct pain,' more precisely conscious ' pain,' calls forth quicker and more positive reactions than would be possible for organic regulation. But then consciousness must be even in its beginning more marked, for a hazy consciousness would not make any essential difference. Nevertheless, one factor appears to be contained in the idea of the " dazed consciousness " which Stern rightly shows, but it seems to me that it will only be clear when regarded from the angle of the Freudian psychological structure. In the *Interpretation of Dreams* Freud has, as is well known, sharply separated his concept of the system Pcpt.-Cs. (Perceptual-Consciousness) from Pcs. (Preconsciousness) and Ucs. (Unconscious), and has assigned exclusive perceptions, sense perceptions, and inner (pleasure and ' pain ') perceptions to Pcpt.-Cs., while memory traces belong to the system Pcs. This schematization can help us considerably in our problem. For in it, one might say, the exact character of consciousness is stressed, which attributes complete continuity to the systems of the unconscious (Ucs. and Pcs.). That which constitutes the dark background of consciousness, which one calls the current of consciousness, does not actually belong to the system Cs.; for in it there are

---

[1] Koffka comes to similar, partly identical, conclusions from quite other reflections. Kirkpatrick touches the question, if I interpret him correctly, likewise in this manner.

numerous very condensed memory traces which belong to the
Pcs. and which only become conscious in a composite, as it
were, not one by one, and give the impression of a " dark "
background in contrast to the perceptions which belong only
to the conscious (" pleasure-pain " sense perceptions). The
perceptions of adult mental life (determined in some stage of
childhood, but I shall not say here definitely in what stage)
do not come about through stimuli (inner and outer), but are
confused with memory traces which are in the process of
becoming conscious; this complication is mentioned here
merely to avoid misunderstanding. Now it is not very
probable, as we have already indicated, that memory traces
become conscious in the primitive consciousness merely as
the function of perception. For then it would consist of more
or less isolated, but completely conscious, perceptions. The
stimuli are caused internally or by the environment. For an
instant, light, warmth, coldness, pain, and pleasure flash,
only to vanish out of Cs. without leaving a trace. The trace
remains in the unconscious, operating from there in some
way.

All this is, of course, merely speculation. But it is permissible—provided one does not forget that it is not here a question
of knowledge but of assumptions, even perhaps of a mental
game—to make a few speculative strides, when one has arrived
at the end of factual knowledge. There is one more thought
to be added. It arises quite naturally from the Freudian
schematization; it is in fact contained in it. If the energic
conceptions of mental life are treated seriously, as has been
done until now only by Freud and his school, the assumption
becomes unavoidable, that a psychic process to which is added
the quality consciousness, also experiences drastic alterations.
One may form an idea concerning the nature and purpose of
the alterations from a consideration of the Freudian suggestions. And one would be tempted to say, the course of
the unwinding of excitation (*Erregungsablauf*) undergoes a
diminution of its free energy through becoming conscious.
The process of becoming conscious binds a certain quantity of
its energy. Then according to the Freudian system of
ideas which is based on Fechner, a general tendency of the
psychical would be fulfilled, that of keeping the excitation as
low as possible. One must accordingly imagine that the
earliest moments of consciousness were associated with strong

excitation and that consciousness serves to reduce this excitation. The predominantly greater reminder of excitation is discharged through motor activity, by crying, kicking, etc.

After this interpolation which terminated rather theoretically, we can return to the sucking of the new-born. It serves the nutritional impulse just as crying does (frequently); it represents, of course, in contrast to crying, the pleasurable side. Both together overcome a painful state (hunger), and result in sleep. The original situation out of which birth awakes the infant is again attained. Both together belong to the conservative or regressive tendencies. But we feel reluctant to regard sucking as a part of this tendency. One objection prevents us: what is the sense of speaking of a regressive tendency here? Since sleep and being awake rhythmically relieve one another in life, one could view all the behaviour of human beings as preparation for making sleep possible, and in this possible generalization the principle loses all its value. Moreover, if being awake only serves to clear away the disturbances to sleep, how does it happen that the waking periods become longer? For the fact that the child's stomach and functional capacity become greater, and the consumption of nourishment progressively lasts longer, only explains a fraction of the unproportionate lengthening of the periods of being awake. There must exist, alongside of the regressive tendency which explains the short waking periods to us, and alongside of the traumatic character of birth and its results which we can include perhaps in isolated cases, a tendency which impels towards a state of being awake; we might well call it a progressive tendency. It is easy to see it in " pleasure," with which certain activities in the service of the regressive tendency are bound up or were originally bound up. Sucking may be given as an example of this. " Pleasure seeks everlasting eternity "—this characteristic of pleasure makes it suited to serve the progressive tendency. It allows the wish to fall asleep again to be forgotten, and generates the effort to remain awake for its own sake. The processes which keep one awake will accordingly be found under those which run their course with pleasure, and it is advisable to give a survey of them first.

THE PSYCHOLOGY OF THE SENSES

The physiognomy and behaviour of the new-born in a warm bath (approximating bodily temperature) is so marked and striking that one inevitably receives the impression that the child is in a state of great comfort. All observers, in so far as they are not biassed by the theory of the " spinal " creature which is incapable of any conscious processes, agree with this. They count the warm bath among those few pleasant experiences which the human being enjoys in its first weeks of life. And since this applies to the first bath as well as to all later ones, Preyer correctly assumes that for most it is the first pleasant sensation after birth. One must note for later discussion that man is indebted for this first agreeable sensation, the first pleasure, to the skin as a sense organ. The new-born is, in general, very sensitive to cold and warmth. The reaction to warmth has not yet been investigated by the more exact methods. Observation without apparatus has taught us that the infant at any age is very grateful for being made warm and being kept warm.

The effects of cold are shown in varied vigorous movements ranging up to crying, and produce a waking state as all authors in agreement find. Canestrini's investigations, which follow up the physiological reaction, have shown such reactions to every cold stimulus, and he has taught us to classify them under reactions of the ' pain '[1] type: immediate acceleration of breathing, an increase in brain pressure, motor unrest, and occasionally acceleration of pulse. From the first hours of life, every part of the skin surface proves sensitive to touch stimuli of all kinds. Movements of weaker and stronger degree are released through stimuli just as much as the physiological reactions. Preyer was able to confirm the older experimenters in this, and corrects them only slightly, and Canestrini, the newest experimenter in the entire field of the sensitivity of the new-born, was able in the main to agree with the earlier authors. But here several very noteworthy peculiarities of the new-born are to be kept in mind.

1. With the exception of stimulation of tongue and lip,[2]

---

[1] ' Pain,' with inverted commas, signifies *Unlust*, as in the phrase pleasure-pain principle. Pain without inverted commas signifies *Schmerz.—Translator*.

[2] To be more exact, two or more limitations should be made: (1) That we have learned nothing from literature concerning the sensitivity

the experimental subject responds by painful reactions to all tactual stimuli. This is surprising, since it is so different from the adult's behaviour. And yet it is not a problem, at least not specifically for us. The result follows from the method. There are stimuli which occur suddenly and are of short duration: they could simply be called, without exception, waking-stimuli. They are chosen because of their high degree of intensity, or their intensity is increased to a degree which will produce a reaction. But since only pain reactions result, one must really say that the stimulus is increased until it produces pain, testing therefore the sensitivity to pain. This would be only ostensibly contradicted if a correspondingly small sensitivity to pain were established in the new-born.

A needle prick is used to test sensitivity to pain. Genzmer found that one or two day old children react to a prick, which would cause a painful expression in the adult, by slight reflex movements just as to an ordinary touch. Canestrini does not completely confirm this observation. His results always indicate slight sensitivity to pain. But although it is not exactly apropos, one must here insert what Preyer established—that the reaction is obviously dependent upon the number of nerve endings touched. A stimulus applied to an area limited almost to a point records no reactions or very weak ones, whereas the same intensity of stimulus on a more extensive area indicates definite reactions. The new-born generally does not respond to locally defined, sudden and quick touch-stimuli, if it does not pass the threshold of pain. It does not appear to derive pleasure from them—a fact which is easily understood, if our conjecture concerning the waking-stimuli appears plausible.

2. The sensitivity of the high-relief areas of the skin of the new-born differs from the adult's state. Lips, upper lip, eyelashes, mucous membrane of the nose, and skin of the forehead are, in comparison with the adult, over-sensitive; body, legs, under-arm and hand[1] are under-sensitive. The greatest sensitivity is concentrated in the lips (Canestrini). It is as if

---

of the genital parts and of the skin of anal areas, which, since it pertains to the theoretical interest of this question, can only be explained by the prudery of the authors; and (2) that the palms and soles of the feet react to touch stimuli reflexively, a fact to which we shall refer again later.

[1] The fact seems to me indubitable for the hand; but I find no notes about it in the literature.

the mouth (the snout, one might say, since the tip of the nose and nostrils also enjoy considerable sensitivity) was the actual tactual organ of the new-born (Sully), and, one might add, its pleasure organ.

3. " The variations in the sensitivity of various parts of the body to touch impressions are at the beginning not as great as they become later " (Tracy). On the whole, the skin surface of the new-born is not marked off, as it is in the adult, into many seemingly restricted zones differing considerably in sensibility, but presents a more homogeneous, undifferentiated surface in which the oral zone stands out as the most sensitive. The two principal, indeed the only ascertained, pleasurable states which comprise the waking life of the new-born originate from these relationships: the pleasure of the whole undifferentiated skin surface derived from the warm bath; the pleasure of the oral zone in sucking.

The older observers were well acquainted with the fact that taste is one of the very earliest sense organs capable of functioning. The experiments of Kussmaul, Genzmer, Preyer, Sikorsky, and Canestrini have proved it. Sweet, bitter, sour are clearly differentiated during the first days. The mimicry which almost always takes place corresponds to the typical facial expressions which appear even in adults for these three qualities of taste. The remaining movements in response to bitter and sour are of a displeasing nature, sometimes defensive, to the extent of choking and spitting (vomiting); in response to sweetness, sucking or licking, which at the beginning should only occur in response to obviously sweet tastes, begins (Preyer). These reactions, of course, appear only in response to a liquid of a definite concentration; there is scarcely any cause for saying that, therefore, taste sensitivity is slightly developed, as some authors have done (Stern, Perez), because " of all the senses the taste stimuli certainly yield the promptest reactions " (Canestrini).

It is worth noting that the first taste even of sweets produces a disagreeable reaction: surprise from a new impression, Preyer says, and only when this is overcome does sucking begin. The fact that weak sour and weak bitter solutions are taken without rejecting them has at times caused considerable perplexity; wrongly so, because there is no other conclusion to be drawn except that every touching of the tongue (or within the mouth and lips perhaps) is followed by sucking, but that only certain distinct stimuli of definite strength, bitter and sour, are warded off. If we add that a distinct stimulus of definite strength—sweetness—not only does not inhibit sucking, but makes it more pleasurable, then we have formulated in general the function of the early formation of the sense of taste for the instinctive needs.

One must not imagine that the pleasure of sweets is continued through sucking; on the contrary, we must agree unhesitatingly with Compaire, when he interprets it as an act aiding the nutritional impulse: and " when the nutritional need ' and the regular instinctive sucking movements bind the infant to the breast, love of sweets encourages general taste impressions connected with this effort, and assist an essential act to perfection through the excitation of the senses." But the existence of sucking could certainly not be made dependent upon pleasure in sweetness, and the pleasure of sucking could also scarcely be made identical with sweetness. This would be merely a factor in the complicated development of the pleasure in sucking. That this is not sufficiently strongly stressed can easily be explained by the fact that psychology from its origin pursued the study of elements so exclusively that the pleasure derived from them did not always coincide in principle, but *de facto* with the positive feeling *tonus* of the senses. That there exist beyond this other pleasure phenomena, instinctual-pleasure, as I shall call it now in contrast to sensation-pleasure, is too little observed and still less studied. Now, if we retain this primitive distinction, there is no doubt that the pleasure in sucking is an instinctual-pleasure, in which the sensation-pleasure in sweetness plays a rôle not yet confirmed, but in any event hardly the decisive rôle.

One characteristic of the sense of taste has been observed repeatedly since Sigismund. If a new-born has drunk mother's milk, it very often offers the most obdurate resistance when alien or cow's milk is given to it; thus Preyer reports of the fourth day, when mother's milk, diluted with water, was given to a baby, it accepted only the original milk, or the diluted milk sweetened to taste like the mother's. One concludes from this that the child has a recollection for taste stimuli very early in life, that it differentiates the sweeter milk in memory, so to speak, and therefore rejects the adulterated or foreign milk. This fact is of intense interest, for it forces us to assume a very complicated process for the first days of life. If the child drinks distasteful liquids, then the nutritional instinct and nursing are accepted into its service and no further assumption is necessary. The rejection of bitter and sour is well understood within the bounds of the nutritional instinct, if one—as we are accustomed to do—views bitter and sour as harmful substances. The behaviour described is no longer an inherent or instinctive one, useful as it may be for the physical development of the infant, but an additional one, acquired in the first days, and clearly intended to relish once more the pleasure that has already been enjoyed. Of course, memory is necessary for this process, but it explains nothing.

The remarkable thing is that such a capricious use is made of the memory, that an imperative longing for a definite sweet taste has developed. For longing (the word is, of course, used only analogously) is the descriptive term for the process. That this is imperative is seen from the fact that hunger is preferred to milk which is not sweet enough for its liking or taste. Nothing contradicts our assumption of this desire in the new-born, and we shall show that it appears clearly enough very early, particularly in the·case of taste.

This dovetails fairly well with the other consideration—namely, the assumption of a yearning for the renewal of the specific pleasure experienced in the first days of life. It shows us the progressive tendency very early and powerfully; or the desire to become satiated quickly and to sleep again is here vigorously interrupted by the wish to become satiated in a definite pleasurable way—i.e., not to become satiated, and to sleep, but to experience that specific pleasure. But the fact itself is not demonstrated beyond doubt, I regret to say. Canestrini emphasizes that in his experiments with infants from one to fourteen days old he did not receive confirmation of this fact. And it contradicts the absolutely established fact of sucking the finger and all suitable objects which lack the quality of definite sweetness and all characteristics of the desired milk.

According to the investigations and observations of the older observers—Preyer, Queck-Wilker, Stern, Sikorsky and Canestrini—it appears unjustified to maintain the point of view, deriving from Rousseau, that the new-born perceives no smell sensations. The sense of smell may, however, be the least developed. A final decision would naturally be premature so long as the psychology of smells is for the most part inadequately explained as is unfortunately the case at this point. Smell does not play a conspicuous rôle in the child's development, and we must, therefore, be content with the scanty collection of evidence. Only one fact must be commented upon explicitly. Canestrini found that, as a general rule, of the infants tested in so far as they showed any positive indisputable reaction to smell stimuli, they responded by breathing deeply, which in the adult is interpreted as a form of pleasure reaction. Because the negative reaction was not established, we cannot exclude unconditionally the possibility that the unobserved interference of a traditional valuation causes the belief that the new-born's sense of smell is undeveloped. The observer who, through his own experience, knows a reagent as foul smelling and notices no defence reaction in the new-born, concludes that childish organs are dull, while in fact the infant has responded with weak pleasure reactions; since it perhaps evaluates positively smells disagreeable to us. We shall be able to prove this in one instance; perhaps it applies more generally.

In many cases which observers marked as lack of sensitivity, positive feeling could be assumed, although it is not pantomimically expressed, and is, therefore, overlooked. Nevertheless, there is no reason to ascribe a relatively dull sense of smell to the new-born, although it is certain that human beings in comparison with animals possess a less developed olfactory faculty. Should the suggested possibility be verified, then some understanding of the way in which the sense of smell was dulled would be gained; it might be concluded that first a reversal of valuation occurred, and then debility followed. This is a possibility which coincides well with Freud's (14) idea of the correlation between the repression of smell and upright walking.

The statements of the various observers differ astonishingly in establishing the first hearing sensation of the child. Naturally, we have long since given up the belief that the child is deaf for weeks. Scarcely anyone disputes the fact that normal hearing functions in the first week. In the same way there is unanimity in the belief that the first hours of life are spent in deafness. The anatomical facts of the middle-ear filled with liquid (Vierordt), the thick stoppage of the hearing passages (Preyer), force us to this assumption, which is not contradicted by any findings. For this period of time the estimates vary considerably from six hours (Canestrini) to four days (Preyer, Dix, Queck). This is probably also the normal individual deviation span. One must, however, emphasize the fact that observation is confronted with a difficulty which perhaps is the reason for the contradictions; but in any case the observation that the motor reactions to hearing stimuli are diffuse and occur only irregularly is of great theoretic importance.

The child does not appear to react at all to the various slight and continuous noises which surround it by day in a normal environment. To sudden and loud noises it responds with manifold movements: blinking, quivering, head movements, throwing its hands in the air, contracting, with undifferentiated shock reactions as Stern so aptly calls them. In so far as physiological reactions capable of proof only by experiment are being tested, the previous observations become more clear and intelligible. Canestrini found that none of the seventy new-borns tested on hearing impressions were definitely without reaction. The experimental subjects were from six hours to fourteen days old. He neglected to state the age distribution, so that the question of the beginning òf the hearing reaction cannot be decided from his work. The proof of a clear and regular reaction on the respiration curve and the pulse curve, as seen on the fontanel, permits us to note that the observer's collection of evidence is too superficial, and not of decisive importance. The observer does not primarily establish when the child hears for the first time, but when it is frightened for the first time by sound impressions. For one cannot designate these reactions in any other way than as fright. This expression is justified by the study of physiological reactions, since Canestrini " could often register graphically an increase of the pulse under increased respiration activity after hearing impressions," which indicates a reaction of the " painful " type.

So far as can be seen from published observations, this unpleasant type is the only one besides the " attention " reaction. One may say that a sudden sound-stimulus of short duration and of a definite intensity—and only such are being tested—generally calls forth ' pain,' of which the motor expression contains equal elements of fright. Toward prolonged auditory impressions, the new-born behaves indifferently, as if it were deaf. To say that it is hard of hearing, that it reacts only to strong stimuli, is hasty. Direct observation determines nothing here, and physiological observation has not been undertaken. In addition, some stimuli used by Canestrini and also by Carmaussel may be mentioned: whispering, a ringing bell scarcely louder than the noise of walking backwards and forwards; talking, which is carried on in the child's room, without a noticeable reaction setting in. And finally it has been shown that even in the first days a definite habituation to sudden auditory stimuli is established by the fact that the reaction to short successive whistles becomes weaker.

The exceedingly surprising fact that the new-born already reacts with a kind of attention to auditory stimuli is once again noted. This will become important for us in a future connection.

When one reads in old books and occasionally in more recent ones (Gaupp) that the new-born is blind, it is either a vague statement or else undoubtedly wrong. Anatomical discoveries, as well as the properties of the eye movements of the new-born, completely exclude the assumption that seeing in the sense of adult sight is involved. Wherein the difference lies cannot be precisely stated with complete certainty. Stern's formulation is probably correct. " Colour, form, condition, distance do not yet exist . . . it is not a question of seeing objects." Nevertheless, the definiteness of his view is a little rash, at least in so far as form and colour are concerned. But to speak of blindness is absolutely incorrect. There can be no doubt that immediately after birth—normally—sensitivity to light exists. Strong and sudden light stimuli, almost without exception, are promptly responded to by changes in the respiration curve and in the fontanel curve, and often by shutting of the eyelids, by twitching and other expressions of fright, and at times by crying: and indeed these occur in sleep no less than in the waking state. Observers and experimenters from Preyer to Canestrini consistently agree in this matter.

The same harmony of opinion does not exist on the question of whether the light sensation is agreeable or disagreeable to the new-born. Here there are enthusiastic supporters for assuming a " seeing-pleasure " from the very beginning—Dix, e.g.; whilst others assume a shunning of light from the beginning; photophobia, an " actual antipathy," Compairé, its spokesman, calls it. Actually there is much to be said for this assumption, and we can understand it quite well from the point of view of the progressive tendency. Espinas' remark that the child opens its eyes preferably in the evening (Compairé) is correct; the references to children born blind are easy to understand and evident; and, above all, the results of Canestrini's research favour this conception. These investigations have shown that strong and sudden light stimuli are accompanied by all the manifestations of 'pain.' But Canestrini would construe the curves of the other stimuli, too, as " tension " rather than as pleasure. In contrast to this, it must be borne in mind that Canestrini's method is somewhat uncertain and does not allow for positive explanation of all the curves, and that the responsiveness of the new-born for medium light-stimuli and distant light sources exists beyond doubt very soon after birth. And, finally, after a few days, even stronger intensities do not cause warding-off movements.

Preyer, who is claimed by both parties, differentiates sharply at this point, and finds that moderate light is agreeable, but strong intensity has an unpleasant effect. This conception seems valid, and there is much to be said for it. One point of view can be added which has bearing on our train of thought, and at the same time weakens the above-mentioned contradiction a little. Measured by the adult state, one can easily call the behaviour of the new-born " shunning the light," but in comparison to its foetal state it is decidedly friendly toward light. It is by no means true that light of every intensity incites the new-born to attempt to reinstate the foetus situation. On the contrary, it accustoms itself very soon in the first two days, at the most, to moderate light, that is to say to relatively weak light, but nevertheless to a stimulus state foreign to the foetal life. Many authors (e.g., Sikorsky) assert that they have observed that even in the first or second day the head turns toward moderate light. Nobody denies this for the end of the second week. This signifies not only habituation, but also points towards positive pleasure derived from the light, and even rejection of darkness is found very early in life.

So Preyer writes: " Long before the end of the first few days the facial expression of the child whose face is turned (in the evening) towards the window suddenly changes, as I shade its eyes with my hand. The dusk, too, undoubtedly makes an impression, and, according to the child's expression, an agreeable one. Whether this is actually and generally valid for the first few days is irrelevant to the fact that we are dealing with behaviour for which we find no analogy in the facts previously described: a part of the fœtus situation is rejected as disagreeable, a stimulus completely foreign to the new-born is coveted. This reaction is the exact opposite of what would be expected from the regressive tendency; here a positive tendency exhibits itself: to exchange the fœtus situation for the waking life. If one chooses to express it so, we can say that from the beginning of life there exists the possibility of pleasure from the sense of sight, which was experienced quite naturally in the first days of life, and which gives preference to the waking state in light and resists the return to the accustomed state of rest of the embryonic life. We have seen the predisposition and foundations for such behaviour as this in the sense of taste, in pleasure in sucking, and we have the earliest apparent expressions of the progressive tendency in the eye.

If we organize the facts about the sensitivity of the new-born's senses, the following systematic comments are, it seems to me, made possible with constrictions.

We have at times used the terms, pleasure and ' pain,' in the sense previously explained, in analogy with adult behaviour and experience, when reactions of a physiological or motor nature permitted these terms. We need not depart further from this nomenclature, but we must be all the more clear as to what actual facts it covers. A glance over these reactions as a whole will show that three types have been built up: I. A bright ray falls suddenly on the open eyes. They close energetically. II. A smell penetrates the nostrils. The child breathes unusually deeply. The significance of both these reaction types is directly intelligible: I. prevents the continuation of stimulus; II. promotes the continuation of the stimulus. We are adding nothing new to the facts, only describing them differently, when we say: in I. the stimulus was undesired; in II. it was desired. We understand these reactions immediately. This does not apply to the physiological reactions (breathing, pulse, etc.) which are tied up in the adult with pleasure and ' pain,' and which we—often enough, but not always, connecting these with R.T. (Reaction Type) I. or II.—find in the child too, and which by analogy with adult experience we explain or name. The   explanation of these reactions is a problem in itself, which is still awaiting discussion. It is sufficient for us that the physiological reactions of the aforesaid kinds I. or II. can be added, since we must assume that where Type I. or II. is lacking, the stimulus was insufficiently intense or biologically not important enough to bring about a response.

Group III. reacts differently. The following may be taken as typical of it. A shrill whistle strikes the new-born's ear. The arms are thrown into the air, the face twitches, the body is convulsed in a brief and slight cramp, as it were. We cannot understand these reactions immediately, for they neither hinder the continuation of the stimulus nor further it. They are purposeless. The reaction of the adult is exactly the same, and equally purposeless. And the physiologic reactions are in both instances identical or similar. From this very little is gained, for although we are acquainted with fright as well as with pleasure and ' pain,' we are further from an understanding of it than from pleasure and ' pain,' which we understand little enough. And the fright of the new-born appears even more purposeless than that of the adult. Sometimes one seeks to explain this phenomenon as a deviation from a primary flight-reflex. Now the fright movements are not fright, but at most a paralyzing flight-reflex, which, as Freud so correctly argues, prevents flight. But at all events one can hope for an understanding of the adult fright from this conception. In the new-born a flight-reflex in itself is meaningless. R.T. I. and II. are specific, different for every category of stimuli, and adaptable to the defence possibilities, and to possibilities for advancement. R.T. III. is general and applies to every field of stimulation. This fact is of double importance. First, we must ask if this common reaction is not a generalized one. And there is some ground for admitting this assumption. The skin as a sense organ has no simple mechanism for defence against stimuli. But the body, as a whole, can dispose of skin irritations. They can be removed by the hands, or finally, in˒ certain cases which have played a definite rôle in phylogenetic development, by the twitching of definite sections of the skin. Now all three possibilities are actually combined in the fright reaction: the intention toward flight, the arm movements, the twitching. A frightened infant sometimes gives the impression of rubbing, pushing something off or defending himself with his hands; he twitches as one does when driving off a fly by facial contortions.

One must now assume that this syndrome is a displacement of the skin stimulation to other stimuli. This is plausible for hearing stimuli. The ear has less means of defence than the skin when such activities as holding or stopping up the ears are not included. One cannot close the ear like the mouth or the eye; the noise cannot be blown away like odours. There may be a way of explaining that this unprotected organ gained control of the reactions of the skin, of course in a meaningless way; for fright does not ward off the noise. (Nevertheless, it is still striking that the reactions, especially to noise stimuli, are so often and intensively, as we saw, of Type III.) But further generalization of R.T. III. of skin and ear can hardly be understood in all sense fields. Here it is purposeless " plus." Nevertheless, I have not suppressed this reference to the defence methods of the skin against stimuli; for even though it does not enlighten us on more than a minute part, it is still worthy of note in such an unsettled question.

Secondly, the universality of R.T. III. makes it necessary to conceive it as primitive, undifferentiated. I have already cited some facts to show elements in R.T. III. which arise from the birth situation; other facts will be brought forward later. It was Freud's ingenious idea to connect fright with the reactions to birth. In any case birth is the first experience in the nature of a shock in the individual's life, and if the child experiences anything during its course, then certainly it must be a kind of fright. For the present we agree with this conception, promising further proof in a later discussion, because it is the only one known to me which encompasses a great many facts and covers developmental psychology. Accordingly, we connect the R.T. III. phenomena to the traumatic results of birth.

Any stimulation of the senses can produce fright reactions. Their conditions are not known, but obviously intensity and suddenness (unexpectedness) play a large part. One can indeed say that at the beginning every sense stimulus which does not correspond to the fœtus situation is responded to by R.T. III. The foregoing statement sums up the observed facts. These facts are unproved for the sense of smell alone—perhaps merely because this sense has hardly been studied at all. But it is certain that no proofs to the contrary can be found in this field. A certain time must lapse before this fright response, which started at birth, disappears and makes room for responses of R.T. I. or II. The overcoming of fright is not attained simultaneously in all stimulus fields; it seems to occur first in the mouth and last in the ear; nothing more definite can yet be said about this. In any case the child during the first days of life is quite completely in the " over- coming phase "; it is generally fearful; it is still completely under the influence of the results of the birth trauma.

Man is indebted to the oral zone, the entire bodily surface, and the eyes for the earliest clearest reactions of Type II. The sweetness of the milk and its odour, the taste sensations during nursing, the warmth of the bath and the moderately bright light, are the sense stimuli from which the new-born very soon, in the first hours and days, has the ability to derive pleasure, from which it does not withdraw its organs, but to which it offers them. We understand this behaviour most easily in the case of the warm bath. Here a situation in which it grew from the beginning, and which it lost by birth, is repro- duced for the organism. The conservative or regressive tendency, which applies to all organisms, shows itself clearly in this instance, and such leading back of a phenomenon to an organic law solves the psychological problem, and replaces it by the biological problem which is no longer within òur province. This is not valid for the eye and the very early pleasure of seeing. On the contrary, it is an astonishing fact that a condition, which was in no way possible before birth, should give rise to pleasure so soon after birth. We cannot yet suggest an explanation for this. We must submit to the fact, and end psychological theorizing by fitting it into a fundamental organic law—namely, the progressive tendency. This term gives scarcely more than the merest description of the facts. Just as the germ cell, in spite of the conservative tendency—at times making compromises with it—changes progressively, so the new-born also changes progressively in spite of the tendency, so clearly exhibited in it, to return to the fœtus situation, and at times forms compromises with this tendency. We see very early the effects of this tendency in the behaviour of the eye in response to light stimuli; still earlier we see the effects of the tendency of the oral zone in relation to taste, touch, and perhaps smell stimuli, which are bound up with nourishment and suckling.

The reactions of Type I., after all is said, can be understood clearly enough as an expression of the regressive tendency.

One form of reaction (Type I.) has been left unconsidered:

attention. Canestrini tries to interpret attention from his hearing-stimulation curves. The phenomenon of attention will occupy us later. In the infant attention is too vague and undifferentiated to make any statement valuable. But we wish to note that it seems to make its appearance by means of hearing, that organ which has neither R.T. I. nor II. at its disposal to any evident degree.

DISCHARGE MOVEMENTS

We have already spoken a great deal about the movements of the new-born, because they are, in fact, the object of the psychology of early childhood; and because of this an organized discussion is desirable.

Preyer has classified the vast number of child movements into four groups: into the impulsive, reflexive, instinctive, and ideational (*vorgestellte*) movements,[1] in which he includes the expressive movements. In the main this division has been retained until to-day, in spite of the fact that the boundary between the groups has become so problematical. We shall ourselves make use of it because it is convenient, not only through habit but, above all, because by establishing the category of impulsive movements it delimits an important set of facts.

The impulsive movements really begin months before birth at a time when the reflexes are not yet acquired, when the anatomical development has not yet made them possible. They are, therefore, independent of all peripheral stimulation. A complete inventory of the earliest movements after birth does not seem to have been compiled. The processes, however, to some extent important, have been described, especially those which are beyond doubt impulsive. The following are considered among these: stretching and bending the arms and legs, which the new-born very often exercises without our being able to determine the external cause; spreading and bending the fingers; stretching the body (often after waking); some eye movements during the first day; the manifold movements in the bath; sundry grimaces, especially, of the lips and eyelids; certainly also the back and forward movements of the hands, particularly in front of the eyes, which Preyer includes

---

[1] Preyer says the lowest kind of ideational (*vorgestellte*) movements are the imitative.

among the instinctive movements. (This classification is not very enlightening. The reason for this is obvious, since out of those movements grasping, which Preyer could scarcely consider anywhere else than under the instinctive movements, develops. But by the same argument all the impulsive movements must be added to the ideational (imitative) movements which, as Preyer shows, develop out of them.)

We are very far from an understanding of this group, so much so in fact that, as far as I can see, after Preyer, no one realized that there was a difficulty here. Preyer sees their cause in instinctive and other organic processes, which take place in the motor centres of the lowest organization. To explain them, "nothing remains but to assume an inner reason for the impulsive movements, which is given by the organic constitution of the motor ganglionic cells of the spinal cord, and which is bound up, in the early embryonic stage, with the differentiation and growth of those formations and of the muscular system. A certain quantity of potential energy must be accumulated with the formation of the motor ganglion cells in the spinal cord and medulla oblongata, and this potential energy is already very easily transformed through the blood-stream, or through the lymph-stream, or even through the rapidly progressing tissue formation, into kinæsthetic energy."

How far this assumption will satisfy modern physiologists cannot be discussed here. But psychologically some objections ought to be advanced, since the assumption contains elements which are well suited for the disclosure of more important relationships. At first it is not quite clear whether potential energy is received only by the growing motor ganglion cells, or whether at their formation it originates in such quantity that it is sufficient for years. The lack of clarity lies in this, that Preyer says that the impulsive movements disappear almost completely and come to pass in adults almost solely in dreamless sleep. One must completely exclude this possibility. Furthermore, these impulsive movements exist only in the fœtus state and for a short time afterwards, without our being able to determine exactly where the transition occurs. If the ganglionic cell has stopped growing or has used up its potential energy, the impulsive movement is transformed into another category; it is not easy to say into what category. This category certainly cannot be definitely specified beyond saying that it differs in some way from the impulsive. It

4

could, for example, serve the pleasure gain of a kinæsthetic type. Of course, in Preyer's scheme of things, there is no room for this conception. But, as always, if one shifts the criterion into the "stimulation of the motor centre of the lowest organization," one deprives oneself of all other than purely negative possibilities of differentiations: since bending the arm can be neither intentional nor stimulated peripherally, nor does it pertain to an instinct, it is, therefore, impulsive. One difficulty is increased, since all impulsive movements can also appear equally as reactions and unobserved effects of stimulation, and stimulus changes can be avoided at best, only under the most accurate experimental arrangements. If, like Stern, one summarizes all the movements without relation to external causes, and "therefore from internal causes" as impulsive, one enlarges Preyer's group with some degree of justification, but not in his sense. And one succeeds finally in adding the hunger cry to them (Stern), or one says with Bühler: "We can say that all movements of the new-born are either impulsive or reflexive movements in the broader sense of the word (inclusive instinct-movements)." It is plausible to classify them thus,[1] but Preyer's emphatic statement, that not all movements are direct reactions to inner or outer stimuli, is thereby lost. And, as I should like to show, a significant suggestion is contained in this reference.

The expressive gestures are similar to the impulsive movements, at least in this respect: that the grouping and organizing of both create considerable difficulties. Preyer built up a group that obviously resulted from practical considerations, which he classifies as instinctive movements, but to which they belong only partially. Later authors have extricated themselves in various ways, for they have not found the question of great importance. The following expressive gestures can be attributed to the new-born: crying, defence-movements of the head, pouting of the lips, wrinkling of the forehead, head movements, grimaces in reacting to sweet and sour, fright. One sees that this group, gained from Preyer and Bühler. is very varied. Crying, I have attempted to show, is to be eliminated. It is undoubtedly an instinctive or impulsive

[1] Of course, it means a great deal to maintain that the defined, impulsive movements "are not carriers of some kind of mental processes."

activity; the well-known first cry is a reflex. There are still other movements not mentioned here, which become more numerous in the first weeks of life. These we shall treat later. But some critical comments must be made here concerning the classification and explanation.

In contrast to the impulsive movements the expressive movements are dependent upon a stimulus, either upon definite internal or external stimuli, or upon a general condition. Their common characteristic is that the movements belong regularly to a definite stimulus-situation, and that they cannot be completely understood out of this situation; they seem to have a relation to other individuals, and they are simply communications to them.

1. Considering the social function of these movements first, we in no way deny it, although it seems rather questionable whether it can explain anything and what it can explain. In countless single instances this function of communication is unwished-for, and it is embarrassing that the suppression of expressive gestures is so difficult. This is certainly valid for the complicated social relationships of people. In the more primitive animals it is striking that the expressive movements are not lacking, even in essentially isolated functions, as, for example, when a cat or dog gives chase. Finally, what can the expressions of pleasurable states convey? It is from such instances which we do not understand that we construct the most ethical and altruistic motives for these insignificant and primitive phenomena. I mean that the social function cannot be the cause of these movements.

2. The expressions are not always, and not completely, comprehensible with reference to their stimulus: they are often purposeless in their relation to society, and when one disregards society, they seem completely purposeless. Now this is not quite correct, for some of the expressive gestures are quite comprehensible as R.T. I or II, and adequate, whereas for others, such as pursing the lips, frowning, crying and laughing, it is in the strictest sense literally true. It would be wrong in child-psychology to consider only the visible expressive gestures, the pantomime. We must also include the physiological movements which can be registered pneumatographically and sphygmographically, which regularly belong to certain stimulus states even more strictly than do the pantomimic expressions. And in this

case, and in the majority of cases, we are, of course, compelled to admit the purposelessness and inadequacy of the expressive gestures in relation to the stimulus. But here also the possibility of establishing a relation with the environment is absent, for these reactions are imperceptible without scientific investigation and are far from being readily intelligible expressions. The phylogenetic development of expressive movements has been only slightly understood, and Darwin (1) shows that some might have had a function, which conformed to their stimuli—about which we shall report later—but why they have been preserved without function remains unexplained.

And this again connects them for us with the impulsive movements, whose function is entirely unexplained in so far as it is not derived from the growing ganglion cells. This means that, excluding Preyer's, not a single attempt at an explanation has been made. But instead of that even here a relationship is established which corresponds to that of society. Many authors emphasize the value of the impulsive movements as exercise (e.g., Stern). Here, too, a misunderstanding must be avoided: the value as exercise exists, but the question remains whether it explains the existence of the phenomena. The warrant to assume a purpose in the psychical and to work with this as an explanation cannot generally be disputed, but deserves conscientious consideration, which we should like to give to more suitable material. But to say in all seriousness that the impulsive movements exist, because later they will make learning to see easier, would bring us critically near to the logic of the biology primer, which asserts that man has one mouth and two hands in order that he may speak little and do much good. I realize that no one says this in all earnestness, and yet the reference to the exercise-value is not always made merely as reference, but is also an attempt, even though inadequate, to diminish part of the senselessness of these phenomena. Lengthy criticism of all this is not justi fied by any abundance of material which I am about to bring forward as explanation. This is only a little and not completely new. But the criticism seemed to me important principally on one ground, which certainly is not very important, but which is treated even more slightly and transiently than it deserves.

Questions of movement are necessarily questions of psychical energy. They are therefore very insufficiently investigated, and considered very theoretically and hypothetically. Of the newer psychologists, Freud above all has given attention to them, and has tried to make use of as simple and as few hypotheses as possible. And since they cannot be completely avoided, the most circumspect and the least sweeping recommend themselves. We have already made use of Freudian concepts in the foregoing, and here we must again link up to them. We assume with him that the state of equilibrium can be so distinctly differentiated from the state of excitation that we say that the balance of energy is disturbed and aims to reestablish itself. The " bound " energy in the state of equilibrium was freed by a stimulus. This state of excitation must be overcome by again binding the free energy. In principle these are assumptions which were not alien to psychology, but those unexpressed ideas which every discussion of movement processes hinted at are here expressed in specific terminology. This is approximately what Preyer vaguely perceives as " potential energy." The localization in motor centres of the lowest organization and the conception that potential energy originates during growth are two assumptions contained in " potential energy " which are not controllable and are unnecessary. We limit ourselves to assuming that a quantity of energy is at the disposal of the organism as a whole. Nothing compels us to express an assumption concerning its localization or origin. But we must expressly assume that the energy can be transformed: bound—free; Preyer says potential—kinæsthetic. These assumptions are scarcely surprising or ineffective in themselves. One way of binding free (freed) energy is by transferring it into " kinæsthetic energy," which is the motor discharge of excitation.

Accordingly we would say that the impulsive movements are discharge movements. This is certainly nothing more than a change of name, implying no greater depth of understanding than Preyer's. Since we are now freed from unnecessary suppositions, we are free to extend his conception actually to all impulsive movements, not only to those which are due to the stimuli of growth. Every release of psychical energy can lead to impulsive movements, even in adults. It need not happen, if there are ways of binding free energy other than through discharge. It is quite probable that growth phenomena produce such discharges of energy, in the forms of hunger, temperature, stimuli, the peristaltic movements, and other similar ones. They can then discharge themselves into impulsive movements. By this we have enlarged Preyer's group of the impulsive movements somewhat in the sense of the above-mentioned classification of Bühler and Stern. But the criteria have become more precise. The discharge movements have no relation to the stimuli. They can be released by outer or inner stimuli, or by processes which we generally do not call stimuli at all, but they have no relation to the stimulus; they do not avert it, do not further it, but are purposeless in relation to the stimulus, one might say neutral to the stimuli. They serve to master the existing energy situation created by stimuli—if there are any—by decreasing the energy level, the quantity of free, released energy.

If the absence of peripheral stimulation as a basis for classification is abandoned, there is no longer cause for ignoring the persistent similarity between the impulsive and expressive movements. Obviously a good part of the so-called expressive gestures is nothing other than discharge movements; not all, of course. We have seen this in crying, for example; we shall explain it more carefully in some other examples. But the temptation to classify all movements as a whole as discharge movements must be resisted. Perhaps every movement without exception is discharge of free energy, but there is no need to make a decision at this point; in any case we have given a general, accurate description of the energy process. But we question the energy process only where it itself represents the function of the phenomenon—that is to say, those instances where, or in so far as, the movement runs its course unrelated to stimuli. We shall meet cases in which decision will be difficult; but in contrast to these there are a great many in which there is scarcely a doubt. And this applies to the impulsive and to a certain portion, as yet impossible of exact determination, of the expressive movements. We shall, therefore, combine both these groups as discharge movements, by which we mean movements or the components of complex movements neutral to stimuli. The movements of R.T. III are in essentials to be added to these.

THE REFLEXES

Preyer's second large group of movements is the reflexes. Varied though the conception of the reflex phenomena may be, there is still scarcely any variance of opinion concerning this group. These simple movements, which are bound to a strong and fixed stimulus, of course exist and form a definite group in themselves. The explanation of this group is uncertain, but it is not important for mental development. The reflexes of the new-born likewise do not seem to have been thoroughly described. Research has not, however, omitted any important reflex.

The established ones are: pupil reflex, the first cry, sneezing, breathing heavily, yawning, coughing, sobbing, hiccough, extension of the great toe when the sole of the foot is touched (Babinski reflex), the knee-jerk, clasping with the hands. In the above, only those which have some definite relation to the mental are named, whereas the physiological ones are not mentioned, although the boundary line between the two is very difficult to determine, the more so since the reflexes are without independent mental significance.

They are of importance for the motor development of complicated processes (for the development of sucking-movements —e.g., compare Popper). Their relation to the stimulus is a double one: they are dependent upon it—no stimulus, no reflex; and they are understandable from the stimuli. They are reactions to the stimulus; they ward it off (for instance, sneezing), or accept it (widening of the pupils in the dark): they could therefore be included either under R.T. I or R.T. II. For some reflexes, classification as R.T. I or II is difficult—e.g., spreading the toes and clutching with the hand. In these cases one can think of reflexes which once were significant. One can assume with Kirkpatrick " that probably they were of use during some phase in the antiquity of the race, in so far as they assisted the mother when carrying the children." The same might apply to the toe reflex, for the primitive posture of the infant—corresponding to the posture of the anthropomorphic ape—was perhaps as follows: to cling with the hands to the mother's skin, and to support itself by its legs against her belly (Moro). We should then have before us instinct-movements which no longer have a biological purpose, and are therefore regarded as reflexes.

ACTIONS

Ideational or voluntary movements do not exist in the new-born; at least we have no grounds for assuming them. But there certainly exist movements which cannot be differentiated from the ideational—*i.e.*, movements to stimuli (inner and outer)—relatively purposive movements of which it is assumed that they run their course without consciousness, an assumption with which we could agree, because it is immaterial for these movements whether they run their course with or without consciousness. Such movements are called instinctive. When the chick just out of the egg pecks for grain, it is a purposive movement with reference to a stimulus. They differ from the reflex in that they are not so fixed, but are, to a certain degree, dependent upon factors which lie outside the stimulus, perhaps dependent on the degree of hunger, and dependent also on the fact that they are capable of a certain adaptation to stimulus variations and capable of skilled perfection. This instinctive action, whether it is accompanied by consciousness or not, differs from voluntary action in that it is not due to thinking (*Überlegung*), to the knowledge of the requisites and the consequences of the act. It is innate. And this inborn purposiveness in relation to the stimulus characterizes the instinctive. Concerning this, general agreement seems to prevail in literature on child-psychology, even though many writers consider the unconsciousness of the act as the more important criterion. Such instinctive-movements can be classified: movements which subserve the taking in and digestion of nourishment (sucking, biting, licking, chewing, swallowing, choking, vomiting, belching, defæcating, and urinating); normal breathing movements, and those which are connected with breathing faculties (sneezing, yawning, coughing) (Bühler); movements involved in the carriage of the head and body (Preyer). According to our previous exposition, crying should be added to these.

Actually, the understanding of instincts is one of the most difficult chapters of child-psychology, and there is no hope of furthering this understanding at this point in the description of the new-born, since its processes are so undifferentiated that the more exact relations cannot become clear. A critical discussion of the question would, therefore, be premature, and I must be content simply to put forward a point of view, the justification for which can be completely set forth later. I shall try to place the emphasis upon the action-character of the instinctual movements. In any case, the word instinct-activity is more euphonious than instinct movement; thus Bühler speaks of impulsive, expressive, reflex movements, but of instinct-activities.

The action is not an isolated movement, but even in the most simple instance a system of movements, because even when it consists of the most simple, single movement it is related to an aim. It has an intention, it serves a need, and is intelligibly determined by this its " purpose," and by this its need. When I move my left hand over the paper in front of me, I perform a very simple movement, but because I happened to brush away a speck of dust, which was in the path of my pen, I thus executed a perfectly valid action. If there was no " purpose " of any kind for this movement, then I can call it a " discharge " phenomenon, or whatever else it might be named. But I am not concerned about whether the whole process was known to me, or what part of it or how much of it. I can execute that movement without the speck of dust, without having noticed it and its intention, and observe all these only later after it is completed. I can make the same movement and be conscious of it, and also be cognizant of its intention. Let us suppose that I am dissatisfied with what I have just written and wish to repudiate it. It would be advisable, then, not to speak of an action, but of a symbolic action, if one wishes to, or whatever one wishes to call it— for this brushing movement is not directed seriously towards the change of the written matter; if it were, then it would be evaluated as an action and, moreover, a false action, for it cannot attain its end. But this example cannot be developed, for the movements of adults are too complex to throw further light on the matter. An action, therefore, is a movement which is determined by need and intention. It runs its course always in such a way that it can be interpreted by a chain of reflections, even when we know beyond doubt that these deliberations have not taken place. The pecking chick behaves as if it knew that grains of a definite kind are palatable and nourishing, and as if it had deliberated as to how it could, with its given body, introduce the grain into its stomach.

Since we are convinced that in the case of the chick neither the knowledge nor the deliberation was present, we say that its action was an instinctual one. And by that we indicate the surprising fact that activities which are not deliberated upon can terminate as if they were. Perhaps it is not useless to remark that one can deliberate incorrectly; there are instinctive actions that go so far astray that it seems as if the animal had deliberated wrongly. It is one of Köhler's important contributions that he shows that apparently " irrational " activities of some animals are capable of the interpretation of having been wrongly " deliberated upon."

Accordingly—omitting the reflexes—we shall construct two large groups of movements: the discharge phenomena and the activities. The activities of the new-born are instinctual: they come to pass without experience, knowledge, or reflection. Above all, there are four important groups of activities of the new-born: crying as its universal activity; sucking activities from swallowing, etc., to defæcation; all the movements, which wish to " reinstate " the fœtus situation (closing the eyes, embryonic hand and feet positions, etc.); those movements which seek pleasure " from themselves," so to speak: pleasure-sucking, gazing into the light, etc. The activities serve the regressive or progressive tendency and the nutritional instinct, if one prefers to separate the nutritional instinct from the regressive tendency. The R.T. I movements could be quite generally classified as defence-activities, the R.T. II movements as offence[1]-activities.

THE STRUCTURE OF THE NEW-BORN

A comprehensive presentation of the psychic phenomena of the new-born, one by one, is justifiable, because these are the starting-point of its development. My task will be to describe these phenomena in the following chapters and in later books, especially since they have been so much neglected in the previous explanations of child-psychology. Such a presentation of the psychology of the new-born contains a considerable difficulty—namely, that its subject is in the highest degree undifferentiated, so that the descriptions will appear in some places subtle, much too interpretative, and theoretical. But this difficulty makes more cogent and obvious a demand which is slowly beginning to filter into the psychology of

[1] *Zuwendungshandlungen* in contrast to *Abwehrhandlungen*.

all stages of development, but which seems essential for the new-born. The demand is for a consideration of the whole after the investigation of the parts, for the observation of the relationships of all those phenomena which the investigator must study separately for a long time in order to recognize them. He misses the full recognition of them if he does not eventually appreciate that isolation is only an economical device of investigation, if he does not remember that perceptions, conceptions, movements as such do not exist, and that the fruit of his method only ripens when he destroys this isolation as soon as it has served his purpose. The new-born is as little as any other living creature a mere sum of sense stimuli and reactions; it is a self-contained organic whole. The whole is not intelligible from the sum of the parts, but rather every part is intelligible in the light of the whole. Such methods for psychological study are becoming more and more recognized. It is a fundamental idea of this book, and I close every chapter with it. Nevertheless, an analysis of the very different ideas and tendencies, which are generally designated as structure, will be necessary. At present I shall term " structure " only the reciprocal relation of the separate phenomena to each other, a feasible and much less pretentious task even so than Spranger's idea of *Struktur* or the notions of the *Gestalt* psychologists. When I say that the new-born itself is in isolation it is meant in this sense only : the natural whole to which we must relate the phenomenon is the new-born and its mother. Birth, indeed, signifies the physical individuation of the child, but not its biological and social individuation, and in a certain sense, therefore, not its psychic individuation. Moreover, we have several times shown —in agreement with all the authorities—that the new-born is obviously incapable of satisfying its own needs—even its most primitive needs, or indeed these least of all.

The new-born is, moreover, completely dependent on its environment—in short, on its mother. This is not merely a defect of its form of existence; on the contrary, it is adapted to this condition. Its structure responds to definite conditions in the organism of the mother, or in the very composition of society. And that gives us the right to call the subject of these interdependent functions or conditions a unity. The new-born itself exercises only a relatively small fraction of those mental and physical performances necessary for the gratification of its needs. The rest the mother (society) performs.

This fact, the special social structure of new-born and infant, needs clear formulation. We inquire into the conditions under which a person performs work for the gratification of others, and we can say that this takes place in two instances. First, when the subject " waited on " is loved. For this is the paradoxical social result of every love, that its object is the accomplishment of a great number of its demands, so love necessarily must behave " altruistically " to a certain degree. Applied to our theme, this is a diffuse paraphrase of banal wisdom: that it is mother-love upon which the child depends, and upon which it reckons because it is never lacking. But the last statement is not correct. The absence of mother-love is not at all rare. This has already been spoken of, and there is still more .to be added. But the child's existence is connected not only with the corresponding existence of mother-love, but with a quite definite and not inconsiderable measure and specific kind of it. And it would be too much to assume that this measure is never short, that the love is always such that its subject is prepared to endure the full measure of work and privation in order to receive compensation from the gratification which work and privation as love activities offer. And here the second instance appears, in which under normal social conditions " altruistic " action is possible. This occurs when the object of the service rendered exerts mastery over the performer (Weber). Strange though it may sound, the infant exerts not only love domination, but also overlordship over its mother. Of course, it does not demand obedience to its orders nor personally punish neglect of them, but it always begins to perform that act (principally crying) which would lead to the gratification of its needs, and it finally dies if no one responds to it. But a mother who neglects her child feels the disdain or punishment of society, which makes itself in some way and in a varying degree the guardian of the child's overlordship, and which thus protects and assures it the gratification of its most important needs. The extent of this protection, its forms, its guardians, are all subject to much variation. We shall concern ourselves with these in a later section. Some manifestations of this actual fact, however, are nowhere absent.

We have named only one important pillar of the social

structure of the new-born when we have shown that the new-born is not an individual, that all its most important activities are not self-concluded, that it is, therefore, absolutely dependent upon the mother, and when we said that the corollary of this state is the infant's love-domination and power which it exercises over the mother and the community. How the love-domination and mastery of the infant came into existence is, however, not explained, and it is perhaps as yet inexplicable. But in any case, until we attempt in its proper place to wrest from this problem what it can yield to us today, we are content with the banality that the overlordship of the infant is irremissibly necessary for the maintenance of society, so long as its love-domination is not strong enough to assure it the fulfilment of the correlative acts.

An isolated suckling would be in an unhappy state: it would be as good as dead from the very beginning. But normally it is as little isolated as any other part of the mother's body, though this does not exclude the fact that occasionally it is so isolated, somewhat analogously to an amputation. (It is important to be clear on this point, because it safeguards one against distorted mistakes in our observations: that the new-born seems to be worthy of sympathy and in need of help is one of its despotic methods, but it is not worthy of sympathy merely because it appears so.) The new-born seems incomplete when we view it alone; it becomes complete immediately when we consider it together with its mother who is dominated by the new-born's love and mastery. But the correct evaluation of the structure of the new-born requires not only the mother as a supplement, but also some attention to the new-born's history. The new-born is the starting-point at which we begin the study of development, but it is not the initial point of the development itself. We know very little about the psychology of the fœtus: nevertheless, the assumption ought to suggest itself and go unchallenged that the fœtal state is structurally characterized by a maximum of " bound " energy, and therefore it expresses the greatest external rest and balance of which we are empirically capable. The mental life of the new-born consists partly in this—namely, the reinstatement of this state of rest as soon as it is disturbed by birth, and after birth when it is recurrently unbalanced through inner and outer stimuli. The most essential element of the psychic structure of the new-born is the conservative tendency.

A whole series of mental phenomena refer to it—we have previously described them one by one—which we represent by saying that they serve the conservative tendency. The remarkable facts concerning the states of irritability of the senses which appear the more contradictory the more exact the methods of investigation are, can be understood from this point of view as positive and significant. If one does not recognize the conservative tendency, then one must say that the functioning of the sense organs is defective: moreover, one cannot account for this fact—that the sense organs nevertheless do function or occasionally can function. But this contradiction can be solved in relation to that tendency and, indeed, on a purely mental level: the sense organs do not function, no use is made of them, in so far as the conservative tendency is effective, which is generally, but not always, the case with new-borns.

One group, however, which is included under the phenomena of the conservative tendency in its broad meaning, can be very well considered by itself, and as an expression of an instinct— namely, hunger and its gratification. Here we can exchange the uncompromising term ' tendency ' for the more precise, more prejudiced, term instinct, even if we wish to avoid, for the present, the discussion of the conception of the instincts. Hunger-cry, head movement, grasping objects with the mouth, sucking, swallowing, are the phenomena which refer to the nutritional instinct. This instinct itself is undoubtedly ultimately classifiable under the conservative tendency, but it deserves none the less a separate category for itself.

These processes have also an historical reference which we must declare as unclassifiable unless we conceive of them as consequences of the traumatic mode of birth. The conservative tendency does not inhere in them; at first they show no tendency at all, but are reproductions whose cause and whose mechanism are comprehensible to us, but whose economic functions are not yet so.

And, in conclusion, even in the phenomena of the first few days, there becomes apparent the beginning of a new structure-group to which, until now, we have attributed a progressive tendency in contrast to the conservative tendency, but whose essential core has a relation to pleasure which is not yet clearly determinable.

B. THE FIRST PROGRESS

SEEING

THE structure of the new-born very soon experiences a series of essential changes which are designated as developmental progressions. The word progress is not entirely a happy one. It is not used to express any judgment of values, but as a descriptive term for phenomena which the new-born still lacks and the appearance of which makes the infant more like the adult human being. But one must remember that development does not run its course uniformly, and that, therefore, some phenomenon foreign to the new-born's structure, or scarcely indicated in it, nevertheless forms itself clearly in the next developmental period, though it is at first very dissimilar to the norm-structures of the adult; so that it is difficult to decide whether the earlier or later stage is closer to the adult, although they differ from each other so greatly. It would be well if there were a suitable word to designate such changes which, in the circuitous route of development, deviate from the starting-point of development without approaching directly the end-point. There is no such term; we therefore use " progress " more unconcernedly than we should if we knew that such roundabout ways as these were necessary steps.

The first progress of this kind demands our special attention for the same reasons that direct us towards a detailed study of the first weeks of life. Manifold as they will prove to be, they stand in firm relation to one another, and give a precise stamp to a definite developmental span. It is, indeed, approximately the first three months which can be considered collectively as the period of the first progress. Naïve observers have been inclined to assign a unified, unique position to the first quarter of the first year. Sigismund calls it the stupid quarter. This name has not persisted, but the separation which it suggests was widely accepted, and, moreover, it vindicates itself on deeper grounds than the convenience of counting by the calendar year.

This phase can be briefly, easily, and clearly characterized.

Child psychologists are scarcely at variance upon the fact that the active use of the sense organs and the appearance of the effects of memory in the emotional life and in the will of the child—as, *e.g.*, Bühler formulates it—are the first important steps of development. Actually both of these do not exist, or are so indifferently indicated in the new-born that the unfolding of both these phenomena must produce a very essential changed structure in the child of three months. In order to perceive this clearly the established facts must first be presented collectively.

A priori it is apparent that the first developments will be phenomena classifiable under the progressive tendency, the tendency to make mental progress. One can therefore expect them to be especially clear in the field of the sense of sight, which from the very beginning—as contrary to anticipation we found—behaves progressively. It is advisable to begin with them.

The eye is from birth very sensitive to light, and moderate light stimuli release manifold reactions of pleasure: opening the eyes wide, turning the head towards objects, the breathing and pulse curves, are all more of the ' pleasure ' than of the ' pain ' type. When the light is agreeable to the new-born, it can still do very little to obtain this pleasure or to ensure its continuance. The movements towards light are at the beginning seldom—though this is not positively established for all cases—of long duration or much consequence, and occur only in response to diffused light from large surfaces. In spite of the manifested attraction to light, there can be no talk of the infant seeing in the sense that the adult sees. Though it is in general debatable whether in the first days small lighted objects (candle-flame) as well as a large bright surface (window) are noticed, it nevertheless is certain that the direction of the glance towards the object and the accommodation to its distance do not exist at the beginning. On the contrary, the capacity for both is gradually acquired in the course of the first three months. The older child-psychology, with Preyer at its head, has devoted conscientious study to this question, with the result that we are well informed on some important questions in this connection.

Focussing the gaze perfects itself in four stages (Preyer, Bühler): (1) The glance wanders aimlessly about; if it accidentally falls on a distinct object sufficiently near, the pleasure reactions already named may appear—or the infant gazes straight ahead and depends upon an object being or coming by chance into its line of vision. (2) About the second week bright surfaces are actively held within the line of vision; turning from one bright surface to others has been observed (eleventh day, Preyer). At this point a kind of real seeing of stationary objects is attained, a stage which provides the infant with considerable pleasure. The next important step—the decisive step, if you will—is (3), which is made in the third week. Then the eyes can follow slowly-moving objects, and they take on a " new, contented, intelligent expression " (Preyer). The pleasure, or at least its expression, increases up to loud " joyful exclamations " (Preyer). Thus the child has attained a certain degree of independence from the accidental appearance and disappearance of light stimuli, in addition to achieving the preliminary condition for actual defined seeing, which is the fixation of stimuli within the retina. With the acquisition of capacity (4), " seeking," the infant has attained that degree of activity and independence which can generally be acquired only with the aid of the head muscles. This seeking usually begins at the end of the third month, and regularly in the following way: the child seeks for the cause of the sound and turns its eyes or its head in different directions, apparently carefully and intelligently planned, often quickly in the correct direction.

Simultaneously with the acquisition of these capacities the convergence of the axes of both pupils develops. At the beginning divergent atypical movements of both eye-balls or movements of one by itself are very frequent. They are by no means exclusive; at the beginning, although rarely, convergent movements occur. These very soon predominate. More exact data cannot be cited, but, in any case, this stage is already reached before the expiration of the first month. After the third month these atypical movements do not normally recur.

Accommodation behaves similarly. It, too, is noticed in the first days, but it is scarcely regulated with regard to accuracy, certainty, and speed. More exact reports are not at hand, but there is nevertheless much to support the belief that at the time of " following " accommodation already functions with some exactness and regularity (Bühler): that before the

5

end of the third month, the development of accommodation is not complete (Preyer), and reaches completion perhaps only at the end of the twelfth.

These facts have become the starting-point of two ardent discussions: first, the question was raised as to whether they cover the nativistic or empirical conception; and, secondly, an attempt was made to formulate from them a suitable conception concerning the nature of the infant's perceptions and of primitive perception in general. The first question could hardly be more in dispute at present. The mechanisms of convergence and accommodation are undoubtedly inherent. This means that the system of muscular movements, which is necessary to perform an act of seeing in the true sense, is prepared by birth. It need not be discovered by the child, and is not " taught " as piano-playing is. On the other hand, it is not completely developed from the beginning, and the co-ordination of muscles which constitutes seeing is not the only kind of movement of which these muscles are capable. Not so in the case of sucking, which is not merely learned, but is at the new-born's disposal from the first day as completely formed co-ordinations of various muscular movements. The motor system of " sucking " is, of course, just as little as " seeing," not the only one which is possible with the respective muscles, but it forms automatically and from the beginning in response to definite stimuli, while in the case of seeing, not only is a more precise co-ordination of the parts generally necessary and gradually develops, but, above all, the condensation as a regular reaction to one stimulus must first be " learned " little by little. This difference appears greater than it actually is, because normally the eye muscles only make more " seeing movements "; because, in part, they are only able to make more such movements; because the lips, tongue, and palatine muscles co-ordinate for various functions for the rest of life. The problem cannot be one of heredity or of acquisition, but, according to Stern's general formulation, it is, " What is inherent, what is acquired ? " And this seems to be the answer: The eye muscle movements are in part inherent (co-ordination, accommodation), in part learned; precision and subordination to the stimulus are acquired; if one can express it so, the combination as sole reaction. It does not have to be expressly mentioned that we are dealing with a reaction of R.T. II type, for the seeing movements serve to admit light, to permit it to act to the greatest degree; it is thoroughly intelligible from this function.

But what does the word " acquired " mean ? How is a thing acquired ? is the question which immediately follows from the answer to this. The second question is important for the clarification of the idea of mental gain: revealing the mechanisms of acquiring is a principal task of developmental psychology. Before approaching the question a few distinctions must be made. Looking consists of a series of unequal psychic movements. The statement that the eye movements of adults are not of a psychic nature at all is hardly too sweeping. They are physiological movements, similar to the movements of heart, lungs, stomach, and inner secretions. There is little reason for separating those movements from these on principle. The physiological movements can very often for a certain period of time become conscious, can be perceived, in the same way as the outer surfaces of our body; they often have psychic results—at times very considerable ones: they can be psychically influenced, sometimes very energetically and lastingly. We have, however, no reason for classifying the peristaltic movements in the field of psychology. And what is valid for this could be equally valid for the eye movements, if the eye movements of adults were identical with those of the new-born. The facts of their development give them a certain place in psychology. Eating is certainly a psychic affair, but the movements of the chewing muscles and tongue are not in themselves psychic but physiological processes. Undoubtedly movements become psychological when they are " discharge phenomena " or " activities." Since the eye movements in the first quarter of the first year are precisely of those categories, they must necessarily be given a somewhat different position in psychology, regardless of the extent to which these genetic facts offer them a kind of midposition between physiological and psychological phenomena.

Koffka alone, as far as I see, remarks that it is to be assumed that by no means all the eye movements of the first days are connected with seeing, but that many are to be conceived simply as impulsive movements, and, therefore, according to our nomenclature, discharge phenomena.

This interpretation seems plausible and justifiable throughout. One cannot sufficiently emphasize that every single undifferentiated state of the early psychic phenomena can have various meanings. If many of the eye movements are discharge processes, it is not surprising that they run their course atypically because the co-ordination of the pupils is not a fixed reflex, but becomes capable of almost every possible kind of movement only later during the course of life.

Above we have classified the psychically relevant movements into two groups: defence-phenomena and activities. If this division is to be maintained, the co-ordinated movements and, in general, all those which are not merely discharge phenomena, but have something to do with seeing, must be regarded as activities. This somewhat contradicts the customary usage of language, but it seems to me it contradicts usage alone. For this classification is in essence justified. We need only make it clear to ourselves that the various eye movements are significant in order that the light stimuli make clear pictures on the retina, and we must be content with the proposition of a " need for seeing." This can easily be done if we consider those facts which have been ascertained concerning the pleasure during seeing and concerning the intensity of this accomplishment.

No observer has neglected to mention the " high pleasure tone " (Bühler), the " great joy " and " loud cooing " (Preyer) of the child, which occur not only at the first seeing or during the first successful stage of the act of seeing, but which accompany seeing in general, and which are especially gleeful and continuous during the first three months. A striking visual object arouses every expression of pleasure, of which the child is capable at the time, even to laughing, kicking, and " screeching." At the beginning the expressions of pleasure are, in general, only slightly in evidence (in contrast to those of displeasure, of which more will be said later), but even the one fact that the child in the first weeks gives his attention to seeing demonstrates a certain degree of pleasure in seeing or compulsion to see, even where the light stimulus can be easily avoided: it needs only to close its eyes, a reaction which the new-born already controls. The following is remarkable, and, in this connection, proof of what Preyer refers to: Wide open eyes, thus admitting the light, is a common never-failing symptom of pleasure; closing the eyes, " not-wanting-to-see," is a symptom of displeasure. It is as if the expression of the pleasure of seeing were typical for every pleasure, which would speak well for the intensity of this delight in seeing.

But being able to see something may also be a compensation for some pain; often, and very early in fact (*e.g.*, the second week in the case of Scupin's boy), the infant stops crying when it is given something luminous and multi-coloured which it can see. It is diverted, not merely for the moment of surprise, but for a longer or shorter period. This behaviour can hardly be interpreted otherwise than as a probable indication that the pleasure of seeing is stronger than the ' pain ' which was the cause of crying.

Seeing is an active process, and is bound up with effort. All signs of attention are connected with seeing. If there is still doubt that the attention of the child in the first few weeks is not passive and extorted, there can be no possible doubt at a latter stage of development. Scupin thus graphically describes the fourth week: " The wakeful child was placed near a many-coloured silk cushion. He gazed at it in sustained attention, dilated his nostrils, and pouted his lips; so that his little mouth was quite pointed. . . . The activity was so apparent that one can only describe the child's behaviour with the words, he wants to see something. Thus, Queck-Wilker writes: ' (Forty-second day) glued his eyes at a point on the ceiling and the head and eyes move backward as the child is turned away from the point. . . . In the seventieth day he follows the lamp light, turns his head after it, and becomes restless when he is shaded.' "

Of course, these developed visual processes are activities. Why should not the attempt to follow a moving candle flame with the eyes four weeks earlier be interpreted in the same way ? But this cannot yet be done, because the latter necessitates head movements, while the former requires only eye movements; the eye movements, moreover, are still unconscious, while the head movements were already conscious. We know that one is exactly as uncertain as the other, and we are not concerned as to whether a process is conscious or not when we wish to classify it as an activity. The decisive reason for opposing this position can only be that the activity is accomplished by an organized psychic factor in the sense of its needs, and it is not easy to assume this need of seeing for the earliest suckling period. But just to prove the assumption of the necessity of such a factor I shall devote some space to the apparently purely terminological question.

If we could assume a conscious ego, which wants to see

we should naturally say that its seeing is an activity. But since we cannot, we must substitute a need, which impulsively or instinctively produces complex movements: activities, or more exactly expressed, instinctual activities. And, in my opinion, that view recommends itself. There exists from the beginning a need to see; instinctively the child performs movements to gratify this need. The term activity expresses the relation of the movement to the need.

Nevertheless, the desire to understand more clearly the "need to see" is conceivable. The first possibility which presents itself is to give this necessity the name of seeing instinct. But we shall not yield to this temptation. In this case the new name adds nothing, and we must avoid the designation, convenient though it may be, of need by instinct, for it is one of the tasks of this book to treat instincts and instinctual life seriously.

Claparède (2) says that the perceptive interest is dominant in early childhood, and that a considerable amount of this interest is devoted to the seeing instinct, for it is more than mere nomenclature. It classifies the need-to-see in a larger relationship, in the established perceptive interest generally. It can, indeed, go yet a step further and explain this interest biologically: interest appertains to that which is biologically important. The consideration of mental development from this angle of interest is related to the one here presented. And one could be satisfied with it, if this interest were not a very puzzling one, and, in the hands of Claparède at least, not a sharply expressed idea. Besides this, the need for seeing is so closely related to pleasure, that one very unwillingly accepts the reversal of the relationship that results from the theory of interest. On this theory the biologically adequate interest, when exercised, produces pleasure. The need to "see" comes from the common perceptive interest; this interest is of biological advantage; it is therefore combined with pleasure. It seems to me simpler to think of the reverse: the need to see is an instance of the general desire for pleasure. Because seeing brings pleasure it is exercised, and so intensely used, that it appears as if a need to see existed. And we have named such ways of behaving, interest. Thus, seeing is simply an activity, whose purpose is pleasure-gain. The fact that seeing brings pleasure and that in any case pleasure is enjoyed is immediately conceivable. Everyone is free to be satisfied with this way out—that seeing is connected with pleasure, and thereby the perceptive interest, the need to see, is aroused, and thus the biological purpose is positively assured.

From the beginning pleasure exists in response to certain light stimuli; there are very early exertions which lead to the formulation of a compulsion for repeated, insured, light experiences, but only after a few weeks (at the end of the first three months) can the act of seeing be more or less completely carried out. A number of movements, important up to this point, are from the start performed as discharge or reflex movements; very soon the rest are also. The substance of the process of completion is as follows: the pleasure instinct gradually gains more control over the movements, they become more and more extensive, are placed more exactly and wholly in its service, and the discharge and reflex processes lose their autonomy; pleasure becomes the exclusive aim, and is more effectively attained. The movements are "innate," the pleasurable tone of light stimuli likewise, and the general instinct to gain pleasure certainly not the least. Control· of the motor apparatus by the instinct is acquired in phases. Of course, this happens in such a relatively short time, that one has no choice but to suppose that the process of acquisition itself is to a certain degree innate, which Koffka (in accord with Stern) has happily termed "maturation" in contrast to learning. This course of behaviour we shall recognize in various phenomena as a typical one. Of course the question as to whether, instead of a growth in the capacity for control, there is not a growth of the pleasure in seeing, or (perhaps dependent upon it, too) a growth of motor power, cannot be rejected offhand. The latter is not valid without qualifications; for if one hopes to obtain any clarity in the problem of psychic energy, one must, as long as it is possible to do so without straining a point, work on the assumption that the quantity of energy is constant. Nevertheless, it is striking that the energy utilized in seeing increases, and one is tempted to say an ever greater quantity of energy (instinctual force) is gradually allotted to seeing. At the same time one obtains a viewpoint for understanding the increasing dominance, the maturation of the act of seeing. It is, figuratively speaking, the result of the flowing of motor power into an inherited apparatus. But where does this plus of energy come from? We do not see a reduction of intensity at this period in any field of the child's life manifestations. If we maintain the principle of constancy, hardly anything remains but the view which Freud (9) represents, that the energy in the organism at the beginning is almost completely bound, and only by degrees becomes free for diverse mental applications. The development of sight is one symptom of such freeing of energy. From this theory a possibility of organizing the pleasure in seeing offers itself logically. It would then be the result of new binding of energy by the discharge in the activity of seeing and its various movements, and perhaps, to anticipate somewhat, by ' perception.'

By this speculation we unfortunately cloud one clear explanation for ourselves. First, we wished to explain the pleasure offered by vision, which we claimed as inborn, as the motor for the development of seeing, and now we say it is the result of that freeing process which seems exceedingly obscure and artificially constructed. This is a contradiction which is not easily solved, especially at this point. We will postpone its discussion, noting meanwhile Freud's (9) assumed repetition-compulsion which, extended into the organic, states that development according to a certain law has been without doubt taking place for unknown reasons, in every single genesis, for thousands of years. In our case the repetition-compulsion is exhibited as follows: the individual begins his life with his energy almost completely bound; it becomes partially free in the first weeks, and binds and discharges itself anew by way of the greatest pleasure possible through the seeing apparatus.

We can better pursue the above discussion concerning the kind of perceptions the eye develops in the child if we consider them in relation to perception in general.

THE ORAL ZONE

Sucking makes its appearance as such a precise mechanism' so soon after birth that one cannot a priori expect any growth of that function. Nevertheless, distinct and significant development of the activity of the oral zone already occurs in the first weeks, a development which, perhaps, can be inclusively characterized by saying that the phenomenon becomes more intensive and more differentiated. The longer the periods of waking become, the more continuous becomes the sucking activity. This occurs in two modes. Not only does the child drink for increasingly longer periods, at times with short interruptions, and towards the end of the meal in what might be termed a playful manner, but it sucks more and more often when it is not hungry and when there is no possibility of satisfying its hunger, its finger or any suitable object which comes into its mouth. Scupin describes very vividly the greater variety of the drinking process from the beginning of the second week:

" As soon as anyone stops near the bed of the crying child, it becomes quiet instantaneously and surveys the bystander. When it is hungry it sucks loudly on its fingers, but this pacifies it only for a short time. Before it is placed at the breast its head rolls back and forth restlessly, the mouth seeks eagerly, and the eyes are wide open. When it finds the nipple it utters satisfied grunting sounds, sucks hastily till it chokes, and sighs as if it were doing the most strenuous work. Then the sucking becomes sluggish and is frequently interrupted, the eyes close, the child purrs like a kitten for a while, and finally expels the nipple by sideward movements of the head."

Though doubt may exist as to whether the new-born makes sucking movements for their own sake, all doubt concerning the regularly-established fact that all children suck their fingers even without being hungry is absolutely excluded during the first three months, and it has actually, therefore, never been raised, although difference of opinion in the occasional interpretations of this fact was very vehement. A note by the Scupins may again serve as illustration (tenth week): " The child preferably sucks its fingers, and sticks the whole fist into its mouth, even when it has just drunk. To wean it from this, a cloth was spread over the child, and it then put this into its mouth with its hand. This proved distasteful, if one may judge from the child's sullen face. After a few attempts it generally stopped sucking." But it stopped only until it learnt either by accident or by trial that the road was clear; for ten days later the parents noted: " The child scarcely takes the finger out of its mouth and bites it zealously with its toothless gums."

This is typical throughout. No method is successful in weaning the child from pleasure-sucking at this age. It is continued with the whole obstinacy of which the child's primitive will is capable, in spite of all obstacles. And pleasure-sucking obviously is a means for a considerable degree of pleasure to the child. It is, therefore, called with justification ecstasy-sucking (Lindner). Not only the obstinacy with which it strains and holds the object it is sucking bespeaks the high pleasure character, but the sucking child's expression is one of greatest satisfaction. The restless crying child can, as every nurse knows, be pacified immediately and often for a long time if a pacifier or other suitable instrument is placed in its mouth. The child often calms itself in that it, after crying for a time, unmistakably gives up its purpose formally, resigns itself to sucking its finger, and thus succeeds in attaining certain gratification. If the nursing has lasted long enough it produces sleep, and, according to all appearances ("blissful smiling"), very satisfying sleep, as after an agreeable exhaustion.

There has been no thorough study of pleasure-sucking, it seems, with the exception of Lindner's work made famous by Freud (2): "Ueber das Saugen an den Finger, Lippen, etc., bei den Kindern (Ludeln)"; Lindner's essay treats the sucking age incidentally. The numerous scattered comments in child-psychology and biographical diaries are indeed sufficient to give an idea about the essential nature of this process, as we have described it above. Unfortunately the comments are not sufficient to extend our knowledge of individual variations. Indeed, the existence of pleasure-sucking seems to have escaped the observers, or seemed too insignificant to be expressly noted. And yet I am of the opinion that it would be worth our while to pursue this question a little. All the phenomena which have occupied us to this point, and all which we shall treat of in this chapter, are normally legitimate; they repeat themselves in the genesis of every single person in essentially the same way. Individual variations in the realm of the normal, of course, scarcely exist. They are really only discernible in one relation: the time of the first appearance of the phenomena; all their later developmental progressions differ considerably in every case. Perhaps, however, an intensive study will teach us to understand these apparent individual deviations as typical, as group phenomena. In spite of this, it is astonishing enough to every one who has observed more than one infant, that each one is an individual and expresses its individuality very early, although it would be difficult to estimate the earliest point of time at which an individual peculiarity appeared, or to analyze its general impression more, closely.

In the face of this difficulty, if we wish to hold on to those facts that to some extent are true, if we wish to retain the dominating factor of that clear but still very general impression, the result in any case will be that the behaviour of the oral zone gives rise to the earliest observations of individual tendencies, as early as the first three months.

Infants differ in the oral function in every conceivable way. Some present a picture of a suffering, impatient, greedy imbiber, while others indulge themselves in the realm of the ever-existing "animal gluttony" (Perez), ranging up to the relatively indifferent, calm, real, and may one say, joyous activity. The accompanying motor processes of drinking, pressing, hitting, holding, scratching the breast with the hands, may be dependent upon the intensity of hunger, and differ according to the momentary mood. Nevertheless, here also some of the characteristic habits seem to develop early. In pleasure-sucking particularly sharply individual behaviour habits develop. Lindner enumerates a surprisingly rich, well-organized though by no means complete, catalogue of behaviour characteristics for later childhood. It ought not to astonish us if an attempt—not yet undertaken—covering the earliest phases of childhood should disclose a considerably smaller variety. Furthermore, this smaller variety will certainly prove to be individually determined. All children, indeed, suck for pleasure just as all children drink. Some begin to be persistent very early, almost unceasingly, and apparently with the greatest straining of attention to procure the pleasure from sucking; others begin later, more intermittently, and less frequently. Certain preferred methods and habits also begin to develop individually rather early and not infrequently in the first three months. In general, the pleasure-sucking of this period differs from the later one in some general characteristics. At the beginning the sucking object is not the finger but the fist; the pleasure-sucking takes place not on the lips but in the mouth, presumably within the region of the Magitot membrane. The change from fist-sucking to finger-sucking, the preference for the thumb, the use of the back of the hand, the fist, the mouth, are active assistance, as Lindner says, which the other organs, the other hand, nose, etc., proffer, and the movements of the arms and many factors could very early become individual habits, personally differentiated ways of behaving. It is very significant how seldom and superficially these phenomena of the oral function become the subject of careful research. The insignificance of this subject can hardly be the reason and the excuse for this singular gap in child-psychology. But it is still more surprising that assertions once made are not further appraised and tested. The poverty of our knowledge about the details of nursing justifies my reference to Herz' works ' which, so far as I know, are the last to give detailed attention to the Magitot assertion regarding the gingival margin. This membrane, also called the Magitot (Vierordt) membrane, appears on the mandibles of both jaws in the region of the eye teeth: it is on both sides as a membranous projection which can be seen more clearly on the under maxilla. The organ is an extensive bloodvessel; it is movable backwards and forwards, and swells during nursing. In case of good development one can speak of very clear papillary protrusions. At times they are connected with each other by a seam, and " it consists of a kind of very small, thin outer lip which extends from one canine to the other, and is capable of some kind of erection " (Herz). The Magitot membrane facilitates nursing in that it is hermetic, and it assists the embrace of the breast nipple. It obviously functions in pleasure-sucking too, because, as I have mentioned above, this takes place not on the lips but generally in the region of the gums. Even when there is sucking without an object, it seems to be an irritation of this membrane; at least, the empty sucking is so employed at a somewhat later period, the tongue being rhythmically rubbed back and forth on the inner part of the upper lip or lower gum. It seems to be in agreement with Herz' observation, that the Magitot membrane on the under maxilla usually develops more pronouncedly. Whether the membrane can be found in every instance is not established. Herz assures us that it certainly exists in very many cases.

The wish to be as thorough as possible in cases where research hitherto has described insufficient material was not the sole reason for the statements concerning the discovery of the Magitot membrane, for it also offers an important point for our method of observation. For obviously the membrane—next to its hermetic function as the piston of the pump which the mouth represents during nursing—offers the infant a surplus of pleasure. Undoubtedly the pleasure which the mouth gives without this organ is sufficient to make the trouble of sucking worth while, for otherwise pleasure-sucking (from the third to the fourth month) after the regression of this membrane would cease, or at least become much less frequent. It is interesting that in the first three months a specific sucking organ exists, whose value as a pleasure organ is not yet confirmed, and it is not insignificant. No histological finding is known to me. Nevertheless there is no doubt of the existence of nerve endings in the Magitot membrane, for it must be capable of feeling. It serves, therefore, as a source of pleasure in continuous rhythmic stimulation, a condition under which every part of the skin surface, and certainly one capable of erection, can give tactual pleasure. To organize our ideas of the function of the oral zone involves a few difficulties at the start. Sucking creates pleasure in any case; obviously enough since it is practised devotedly. Gratification of the nutritional instinct occurs, therefore, from the beginning during pleasurable experiences. One might very well interpret this fact biologically as if the function of this pleasure were the ensuring of the nutritional instinct (Compaire and Friedjung). One could express it somewhat as follows: Nature gives the tactual pleasure as a reward for diligent imbibing, and thereby attains its end in that the child inevitably drinks. This conception does not tell the psychologist very much. He would rather assume that the nutritional instinct—as an instinct—gratifies itself, in that it relieves discomfort, and thereby again brings about a state of equilibrium. But the phenomena described show that not all activities of the oral zone can be caused by the nutritional instinct. We see here plainly that in the first weeks a differentiation appears which was not perceived clearly in the new-born: which was, in fact, scarcely indicated. Pleasure-sucking does not serve the nutritional instinct by the acquisition of pleasure for its own sake. It is tactual pleasure, and is experienced during the satisfying of the nutritional instinct. Once experienced, it is continuously sought for, as every tactual pleasure in the simple mental relationship is, since as yet prohibitions, inhibitions, and repressions are not known. We must sharply emphasize this branching off of one kind of pleasure, this detached pleasure which is given by the gratification of the nutritional instinct, even if in reality this deviation does not appear obviously peculiar. The child learns during sucking, which serves the regressive tendency, to recognize a pleasure which, so to speak, is so sweet that, for its sake, the child refuses to follow the regressive tendency, it delays the state of sleep, and pursues the acquisition of this tactual-pleasure: pleasure-sucking. Since sucking occurs with open eyes during imbibing as well as in pleasure-sucking at least in the beginning phases, it offers also increased opportunity to experience repeatedly the pleasure of seeing. And both of these seem to be a compensation for staying awake. At least, this seems to be the infant's optimistic outlook on life. Freud (2) formulates his important contribution by saying that the instinct to experience this pleasure anew, and for its own sake, develops in connection with the vegetative function.

The first refinements of the function of the oral zone are, therefore, not to be found in their essentials in the fact that the instincts learn to control the necessary apparatus, as was the case in the development of seeing, but in their differentiation; in the separation of the pure gain in tactual pleasure from the taking-in of nourishment. With this the infant obtains a first substantial degree of independence from its environment; it detaches itself psychologically from the body and person of the mother. It becomes an individual, for until now it was, as we have shown, dependent upon its mother during the whole waking state for the gratification of its needs, and it still remains largely so for a long time.

Since two different instincts make their appearance in the function of the oral zone, the necessity to name them presents itself; in other words, to classify the one which cannot be the nutritional instinct. The simplest way would be to call it tactual pleasure instinct. This term is, however, foreign to psychology, and I have reasons for not creating this new word, which will be explained later. Lindner stresses the sensual character of pleasure-sucking, and considers it under sexual manifestations. This classification is completely right, for the tactual pleasure is an essential part of all sexual pleasure; it is one of the aims, indeed an inevitable and perhaps the only direct aim, common to the sexual instincts. Nevertheless, this classification of Lindner's is only incidental; it is not exact, and does not refer directly to the infant, whose pleasure-sucking is scarcely mentioned in his works. Freud (2) has expressed a definite conception of pleasure-sucking as an expression of the sexual instinct, and has confirmed it in his own works and through those of his followers by numerous examples and references. Freud's idea of the sexual instinct is broader than that in use before his time. He calls all phenomena which tend toward the gain of pleasure from touching as touching, sexual. The range of the Freudian ideas is, of course, not exhausted by this definition. What one would probably designate as tactual pleasure instinct is certainly identical with the sexual *Trieb* of the Freudian nomenclature. I have no desire to oppose this nomenclature; our earlier assertions must, therefore, be formulated in Freudian terminology. Pleasure-sucking is an expression of the sexual instinct; its aim is to win the sexual pleasure—the tactual pleasure—which the lip, the mucous membrane of the mouth, and the Magitot membrane have to offer; it differs in its dependence on the nutritional instinct. The oral zone is to be designated as erotogenic. Freud considers it, therefore, as part of the body which can serve as a source of sexual pleasure. Of Freud's discoveries and novel conceptions the characterization of pleasure-sucking as a sexual activity has aroused unusually violent hostility. The outpourings of his opponents are innumerable. But one seldom reads an objective analysis, one reads only excessively vehement attacks. Thus, for example, with reference to our topic, Stern (3) speaks of the "height of absurdity," of "clumsy hands" which "transgress upon the growing soul . . ."; "absurdity . . .," ". . . not only a scientific error but a pedagogic sin," etc. This excitement, surprising for objective scientists, has subsided in the latest literature; many investigators agree more or less with Freud. Others hold to their denial, with or without effect. Their reasons for this will soon be considered in so far as they state any. But first, with emphasis on the peculiar way of behaving shown by these objectors according to their reactions, the question of the sexual nature of pleasure-sucking is no pure scientific problem; they are obviously concerned with something else, with more than the establishment of a fact or the simple consideration of whether a term is properly chosen.

It is a strange thing that pleasure-sucking, even where it is not conceived of in Freud's sense, seems to present more reason for valuation than for investigation. For in contrast to the deficiency of scientific attention to this phenomenon there exists a rich abundance of attempts at curing the habit, and ugly threats. We shall find the same thing in aggravated form in connection with another disputed question, masturbation. Accordingly, a few suggestions are here sufficient. The Scupins felt obliged to do something about pleasure-sucking; parents, even scientific ones, are most often of this opinion; the number of doctors who consider pleasure-sucking harmful is likewise very large. The conviction of its harmfulness is upheld in many ways. An extreme but therefore very instructive example is the English physician, Thomas Ballard, " who, from the above-mentioned phenomena, builds a theory on the useless and objectless sucking of the child by which he attempts to explain most of the sickness of infants, and even of the lying-in-mother " (Herz). It is not our task to decide at this point how far pleasure-sucking is unhealthy. In any case, it is difficult to wean the older child from the habit; infants cannot be weaned at all. It is widespread among infants, and the question of its harmfulness remains open. Why do many physicians naturally assume that it is unhealthy? And if this assumption is based, perhaps, on their own experiences of its harmfulness, and these experiences could be considered credible, why, then, is the naïve, educated person *a priori* disposed to attribute all kinds of evils to the pleasure-sucking of the child; whereas the masses and, it appears, primitive peoples consider pleasure-sucking completely harmless? The intensity of feeling towards this problem is not exaggerated, though some, perhaps, are but vaguely aware of its existence. Evidence of acute feeling seems to me undoubtedly present. At all events, there are many people who think it wrong to allow pleasure-sucking, and who would like to prevent it. Their arguments are so varied, their fears so variously named, that one wonders whether these arguments and fears are rationalizations, and whether they are not unconsciously fighting something else besides the harmless pleasure-sucking. Allers, an impassioned opponent of psycho-analysis, is convinced that in adults pleasure-sucking is of a sexual nature. Gross relates kissing and its rôle in sexual life to infantile sucking. Galanth published an interesting confession of a young girl which indisputably shows that the thumb-sucker experienced sexual delight. These few examples show that the adult conceives pleasure-sucking in himself and in older children as sexual; the infant appears to him still innocently pure, far from indecent as the sexual now appears to him. Hence the vehement denial when someone dares to assert that the infant has sexual inclinations, and hence the war against pleasure-sucking, the anxiety as to its results. It is unconsciously conceived as sexual, even when the conscious signs are of another nature.

Freud's views seem less absurd than the basic misunder-standings of his opponents, who do not wish to hear what Freud repeatedly emphasizes—namely, that his term "sexual" embraces more than the current idea, embraces the whole field of tactual pleasure; these opponents wish to lead him *ad absurdum* in that they suppose that he assumes adult sexuality in the infant. The word sexual may be unfortunately chosen—but is the expression kinæsthetic nicer or more fortunate? The Freudian term is well defined; those who judge it must do so on the basis of its definition. We now substitute it for tactual pleasure-instinct, because I do not feel justified in coining new words when there is already a term at hand in scientific literature—although these would, perhaps, be less harmful but lest apt. If the word designating this idea is clearly understood, then there can be only one motive in avoiding the word sexual: prudish considerations, or the reader's hostile view of sexual phenomena. I do not think this consideration useful. Child-psychology is to become the *scientia amabilis* for young mothers and kindergarten workers—at least, the broad outline is addressed to them—and this state of affairs is hardly desirable. Gratifying as it may be that young mothers and kindergarteners find the psychology of children interesting, developmental psychology ought not, however, to be carried on or even written exclusively for them, and certainly not for the prudish type. The pertinent objections which to my knowledge are raised against the classification of pleasure-sucking as an expression of the sexual instinct are well represented by Stern (3) and Allers. Stern, often divagating into emotional outbreaks, makes objection as follows:

1. False analogous conclusions drawn from the adult to the infant. But surely our presentation is to the point, since we speak only of the infant itself, and merely draw the positive conclusion, certainly not a daring one, on which the possibility of all developmental psychology rests—namely, that the rhythmic stimulation of parts of the mouth produces tactual pleasure. That this tactual-pleasure is the same as in the

6

adult is to be assumed *a priori*. Those who will not have it
so must prove it to be an exception.

2. "That the sucking instinct as the *conditio sine qua non*
for the maintenance of life must be strongly developed in
the small child annoyed psycho-analysis but little." Quite
rightly in this case, it seems to me, for how shall we explain
the persistent use made of this instinct which is absolutely
unsuited for the maintenance of life ?

3. The mouth is the most primitive tactual organ. This is
undoubtedly correct. "Even before the development of
grasping with the hand is made possible, the mouth gives the
earliest knowledge of the form and consistency of things."
This is somewhat less certain; we can say very little as to how
far the mouth brings to pass the recognition of which we shall
speak later; but so apodictically explained it is not "wholly
conceivable why the child, even when it is not hungry, sticks
things by preference into its mouth and sucks them." Sucking
is completely unnecessary for perception, and cannot accordingly be made intelligible from that angle; and it is still less
intelligible how sucking its hand in the same place for a quarter
of an hour, and thereby becoming sleepy, furthers perception;
it is only explicable by assuming a tactual pleasure similar to
that of adults, but surpassing it in intensity.

Allers "does not maintain that all these . . . forms of
activity of infants or small children are not, and cannot, be of
a sexual nature." According to his previous statements, it
appears to him even probable. Only "the Freudian proofs
are not sufficiently strong." A basis for the Freudian assumption exists only "when one is convinced of the identity of all
pleasure, at least of all somatic pleasure, with libido." How
Allers himself thinks of it he does not disclose. We have
every reason to assume an identity of all tactual pleasure, and
I agree with the Freudian designation, "sexual." Only one
point of view which here assists us need be cited. If one traces
back the phenomena of adult sexuality in its ontogenesis—and
that is the task of developmental psychological investigation—
one finds as one of the deepest roots of the extensive phenomena of sexuality precisely the function of the oral zone. It
plays in the normal adult sexual life a subordinate rôle—at any
rate, not a disputed rôle: the earlier one goes into early childhood the more important becomes the oral zone. At the end
of the first year, in the second and the third, according to the

interpretation of the investigator, an indubitable pleasure-sucking activity is to be found. From what did it develop? Obviously out of the earlier pleasure-sucking. The sexual character in it may be doubted. But it is difficult to imagine that the asexual pleasure-sucking of the second and the first years is suddenly changed into sexual (I use sexual in its broadest sense). In spite of that, it will be designated in developmental psychology as sexual—since the other quality is not proven—according to the methodological principle of developmental psychology, that different psychic phenomena of the same origin are to be conceived and to be designated as related psychic phenomena.

The first phenomena in which the ways of behaviour differentiated themselves very clearly from the original completely undifferentiated state, and whose characteristics adhere to later sexuality out of which this sexuality therefore develops, are to be found in the oral zone, and, indeed, in the pleasure-sucking of the infant as soon as it has become independent of nursing.

HEARING

The development of seeing and the differentiations in the oral zone are two distinct forms of the "first advances." Neither of these corresponds to the processes which we can designate as the first progress in hearing. The observation of this phenomenon in its first phase of development is, of course, essentially more difficult, indeed, it is in part completely impossible, and the facts which seem established are, therefore, very few in number and partially ambiguous. To establish the main tendency and the decisive turning-point must suffice. The essential content lies in this, that the initial fright—the pain reaction with which the child responds to auditory stimuli, or, at any rate, to loud and sudden stimuli—yields a pleasure in hearing. The new-born's behaviour in response to hearing stimuli, which we have described in its place, displays the following changes according to biographical diaries:

1. The shock reactions become less frequent within the course of the first three months. They do not disappear entirely, for even the adult at times reacts to sudden sounds in a way which is biologically meaningless. But in the adult it is only an instance of fright, which is by no means released

solely by auditory impressions. And so one lists the shock reactions in the child as states of fright when they are found at an age when the mental processes which we ascribe to fright permit us to assume them; that is, generally in the second half of the first year. This is a somewhat inexact procedure which we can easily make precise if we formulate it as follows: the shock-reaction ceases to be the only obvious reaction to auditory impressions. At any rate, this occurs in the first month of life; as for more exact data, the reports of authors are contradictory. This is understandable, for it depends greatly upon accident, even in the case of a child who is observed systematically, whether the new way of reaction is immediately noticed or noticed shortly after its appearance. In Stern we find a note from which another reaction than the shock reaction can be assumed for the first time; this refers to the third week. In Dix the time is approximately the same, in Scupin on the twelfth, in Preyer on the eleventh day, and in Ischikawa on the sixth day. My own observations lead me to believe that Wilker and Preyer establish the actual beginnings, while the observers who report a later time missed the first phenomena— at least, as far as their writings are concerned. The second week might, on an average, end the average first stage of a new reaction to noises and sounds.

2. The earliest form of this new reaction is sustained atten- ˌ tion. Dix described it clearly. " The body motionless, open mouth, brow wrinkled, the gaze turned inward. By the ' gaze turned inward ' I mean the following: when Bubi was dependent only on hearing because he saw nothing at that time, the eyes showed a ' dreamy ' expression such as I later found in him during mental attention. Bubi appeared to see nothing, only to hear, for as soon as he saw the source of the sound, too, and the sought-for object was plain, his eyes began to sparkle !" We shall later occupy ourselves with this phenomenon, but in the meantime we shall proceed to the presentation of the developmental phases.

3. Attention is soon accompanied by lively expressions of pleasure, a phase which is generally reached, at the latest, in the beginning of the second month; thus Scupin's child laughs heartily in the fourth week when its mother speaks to it, shouts for joy in the sixth week in response to a rattle; Preyer's son gives the impression of extreme satisfaction in the seventh week when someone sings; Tiedemann's son showed the same

satisfaction at the age of one month and a few days when he
heard music for the first time (Compairé).

4. Similarly in the second month, certainly in the third, the child turns its head more or less in the approximate direction of the source of the noise: at first, indeed, without looking for the sounding object. Dix made note of this on the sixty-first day, Shinn before the fiftieth day, Scupin in the twelfth week, Preyer before the eleventh week—if I correctly understand the statements of the authors, who scarcely differentiate between attending with the ears and with the eyes.

5. Shortly after this, therefore, in the third month, the child not only turns its ear (head) in the approximate direction of the source of the sound, but searches for it with its eyes, knows where to find it quickly and surely, and fixates on it, even in rather complicated instances. Scupin's observation of the fifty-seventh day gives a good idea of this: Bubi recognized that when sound came from the piano, he must look at the moving keys. Strictly speaking, this phase no longer refers to the development of hearing, but to seeing; it is organically connected with the latter, is the regular consequence of it.

The pleasure character of the reaction begins certainly at the third stage, very probably during the second phase. We need only refer shortly to the second phase, in which the auditory stimuli result in sustained attention. This state need not be accompanied by pleasure at all. Indeed, by itself, it is not pleasurable; perhaps there are indications that ' pain ' is to be assumed in this sustained attention. Yet it stands between both phenomena. But the second phase is characterized not only by this tension, but the auditory stimuli under consideration have a quieting effect on the child; every nurse knows this, and the authors have seldom failed to recognize this. If the noise—sound, chord, etc.—stops, the child often begins to cry again. Here the tension obviously was transferred into a satisfaction at the perception of the tone. This attentive listening to sounds is an adequate reaction of our Type II. It corresponds to the wide opening of the eyes in response to agreeable light stimuli. One " opens the ears " in the same way, though, of course, the process is not visible outwardly concerning the inner motor processes we know little, and that little is doubtful, so that it cannot be brought in here.

The child overcomes the initial fright and ' pain ' character of the auditory stimuli, and transforms them within the course of the first three months into a source of pleasure. Two facts do not easily become part of this general formula.

1. New-born children in general fail to react, as shown, to a goodly portion of the environmental sounds, although it can hardly be understood why they should not perceive them. This is still more valid for the infant. For the effort of the environment to maintain a noiseless quiet ceases as long as the infant is awake, whereas in the case of the new-born people often make an effort to maintain quietness. Nevertheless, the infant is obviously not attracted or frightened by the sounds which surround it, unless they have definite qualities.[1]

2. Now as before, the shock reaction to auditory stimuli is present. It occurs less frequently, but it is not necessarily infrequent. Its continued existence forces on us the assumption that the stimuli must comply with definite conditions, if they are to be perceived as pleasurable. If confirmation were forthcoming for my own impression from observation that the degree of fright increases and decreases periodically during the first three months, it would be a proof that the conditions for Reaction Type I or III lie not only in the stimulus, but in the whole psychic situation. In spite of the obviousness of this, no profound investigation has yet been undertaken and the observations are extremely contradictory. At best the following can be considered valid: sensitivity to sound grows in some manner during the first months, and sensitivity to sound only gradually appears to extend to relatively distant noises; furthermore, sudden, short, distinct and loud sounds call forth the earliest and longest fright reactions; on the other hand, the human voice, music, and singing play a specially significant part; they are enjoyed very clearly as a pleasant experience.

If one checks up in the published diaries of children what auditory stimuli are recorded as being of a pleasurable character

[1] Sikorsky asserts: " If one observes children when they . . . lie in their beds and ' kick,' it is noticeable that they listen to the sounds of their movements, of their clothes, of their breathing, and perhaps even to the sounds of their heart beat. . . . One can say with assurance that the child is absorbed completely in hearing." These opinions cannot be brushed aside: nevertheless, I am of the impression that this applies to the first two months; but it could perhaps be proved as a deepening or broadening of the fifth phase.

first—not a very conclusive test, but nevertheless some kind of test—we find that they are usually the human voice, chords on a musical instrument, or rhythmic sounds of some kind. One must at the outset presume that the second and third phases are attained at first, or perhaps exclusively in response to repeated rhythmic sounds, while the original way of responding to other stimuli is retained if only they call forth a definite intensity, strength, or unfamiliar quality from the sphere of indifference. Joy in " sound as such " (Compairé), in noise and bustle of any kind, is a later stage which possibly begins in the fifth phase or perhaps a few weeks later.

At present, the available material scarcely permits us to systematize the facts concerning this tendency. If the mere organization is unsatisfactory, how questionable must be the comments based on this faulty investigation and the still more faulty schematization which are designed to classify and clarify. Besides this, the fact that the psychology of hearing has remained so completely rudimentary as compared with its psycho-physics hinders us in this organization. It offers even greater difficulties than the psychology of seeing.

It is often said that here there is a specific problem, that hearing is a " more obscure " process than seeing, even extending so far as to include the " mysterious " effects of music. A few examples from very different facets of this general view may lead us to a discussion of the following statements, to be taken up from time to time in the course of this book.

The paragraph from Jean Paul's *Levana* is given intact, although only a few sentences apply in this connection. Thus, certain basic ideas of my book will assume a poetical form in this quotation.

" The first breath, as well as the last, closes an old world with a new one. The new one is in this case the world of air and colour, but still belonging in the realm of emotions, and so it is that birds die in eggs, and soft curled-up silkworms die at bursting. The first sounds, an obscure chaos, fall on the swaddled soul as does the first light. Thus the morning of life commences with two perceptions of distance for the freed prisoner, as does the day's morning with light and song or din. Nevertheless, light remains the first herald of the earth, the first beautiful word of life. Only a loud noise can penetrate into the still dormant ear; but this sound is created by the woman-in-labour through nothing else than child-birth itself, and thus the world of sound begins with dissonance, but the world of sight with lustre and charm." Compairé emphasized strongly the significance of the mother's voice for the child's development; indeed, he becomes almost pious when he speaks of it. " It is the auditory perception which first seems to free the child's intelligence . . . one must reject the poet's verse and say: ' Incipe, parve puer, lingua cognoscere matrem.' The human voice, especially the mother's voice, which, as it were, is the call of active intelligence to one yet dormant, finds its way the most quickly of all the sense impressions to the attention of the child."

The one consideration that goes beyond the facts which are found in the literature on child psychology is Compairé's opinion that the initial limited sensitivity to sound serves to prevent the damage which could be done to the child's ear if it were exposed to the whole force of noise stimuli. The falsity and inaccuracy of this pseudo-biological statement is so obvious that we can omit refutation. Instead of such refutation a statement of principle must suffice—namely, that child psychology must avoid being satisfied with false explanations which use as the basis of an explanation a problem from another science, biology, and at that from its unsolved chapter on the purposiveness of organic phenomena. Let us turn back to our own reflections.

The initial ' pain ' reaction to every auditory stimulus is understandable. It is consistent with the regressive tendency. We have tried to understand its shock-character from the economic point of view—the point of view of energy. If we reconsider the results of our discussion of the discharge phenomena, we conceive them somewhat as follows. Noise as a stimulus increases the level of energy considerably; the reduction of energy generally serves a sudden motor discharge. As such the shock reaction might at first be conceived—without determining its special forms of " running-off." Why, then, is the auditory reaction so general and energetic ? Because it is endowed with an especially high level of energy. This answer affords an important explanation, and one can make it without being too daring. For noise, especially loud, sudden, short, and sharp sounds, is a regular impact. It is to this impact especially that the shock reaction persists the longest. The child starts back, as it does when it is suddenly touched. Why such corporal touching, such a specific re-action, should produce such an increased level of energy still remains to be explained. The auditory reaction is, however, classified in a group of phenomena to which it has similar forms, and with which it can be conceived as identical, and thus loses a part of its unintelligibility. And the difference from the completely dissimilar behaviour of the eye is clear. The ear is really a part of the skin surface which is disturbed during perception by a material part of the outer world. How exact this is can be seen anew in the light of the identical reaction to a sudden and strong touch stimulus. The analogies which we attempted above are actually not merely analogies.

If the contactual character of the noise-stimulus helps us to understand the strength and form of the ' pain ' reaction, it is convenient to use it also for the classification of pleasure reaction. A really astonishing analogy exists here: rhythmic stimuli of prolonged duration, of a certain intensity, call forth vivacious pleasure. The large number of stimuli between the shock form of stimuli and this met with more or less complete indifference. A few characteristics of pleasurable expression can be mentioned here too; it seems as if laughing occurs first as a response to auditory and tickling stimuli, and only then becomes a general pleasure reaction; the extreme fatigue of the psychic apparatus through the enjoyment of the auditory pleasure reminds one of the similar drowsy effect of tactual pleasure. The cradle song is based on the characteristic effect of sound on the childish psyche; Preyer's son in his eighth week fell into a six-hour sleep after his first hearing of music. Nevertheless, I do not wish to over-estimate the similarities; the first occurrence of laughter and the function of laughing are too little known, the nature of fatigue too little understood, for these arguments to be conclusive. But it remains striking—and for those who do not accept my assumptions difficult to explain—that hearing and sucking (especially sensitivity to touch in general) are in many respects more similar than hearing and seeing.

Could one, therefore, conclude and say that hearing is an activity in the service of the sexual instinct ? I do not think so, although to say so is tempting, and many facts concerning the significance of singing and vocalization in animals and human beings could be brought forward. But the last pertains only to adult sexuality and its exceedingly complicated relationships; and the temptation to simplify must be resisted when important reasons, which in my opinion are as follows, are against it:

1. Hearing is not an activity at all—even here it is a complete contrast to seeing. Shocks as well as cooing, waving the hands about for pleasure, wriggling and laughing—all these in the case of hearing are discharged phenomena and not activities, for hearing serves neither to remove the stimuli nor to create the stimuli; the muscular movements of the tensor tympani, which at times we wish to equate with the eye movements, are, in general, questionable with reference to their stimuli, and not proved in the infant (Bühler). The infant can do nothing specifically to remove an unpleasant auditory sensation, cannot fix or bring about an auditory pleasure so long as it cannot itself produce tones and sounds. Whether or not head movements in the direction of the sound really bring about increase in the pleasure of hearing is not certain; if it were so, then this would indeed be an activity—but an insignificant one.

2. It must not be overlooked that hearing is, indeed, similar in many respects to tactual sensitivity, but it is nevertheless not identical with it. It is probable that in the very little differentiated state of the infant the tactual pleasure and hearing pleasure are more related to each other than they are later; because of the absolutely different structure of the related sense organs there is no possibility of assuming an identity. It is, therefore, not advisable to ignore the considerable differences; and, further, a diluted formulation designating hearing as " sexual," although it is not even in the service of the sexual instinct, would lead to misunderstandings. But considering the otherwise obtrusive relationships, I would rather call in the Freudian conception of libido which embraces more, and is more precise from the point of view of energy than the conception of sexuality, and designate hearing as a libidinal phenomenon. In particular, the hearing of infants is still remote from the complications and differentiations of the adult state. Libidinal phenomenon is a designation which fundamentally is only another scientific term for that which philosophies and languages mean when they speak of the disturbing effects of music, which is nothing but pure auditory pleasure artistically elevated.

Sustained attention appears after the shock reaction, and before the expressed pleasure reaction. This is already substantiated in the new-born (Canestrini), although the expressive gestures belonging to it only appear clearly in the second stage. The psychology of attention cannot well be studied during the infant's early development; its problems and manifestations will, therefore, not occupy us in greater detail until later. But an essential sign of attention can be clearly seen in the auditory reactions as early as the first weeks of life; and I shall now begin, therefore, a partial discussion of the phenomena. This method I hold to as a fundamental mode of presentation for this book, although aware of its faults, for the sake of its few but, in my opinion, valuable advantages. Outwardly perceptible in the attention of the infant of this age are: (1) a state of rest; (2) the wide-open eyes; (3) in the beginning, those facial expressions which we call tensions; (4) pouting of the lips (perhaps not in the first month). The physiological signs are principally the stopping of breathing and circulation. Attention and the paralyzing form of fright appear on this ground to be closely related. In the first days of life attention cannot be differentiated from fright, for manifestations (2) to (4) are still lacking, and the state of fright-attention lasts for a short time only; it is released from the shock-reaction by auditory stimuli, which generally call forth a reaction; it is released from the continuation of the pre-stimulus state by auditory stimuli of a neutral character. In the last instance, one might speak of a small degree of fright. And yet the tension is not necessarily a constituent of fright; it is still less exclusively the initial phase of fright; on the other hand two different developments proceed from this point of departure. One leads to attention, the other to fright; the simplest form of attention is when the case of " slight fright " is prolonged; the typical form of attention is really already given when the " slight fright " is combined with the reactions of Type I or II. And, finally, attention is a completely developed phenomenon even without accompanying action, a form of behaviour in itself; or a manifestation accompanying manifold processes.

It is remarkable that the two opposite phenomena, rest and the highest motor excitation, are in their origin so closely connected with each other. This gives the impression that the state of rest—the tension or relaxing before a sudden discharge of energy—is somewhat like the accumulation of energy before a vigorous outbreak. If one wishes to formulate this impression more precisely, Freud's circumspect and yet far-reaching con-; jectures concerning fright and ' pain ' in *Beyond the Pleasure Principle* are applicable. He supposes that ' pain ' corresponds to a breaking through, to a limited extent, of the psychic defence against stimulation. " And what are we to expect as the reaction of the mental life to this invasion ? From all sides the cathectic energy is summoned to create all around the breach correspondingly high energy cathexis. An immense " counter-cathexis " is set up in favour of which all the other psychic systems are impoverished, so that a widespread paralysis or diminution of other psychic activity follows." One may, therefore, assume something reasonably similar for fright. The manifold problems which result from this conception will be better discussed in a more advantageous place. At this point we are only supplementing our division of psychic motor manifestations into activities and discharge phenomena by the processes of cathexis.

Accordingly, fright-attention is a protection against a too sudden and strong increase of energy by certain stimulations from the outer world. It is, above all, significant in the processes of the ear—as if a special danger threatened the psychic apparatus from this organ. And the reaction to auditory stimuli which are stronger than neutral ones is originally the cathexis; if it does not suffice—to name only one possible instance—it is followed by powerful discharge phenomena. That this becomes less frequent during the first few weeks can also have its cause—along with the reasons which we will learn later—in that a certain mass of " counter-cathexis " remained at the disposal of the ear, somewhat as if after every actual auditory stimulus the cathexis is not completely discharged and is not withdrawn, but is held in reserve as a residue for dangerous moments, so to speak. The ear then becomes a zone having a higher level of energy, which should make its adaptation to the source of pleasure thoroughly intelligible, as we shall see later. If the cathexis has become independent of fright (its discharge phenomena), then it is quite obviously, or at least in essentials, what we are accustomed to call " attention." Attention should be added to the cathectic phenomena, and the first advances in the field of hearing consist in certain changes of the cathectic relationships which cannot yet be more exactly formulated.

THE INSTINCT GROUPS

A list of infant activities has not yet been compiled. There is no point in collecting and organizing all the activities given in the observational diaries in the literature of child-psychology; for the actual usefulness of a list lies in its completeness, and in this respect the diaries are very deficient, especially the printed ones. We feel obliged to comment on a few typical instances, and are certain that an intensive study will show that the first beginnings and the advances of mental phenomena began still earlier than the observations at present available permit us to assume. The following seems to me to be a rule for the development of child-psychology: while the naïve observer tends to read adult mental life into the expressions of earliest childhood, the scientist assumed too big a gap between the infant and the adult. Since Preyer the time for the first appearance of the faculties of will and intelligence is being pushed back nearer and nearer towards birth.

The simple defensive or offensive activity becomes obviously complicated during the first three months in two directions: (1) Activities no longer relate exclusively to one stimulus, but to two or more. (2) The activities are accompanied, interrupted by (and, indeed, consist of) a number of movements, whose relation to defence or offence is difficult to understand.

The first is probably the case when the child contemplates the swinging rattle, or when it looks for the source of a sound. A considerable complication enters when the activity relates to the future and past, when expectation and memory influence it. The second complication occurs when the child responds to talking, accompanied by friendly nodding, with laughter and 'A-brrh,' with excited trembling and kicking. Both directions of this development need a more careful presentation than we can give; perhaps it would then lead also to more simple and more conclusive interpretations.

First, the organization of the numerous activities will certainly interest us; to a large extent, our task is to summarize what has been discussed in various parts of the book. The result is a collection of a number of groups, whose range is as varied as their intelligibility.

1. *Defence (Warding-Off) Activities.*—These proceed from a definite, usually localized, unpleasant stimulus. Closing the

eyes; turning the head away; movements of the hands as in brushing something away, are the earliest differentiated ones; crying is the most common defence activity. All of these develop only slightly in the first three months, for during this time, raising the body, purposive mobility of the hands, arms, feet and legs, have their beginnings. And it is these organs, which become the real means of defence against the external world. Above all, it is the slow development of bodily movements that makes crying the only defence activity against all the disagreeableness of the outer world during the first period of childhood, for shutting off the stimulus does not suffice. The child cannot yet independently free itself from its condition, cannot push the disturbance aside. One is almost tempted to say that it would like to do this, but its muscles do not yet respond to its will. In such instances crying seems to take on that differentiated form which all observers, in agreement with mothers and nurses, describe as naughtiness and the result of temper.

2. *The Nutritional Instinct.*[1]—To the nutritional instinct we have added: the hunger-cry, sucking as soon as an object capable of being sucked happens to be put into the mouth, swallowing if the object secretes a fluid of a certain quality, renewed hunger-cries if no secretion occurs after a short time, and perhaps expelling the mother's nipple at satiation.

Movements of the head towards things (offence movements) are noticed very early, when the breast is brought near the face. In the first weeks of life the activities of the nutritional instinct are released by seeing or smelling the breast, Very soon, too, by all kinds of preparatory activities, *e.g.* tying on its bib: usually extreme restlessness takes possession of the infant, which easily changes to a hunger-cry or fingersucking, or causes uncontrolled seeking movements of the head, etc. Very often already at this time there is a kind of holding, hitting, scratching the breast with the hands when the child is placed at the breast and during imbibing. It can hardly be decided whether these are already instinctual activities or defence phenomena, or whether they are absolutely accidental, due to the position of the hands in front of the mouth, which is similar to the embryonic position; but certainly the hands—as we will later see in greater detail—have very early a function in the service of the nutritional

---

[1] *Fresstrieb* usually given as *Esstrieb.—Translator.*

instinct. It is equally difficult to decide how far the pouting of the mouth during attentive looking can at this stage be interpreted as an expression of the nutritional instinct.

This explanation has much in its favour. I have already referred to the explanation—and will return to it again—that it is admissible to ascribe to the nutritional instinct behaviour that can be stated thus: if the individual is hungry—or not completely satiated—every perception of the eyes and the nose may be said, with reservation, to release the impulse to master (possess) the thing orally. Pouting the mouth would thus be not an expressive gesture of attention, but an activity preparatory to eating, to sucking the attentively observed objects; a preparation which, during the period before the child has control over its hands, cannot lead to any results, but which leads to seizing and sticking things into its mouth as soon as grasping is learned. That pouting the mouth is also an expression in response to sweets fits into this explanation very well; for what more alluring expectation can the infant have than that the object seen will taste sweet when the mouth grasps it ?

3. *The Sexual Instinct,* understood in that broad meaning for which Freud is responsible, in which all gain of tactual pleasure is included, causes that complex of activities which we have discussed in detail under pleasure-sucking. Those activities of the infant which may occur, in order to attain or to strengthen and maintain the effects of the warm bath, should be added to the sexual instinct, for the pleasure in the bath is charged with tactual pleasure. It is, however, very difficult at this stage to distinguish the discharge manifestations from activities. The sexual pleasure of the bath is " a gift of the environment " which the child cannot produce for itself, but which it can only enjoy somewhat as it enjoys the libidinal pleasure in hearing.

4. *Visual Pleasure.*—To attain, ensure, and increase the pleasure in seeing leads the infant to perform those complicated movements which constitute seeing. The development of these movements during the first three months we have presented above in detail.

In the study of discharge phenomena, one or another phenomenon will clearly appear as an activity, but really the organization of the activities has been treated exhaustively by what has been said. Out of this organization it is conspicuously noticeable that the chief object and means of the infant's activity in the first three months is its head. In contrast to the head, the hands play a very subordinate rôle; the rest of the body does not come into consideration at all.

To make a separate group of the offence activities is not necessary, because all the offence movements (*Zuwendungsbewegungen*) are included in the groups mentioned, especially in the nutritional-instinctual and sexual-instinctual activities.

It cannot be asserted that this classification will be a completely satisfactory one, and since child-psychologists have until now shown practically no concern with the instincts, success could not be expected in this—almost the first—attempt to organize all the manifestations of the instincts.

Groups 1 and 4 are unfortunate; for they must be classified either as new instincts or among the nutritional or sexual instincts, if the grouping is to appear satisfactory. But before either possibility can be discussed, it is advisable to relate this grouping to the literature on the subject.

Kirkpatrick is the only one of the child-psychologists, in the narrower sense, who assigns to the instincts an essential rôle in child research. He distinguishes five groups of instincts: self-preservative instincts, parental instincts, group or social instincts, adaptive instincts, and the regulative instinct. He apparently finds operative in the infant only the instinct of self-preservation and a primitive form of the adaptive instinct. There is no reason to speak of the latter (imitation) in the first three months; in another connection some criticism will be directed to this idea. Kirkpatrick includes in the self-preservative instincts all that we designated as the nutritional instinct, the group of defence movements, and in truth all the activities that can be seen in the infant. For he defines the self-preservative instinct as follows: " To these belong all the impulses to move which aim at the momentary well-being of the individual. . . . The simplest form of this tendency one sees in the strivings to move so as to increase the stimulus once received if it is favourable, and to decrease it if it is unfavourable." This means that all activities of infants arise from the instinct of self-preservation. It is obviously true that they all preserve the infant, at least under normal conditions. This conception accordingly has nothing nonsensical in it; indeed, it affords a certain amount of philosophical satisfaction which always occurs when very various manifestations are traced to a single principle. But it is difficult to see why it should be necessary to discover further instincts; the parental instinct can also be reduced to activities which try to produce "momentary well-being," and seek to ward off momentary indisposition. This is a common characteristic of the psychic in general, in spite of the fact that occasionally activities occur which produce 'pain.' It is a general principle of psychic occurrences, and indeed a primal principle, that the tendency is to prevent 'pain' wherever possible, and to obtain pleasure wherever possible. Freud (4) has given this general tendency a very appropriate name, the "Pleasure-Principle."

It does not help very much to call this principle an instinct, because, if we did, an impulse embracing the whole process would be established. This would not free us from the necessity of establishing special instincts. It would, however, allow these special instincts to be subordinated to the general instinct, but little would be gained thereby. I shall, therefore, maintain the "pleasure-principle" as an attribute of psychic occurrence distinguished conceptually from instincts; and to establish the relation of the instincts to the pleasure-principle will be a task in itself. One relation is immediately recognizable: in general the instincts adapt themselves to the pleasure-principle; their aims are bound up with pleasure; their ungratified impulses with 'pain.' Nevertheless, this relation is by no means always so simple. Such a conceptual division is suggested by the consideration that the pleasure-principle, pleasure and 'pain' in general, are perceptions of the Cs. system (Consciousness), whereas instincts are attributed to the organic system; thus one excludes important aspects if one makes the theory of instincts dependent upon the processes of the mental system which we understand with certainty only in the adult human being.

Outside the field of literature of child-psychology, occupation with the psychology of instincts is far less frequent or intensive than this important and obscure problem demands. Nevertheless, we could not complete in a few pages an examination of the advantages and disadvantages—for our task—of the various assumptions and classifications. It is, therefore, a happy coincidence that the only theory which regards the problem from the genetic point of view, the only theory of instincts from the point of view of developmental psychology,

7

is the psycho-analytic theory, and that the child-psychologist does not need lengthy justification when he tries to apply it—as the only existing one—in organizing the facts in its fields of research. Freud's theory of instincts finds two sufficient. At this point one must distinguish the older phase of the theory from the newer one; the turning-point is obviously Freud's small but profound book, *Beyond the Pleasure Principle*.

The differentiation of the sexual instincts from the ego-instincts belongs to the older phase. The sexual instincts have been carefully studied from all angles, and have been made intelligible in their development; in Freud's *Three Contributions to the Sexual Theory* the first developmental psychology of instinct is given—though only of the sexual instincts. The ego-instincts do not receive any intensive treatment, they are only postulated, and merely separated from the sexual instincts; under ego-instincts, then, are included all those which are *not*-sexual instincts. The new phase of the theory leaves the conception of the sexual instincts untouched; only sadism receives a fresh interpretation, but not, after all, a fundamentally new one. The earlier interpretation of sadism, as a partial impulse of the sexual instinct, no longer applies in the same sense; its relation to the sexual instincts becomes more complicated; it is credited in its " defused " form to its opposing instinct. But the ego-instincts are fused with the sexual instincts into a further unity: as life-instinct or Eros, in contrast to the death-instinct, of which it was or is impossible to show an indisputable psychic component; but the defused conception of sadism can serve as an instance of this type. Eros and the death-instinct attain a further unification in essence, and in the aim of the instincts in general; thus Freud's (9) formulation is: " An instinct, therefore, would be a tendency innate in living organic matter impelling it towards the reinstatement of an earlier condition, one which it had to abandon under the influence of external disturbing forces, a kind of organic elasticity, or, to put it another way, the manifestation of inertia in organic life."

What profound relationships and far-reaching explanations these constructions make possible Freud shows in *The Ego and the Id*. Nevertheless, I shall confine myself only to the assertions of Freud's earlier theory of instincts. The new theory is built up from a point of view which offers no important advantages in our task, since our material is neither rich nor lucid enough. The life- and the death-instincts are biological forces, they are beyond the conception of the individual. The explanation of the mental phenomena in the infant requires more concrete statements. The instincts are forces within the individual which determine its activities and behaviour in a typical unified way. The aims of the instincts are not known; they must be inferred from the actions; the more closely the aim is defined, the more concretely and the more inherently it is assigned to the individual, the more surely fitting is this conclusion. The instincts are obviously, moreover, forces which extend beyond the domain of the individual; and Freud in his newer formulations keeps this in mind. But at the same time they make certain aspects less clear; they are biological, philosophical; as far as they apply to psychology, they belong to metapsychology, with which the present psychology of infants had better not concern itself yet. We do not fall into any disagreement with psychoanalysis, or even with some of its assumptions, if we hold in essentials to the differences of the old theory of instincts, since the newer theory does not contradict the older theory, but only elaborates it, carries it further biologically and metapsychologically. This is evident in the separation of the sexual instincts from the ego-instincts. Their fusion with Eros does not remove the differences so conscientiously investigated in the early days; it is only that they no longer appear so final, because the common qualities of both groups, as opposed to the death-instincts, are so conspicuous and important. But for understanding the child, it is more important to separate these two groups of instincts than to relate them.

To relate these two separate instinct groups to the pleasure-principle offers great possibilities. The pleasure-principle comprises two different tendencies: the prevention of pain and the seeking of pleasure. Fundamentally, both are positive ways of behaving, not only the striving for pleasure, but also the preventing of ' pain,' for this is a striving for a state of definite balance and rest, which in a certain sense can also be called " pleasure." We have already seen in many instances how prevention, warding off of ' pain,' can be interpreted as an instinct to return to the situation which existed before the stimulus, to a situation of psychic rest and absence of stimulation—in the last analysis a return to the embryonic situation which was disturbed by the first durable stimulus, birth. Nevertheless, this " pleasure," the absence of stimulation, is obviously of a different quality from pleasure which is sought, for instance, in thumb-sucking, and it is scarcely advisable to include birth under the same designation. On the other hand, one can justifiably emphasize that striving for pleasure finally merges into absence of stimulation—for example, sleep follows pleasure-sucking. One should not, therefore, conclude that the aim is not striving for pleasure, but that it is the state of absence of stimulation which follows it, and pleasure is merely a means of attaining it. This is, too, contradictory to the nature of pleasure, which tends to maintain itself, the ending of which is regretted if the intervening fatigue has not made such regrets impossible, and which is again immediately strived for as soon as the fatigue has passed and the necessary conditions are given. To consciousness, in the simple case, pleasure itself is indeed the aim of the instinctual activity. The psycho-analytical investigation of the *Unconscious* reveals no other aim than this—*e.g.*, it reveals the substrata on which pleasure should be experienced, but it certainly does not reveal the state of rest after pleasure has been experienced. So that pleasure—which is, of course, an insufficiently understood stimulus-situation—and undisturbed rest are two distinguishable aims which pursue two differentiated instincts: pleasure adheres to the group of sexual instincts; absence of stimulation adheres to the instincts of self-preservation. The name instinct of self-preservation is not free from ambiguity. We have already indicated that self-preservation is the result and not the aim of this instinct. Its aim is a state of absence of stimulation—and I shall later show that under certain conditions its aim is " mastery." It would be less ambiguous to apply to it the name death-instincts, and it will occasionally be advisable to do so if this tendency toward destruction and toward the return to the embryonic quiet should be especially stressed; in general, this nomenclature in Freudian terminology does not contradict our classification, but only partially covers it. This group of instincts of self-preservation adheres to the " ego-instincts," which Freud (9) differentiates from the object-instincts (the sexual-instincts). This is the essential contrast between the two instinctual groups which we see sharply indicated in the infant: the libidinal turning-toward the world, and the narcissistic withdrawal from the world. Nevertheless, applied to infant psychology the term ego-instincts would lead to constant misunderstanding. At this period the ego develops very slowly, and is at the end of the period still quite undifferentiated. Whereas the adult sexual instinct develops in essentials out of those still insufficiently differentiated instinctual-sexual-activities—and because of this continuity named rightly—the gradual growth of the ego out of the primitive expressions of the " ego-instincts " does not take place in so direct a way. On the other hand, more complicated but still little known relations predominate here. To clarify them would be the task of the psychology of infancy and early childhood, and a more precise nomenclature is therefore advisable. In order, therefore, to define this task and clarify other existing obscurities, the group of instincts of self-preservation, the ego-instincts, will for the present be designated as R.-instincts, wherewith the R. will call to mind the state of rest (*Ruhezustand*), the absence of stimulation (*Reizlosigkeit*), the pleasure-in-rest (*Ruhe-Lust*), as well as the regression, the regressive tendency, into which the conservative tendency changes more and more obviously as the new-born grows older.

It must not be overlooked, and therefore it is repeated, that the relation to the pleasure-principle is not necessarily so simple as the division attempted above would lead one to assume; particularly because in reality the instincts appear in a variously condensed and fused form, and because our distinctions are still only scientific abstractions. The relation to the pleasure-principle is not less simple, because the pleasure-principle has its origin in the economic viewpoint, and because the conception of both instinctual groups originates in the dynamic viewpoint of psychological ways of thinking, and both viewpoints—as different ways of considering subjects which are in part the same—stand in a relationship to each other which is not entirely simple, Freud (7).

Returning to our organization of activities, we can improve the unsatisfactory points to a certain degree. From 1 (discharge activities), and 2 (nutritional-instinctual activities) we form Group I—namely, those activities which are attributed to R.-instincts. They strive toward the narcissistic state of rest, and try to re-establish it when it is disturbed. They represent the Freudian ego-instincts and partly also the death-instincts. Group II: in contrast to the R.-instincts, the sexual impulses have as their motive to activity the winning of pleasure; and, indeed, not that " pleasure " which the state of rest without stimulation may offer, but pleasure which is won from manifold stimuli, " objects." The visual pleasure activities (4) are more closely connected with this Group II. To examine the details of this relation will be easier and more fruitful in phenomena which appear later in infancy.

It is impossible to speak of instincts, indeed even of development, without soon arriving at that limit of psychological insight which runs through all those phenomena included in the word "heredity." The inborn mechanisms, the tendencies of the instincts themselves, and of the activities and potential forces inherently dependent upon them, the succession of manifestations (Semon's *Recurrence of Memory*), the regular maturation of motor apparatus and of mental capacities, are behind the two instinct groups, behind the pleasure-principle, and outside our task. Freud's death-instinct and Eros, his repetition-compulsion and his definition of instincts touch these problems. The psychology of the infant, child, and youth must not neglect to indicate the connection with these. Psychology cannot neglect this, for the repetition-compulsion is scarcely differentiated from the earlier expression of the conservative tendency of the instincts of self-preservation (our instinct Group I). Even a venturesome author will be unable to relate these at this time, if he wishes to offer more than mere subjective ideas.

LAUGHING, WEEPING, AND FRIGHT[1]

The considerable changes which the discharge phenomena, especially the so-called mimetic expressive gestures, undergo during the first three months are very complicated. The differences between these manifestations in the new-born and in the three-months-old child are more fundamental than between those of the three-months-old child and of the adult. For into the first developmental phase fall the development of all the indications of movements expressive of feeling, the body pantomime, and partly the facial expressions of feeling, whose development is, in the remaining course of life, really only modification and diminution. What we assume to be,

---

[1] Translated: *Weinen*, weeping; *Schreiweinen*, crying; *Schreien,* screaming.

in the child, an expression of a weak 'pain' feeling the adult expresses only by very strong overpowering affect: loud weeping. The remaining question as to how this occurs arises during the first three months and is a very puzzling problem.

This is valid at this early period for the most conspicuous expressions, for crying and laughing, both of which are lacking in the infant, but which the three-months-old child has in complete control, and which lend it the occasionally paradoxical expression similar to humans, to adults. To forestall criticism (1) We do not understand crying and laughing in any scientific way. (2) But we obviously understand the crying child and laughing child, or perhaps we merely believe we understand it.

The crying of the new-born becomes weeping when tears appear. The time of their appearance varies apparently with the individual. More recent observers have noted the first tears from the third to the ninth week (Dix), whereas Darwin (1) and his commentators report "one instance at an unusually early age—the forty-second day," but it is generally reported to occur from the sixty-second to the one hundred and thirty-ninth day. Of course, Darwin speaks of the time when first the tears stream down the cheeks, which is not the decisive time for observers since Preyer; nevertheless, it is certain that the time for the appearance of tears varies according to the individual. Of course, tears can be produced by irritating the eye, even before they appear spontaneously as manifestations accompanying crying; and during the time of habitual crying the cry of the infant occurs without lacrimal secretion. More exact observations will perhaps teach us to differentiate; perhaps crying is connected with other causes, with specific situations. If this were true, it would probably give an important insight into many questions, but it is vain to make assumptions where facts have not yet been proved. We do not know why there are variations in the time at which secretion begins. Lehmann has asked the question and supposes that the spontaneous lacrimal secretion must be released by a somatic irritation which dust, touching the eyes, certainly produces in the first weeks of life, but at accidental times.

There is no reason for considering screaming in itself as a discharge phenomenon. It is an activity just like every other early infantile activity, as I have explained above. A fair portion of these activities which were classified as expressive gestures are nothing other than muscular movements which necessarily belong to the screaming activity or become more intelligible in that connection. According to Darwin's careful analysis, the facts can be presented somewhat as follows: Weeping (screaming) is characterized by (i) expiration; (ii) closing the eyes tightly; (iii) frowning; (iv) wide-open mouth; (v) lips drawn back, mouth "four-cornered"; (vi) tears. (i) and (iv) constitute crying; they need no further comment. Frowning (iii) and the peculiar drawing-back of the lips (v) both result from the anatomical situation of eyelid, cheek, and nose muscles; they are consequences of the spasmodic closing of the eyes. These alone are to be found in every violent convulsive expiration and serve to protect the eye from congestion, and from blood clots in its veins, so that all expressive gestures of weeping are part of the crying activity, except the tears. Darwin was scarcely successful in classifying them as the motor manifestation of this activity. The compression of the eyeball may affect the tear glands reflexively, but he must, nevertheless, " consider crying as an accidental result, as much without purpose as the secretion of tears resulting from a blow on the eyelid." As the reason for his opinion, Darwin says that there is " no difficulty in seeing that the flow of tears serves to alleviate the suffering." And we must still today be satisfied with this classification of crying under the discharge phenomena. Nevertheless, we cannot suppress the doubt that this offers even less explanation for the phenomenon in the infant than for the same phenomenon in the adult. For even if we presume to imagine, no matter how, that mental suffering is considerably relieved by such discharge, it is still insufficiently illuminating in the case of the more imperative and physical " suffering " of the infant. But we thereby touch the subject of discharge phenomena as a whole, whose nature and development we still have to describe.

The problem is made much easier by the fact that weeping is not the absolute criterion for ' pain.' Children and adults can cry from pleasure and for joy, which, of course, presupposes a certain complexity of feeling and of psychic structure; on the other hand, hearty laughing—without any psychic complication—results in a flow of tears. From this it is concluded that the tear glands are affected by strong compression of the eye muscles (Lehmann). Yet this interpretation does not touch the heart of the matter; for, firstly, laughing with tears seems not to occur in infants at all, the relation cannot, therefore, be a primary one; secondly, a certain moderate function of the tear glands is very often a manifestation of all pleasure, even those unaccompanied by any visible movements of the eye muscles. The "sparkling" eye—certainly a result of some tear secretion—is a common pantomimic expression of pleasure. There exists, therefore, a relation between 'pain' and pleasure feelings on the one hand, and on the other between pleasure and 'pain' with the activity of tear glands in general; and only certain forms of this secretion are more closely connected with 'pain,' others with pleasure.

If one considers the appearance of tears chronologically one can formulate as follows: moderate moisture of the eyes begins in the first weeks of life during pleasure and 'pain'; stronger secretion occurs only later and in the form of tears accompanied by cries of displeasure. This is the situation at the end of the first three months. The next development is marked by the fact that the connection between crying and weeping is released, that the strong flow of tears in 'pain' becomes independent of crying; that a copious flow of tears occurs as a result of laughing in response to pleasure; finally, that weeping, as an expression of 'pain,' becomes gradually less frequent, actually ceases completely, and only occasionally recurs in moments of greatest affects; and even at this stage weeping sets in in response to pure unpleasant affect, but also in response to one which may be considered essentially pleasure. In the last stage of its development, the convention of the community plays a great part; there were peoples, and there still are peoples, who use weeping as an expression of both pleasure and 'pain,' others who repress it even more strongly than I have described above. To inhibit the expression of affects is without doubt conventional. To interpret the processes of early childhood as Lehmann seems inclined to do, is without doubt incorrect. A more probable interpretation would draw into account the factors of imitation in the laughing of the child and even of the infant. In weeping imitation certainly does not play a part. One laughs with a child in play, but one does not weep with it.

The functioning of glands under different emotional states has been insufficiently investigated in adults, but in the infant not at all. Perhaps an understanding of lacrimal secretion will first result from an understanding of perspiration, perhaps too of bladder and bowel movements. Since such studies are still lacking, we must show by the mimic alone that the expression of pleasure and the expression of ' pain ' are by no means completely contrasted, and that this was originally even less the case than in later life. The facial expressions of laughing are not directly opposed to the facial expressions of crying. If we follow Darwin's analysis of laughing we differentiate as follows: (1) making sounds; (2) opening the mouth; (3) moving the upper lip; (4) slight contraction of the orbicular muscles of the eyes; (5) raising the cheeks from the cheek bones, mostly connected with turning up the corners of the mouth; (6) glistening of the eyes. Even the expressions of laughing contain a complex of movements co-ordinated with, and dependent upon, each other: movements (2), (3), (4), and perhaps (6). This complex is identical with the facial expressions of crying; it is a weak form of crying: it is very often difficult to know whether the mouth grimaces of the infant will lead to smiling, laughing, or crying. The specific expressions for laughing are originally only the fine nuances which are given by the lifting of the corners of the mouth (it is not known when these begin, but in any case they already exist in the first weeks of life), the open eye (the weak contraction of the ring muscles); the unusual sounds, and the lustre of the eye which later become specific. If crying consists of strong-continued expiration, interrupted by short and weak inspirations, then laughing, on the contrary, consists of long, strong inspiration, and is interrupted rhythmically by short and weak expulsions of breath. Laughing is, accordingly, as far as the pantomimic expression is concerned, partly identical with crying, partly (open eyes, inspiration) its exact opposite. Ontogenetically, laughing appears earlier than loud crying. The observers differ considerably as to the time of their appearance: first in their different conceptions of the phenomena. In the first days of life movements of the mouth which seem somewhat like smiling appear frequently, but if one wishes to designate the time of the first smiling as a sign of a feeling of ease and comfort, one must leave out of consideration these early grimaces up to the second week. But secondly, laughing in the beginning of its development is obviously very dependent upon individual factors, so that the time varies occasionally in different children. Preyer " noticed an audible and visible laughing accompanied by increased gleaming of the eyes for the first time on the twenty-third day."

This time, from the third to the fourth week, agrees with most observations; laughing only completes its development, in the matter of the duration, rhythm, and strength of the laughing sounds, at the end of the second month or at the beginning of the third; the differentiations and nuances continue into the fourth year of life.

Laughing grows out of weeping by changes in inspiration, by holding the eyes open, and by the addition of the specific movement of the jaw muscles. This last detail is completely puzzling, for there are no assumptions or speculations about it.

Laughing is not an activity; it has no discernible purpose; not even a biological purpose can be assumed. The function which it exercises in society, its binding psycho-social force is certainly a result, but it cannot be claimed as its determining cause. It is often shown—*e.g.*, by Stern—how the expression of pleasure states follows after feelings of displeasure, and it is shown that this sequence has its biological significance—in human beings we really mean "sociological" significance. The cry of 'pain' summons the mother. This assertion is correct, and we therefore call the expression of 'pain' an activity, but from this reflection it does not follow that expressions of pleasure must always occur. The expressions of pleasure in the adult are generally still more infrequent and even weaker than the expressions of 'pain,' but in the infant they are by no means more subdued, certainly not less frequent and not less conspicuous than the expression of 'pain.' On the contrary, the healthy and well-reared child of three or four months is characterized by few other manifestations as obvious as its manifold and vivacious manifestations of pleasure. There remains, therefore, no other possibility than to interpret laughing as a whole, as well as the secretion of tears from the complex of loud crying, as a discharge phenomena—though this interpretation does not alter the puzzling character of the phenomenon.

Methodologically it is quite legitimate, when we feel limited, to call in the social components of laughter, of the discharge phenomena in general, in order to explain them and to carry this rejection to the point of combating the term "expressive-gesture," which is responsible for erroneous perspectives. The methodological principle which guides us is the same which induces us at times to proceed as far as possible without the idea of heredity, without the phylogenetic point of view. Only thus can we arrive at the deepest understanding of the psychological forces and their manifestations. We must no more overlook the social factor than the hereditary factor. And since, throughout this book, we introduce more historical material into child-psychology than is customary, and consider the relationship of the adult environment to the developmental entity—the infant—we must certainly not neglect to recognize the effects of these relations on the infant itself. If one seriously accepts the term expressive-gestures it might be defined as an inherent psychic residue of a social tendency. Authors have something of the kind in mind when they say that the expression of ' pain ' appears even in the new-born, because it is useful to it. As far as I see no one has given the same consideration to the child's laughter. Since we distinctly separate such social-psychological considerations from individual psychological considerations we must make an attempt to examine them—an attempt which might lead to some slight exaggeration—and thus gain, perhaps, valuable insight.

The consequence of crying is that the mother hurries to the child and removes the disturbing stimulus. From this consequence the social value, the social tendency of the phenomenon—crying—can be inferred: the effect is substituted for the cause. What is the consequence of laughing ? The answer is not easy. The difficulty is not that there is no answer to this question, but that one hesitates to express it because it seems unscientific. Every mother knows well the effects the infant's laughter produces upon her and upon all who witness it : happiness, joy, love, cheerfulness. The jubilant child inevitably calls forth feelings of happiness in the mother, joy—at least—in all onlookers, and the child immediately experiences the effects of its activity: it receives evidence of affection, love, and tenderness. The beautiful family idyll is, of course, not necessarily the consequence of every single laugh, but it is the probable, the usual result if the child and the environment are normal. There is no difference in the case of the infant's screaming. Even this occasionally remains without result, and many a child has grown up under conditions in which this occasional instance became the normal one. It cannot be assumed that the described effect occurs only in our present social relationships. On the contrary, this relationship has undoubtedly always existed in every social structure;

it follows inevitably from the identification which necessarily takes place between the mother and the child. I shall have to devote to this tendency a more detailed discussion in later chapters. It is here supported by very superficial knowledge: the expressive gestures of affects are exceedingly contagious; we understand the laughing child because to see it laugh creates a certain tendency to laugh too; this tendency and its appropriate feeling are almost one and the same. If laughing is more than a discharge phenomenon, if it has any value as an expression, then no other interpretation is possible than that the result of laughing is the mother's love (taking into consideration only these representatives of the outer world), her subjective feelings of love and their expressions, which bring the child love. If there is no objection to substituting the cause of weeping for the effect, one can come to no other conclusion about laughing, and one must say: the child's laughter is an activity of love, it aims to arouse and obtain love by its laughter.

For the present I do not wish to adopt a definite attitude towards this possible, perhaps indeed very agreeable, conception; some of the following material will support this conception, other material will force us to greater precision and qualification. It is by no means a complete solution of the question which we are here discussing. For, besides the question itself, there remains the problem of the form chosen. Why is laughing, why is this characteristic form of inspiration, a suitable activity of love? At least it throws light on the darkness of the pleasure-discharge phenomena in general, for among these there are some which are imperceptible and which can, therefore, have no social significance.

First, let us consider from a developmental psychological standpoint, with the degree of precision which the present situation in child-psychology permits, the ontogenesis of the specific manifestations of laughing: smiling, turning up the corners of the mouth and inspiration sounds. A kind of smiling, an expression of snug comfort appears during the first days. The critical observer, in contrast to the happy mother or proud nurse, will rightly refuse to consider it as real smiling. Yet this slight movement contains signs of smiling; it is described as a broadening of the mouth with slightly opened lips, perhaps from the beginning connected with slight lifting of the corners of the mouth, and it occurs during a state of satisfaction, during satiation, while the child is falling asleep.

Freud (13) shows that this expression is quite intelligible as a refusal of further nourishment. It is the exact opposite of the pursed sucking mouth. The corners of the mouth are automatically turned up—according to the impression I have gained—when the broadening of the mouth occurs vigorously and quickly; this occurs especially when one attempts to make these movements in response to the sensation of sweet tastes; whereas bitter tastes cause the corners of the wide mouth to drop. This is called the preliminary phase of laughing: it might mean " enough of sweetness," and it would then be an activity intelligible in itself. It becomes real laughing with the energetic lifting of the corners of the mouth, a result of using the zygomatic muscles (*Jochbeinmuskels*). Observations which have been made are not exact enough to lead to more definite knowledge. With this exception one must affirm that real laughter occurs in response to certain visual perceptions, above all when seeing moving objects and when hearing the human voice, and is sometimes accompanied by a grunting, gurgling, and crowing sound. It is as if the movement of the muscles of the cheek bones were connected with attention. A glance at the close connections between the muscles shows that attention can be related to the orbicular muscles as well as to the ear muscles, which of course do not usually function in the child, and experiments have given me the impression that very attentive looking, and still more clearly attentive listening, tend to move the muscles of the jaw, and with them the corners of the mouth. If this impression were to be confirmed, the details of the laughing pantomime and the expressions of joy could be understood. The deep inspiration, which is followed by a slight cramp of the diaphragm (fit of laughter), and is rhythmically repeated, remains. Infants probably begin to laugh in this adult manner towards the end of the second half of the first year. Towards the end of the third month they have developed only a short " bleat " (Dix); and in the second and third month the rhythmic, spasmodic element is only indicated. At this point laughing consists of building up short tones during quick, deep inspirations.

If laughing in adults is a form of an agreeable fit of choking, then the earlier laughter of the infant is only the first phase of this: the inspiratory apnœa, whereas the expiratory apnœa is still lacking. This is more likely present in screaming. Later, laughter combines in itself both forms of rhythmic sequence, beginning with the inspiratory phase. Spasmodic laughter can hardly be distinguished any longer from weeping, and shows the pleasure and ' pain ' elements closely intermingled in its expression, much more clearly and more conspicuously, as we have already observed in connection with laughing in general. Diametrically opposed though the feelings which call forth laughing or crying may be, the expression of laughter is by no means the opposite of crying. It is much more a mixture of this with " pleasure movements." The ' pain ' element is lost, is forced into pleasure, one might say. The genetic course of crying led us to the first expiration, to the first cry of the new-born. If we look for the first deep and intensive inspiration, we must go back a few seconds further to the first breath of the new-born, the first post-fœtal act of the human being. This first inhalation is reproduced in any laughing fit, together with apnœa, which follows it and which releases the first expiration.

There is no doubt then that keeping the eyes open, broadening the mouth, and raising the corners of the mouth are connected with pleasurable situations, and that raising the upper lip and contracting the eye muscles are connected with unpleasant situations, and we, therefore, speak of a fusion of pleasurable and painful movements in the act of laughing, but we are still doubtful as to how to classify inspiration. It is certain that if the child at birth had an adult consciousness it would perceive birth as extreme ' pain,' akin to suffocation, spasms, choking, and the affects of loud noises; as an extremely disagreeable state of anxiety. In this state the first breath (*Inspirium*) must seem, indeed, a short but very considerable relief. The first breath itself one might, perhaps, with a certain degree of correctness, designate as a component of pleasure. But however this may be determined, the significance of the reproduction of this moment of the birth situation in exquisitely pleasurable laughter seems clear: it is as if by laughing the ' pain ' (trauma) of birth is overcome. All the ways of behaving which belong to the R.-instincts—contained in that complex of laughter which is identical with weeping—are invested in memory with symptoms of pleasure, one may say are invested with the pleasure enjoyed from oral, acoustic, and visual gratification.   This, perhaps, savours of philosophy. Though I make use of this interpretation, it is not my intention completely to forsake empirical ground; I am merely organizing all the impressions and information which the analysis of expression makes possible.

I agree with the point of view of many psychologists who deem laughter worthy of consideration. Although the points of view deal, for the most part, not with laughter but with the ridiculous, and although the extensive literature has not produced a unified and conclusive understanding, nevertheless opponents otherwise irreconcilable are in agreement on some points. The incongruity of expenditure and result, the resolving of a fear, the economy of psychic expenditure, all these are the roots of the ridiculous, are causes of laughter,[1] and the overcoming of a threatening unpleasant situation is a very common release for the joy of laughing. This does not, of course, exhaust the nature of the ridiculous for the adult, but it is not my task to give a general psychology of laughter. For the laughter of children this explanation contains a very essential factor. Inaccurately reported observations hinder the establishment of a universally valid assumption, but for numerous cases, especially for the first laughing situation of the infant, the following applies: it laughs when it should be frightened; it laughs suddenly in a situation which hitherto frightened it. Here a reversal similar to that in auditory pleasure takes place. This is especially clear with reference to auditory stimuli (the mother's voice), but only at a slightly later period.

From some observations it is easy to see how the child vacillates, how it is frightened at first, then laughs when the stimulus takes on a recognized form, but ends by crying. In the study of the earliest causes for laughter it must be noticed that it is always the mother, her look, or her voice, which draws out the first clear and intensive expressions of laughter; after her come vivid colours or movements (*e.g.;* the rattle). The development of real laughing naturally takes place in contact with the mother, and especially while she is speaking to the child. Recognition, the familiarity of impressions, seem to stand in close relation to laughing. It is the new reaction to stimuli. At first they are repudiated by defence activities

---

[1] See Freud (13) and the presentation of opinions of others contained therein.

(R.T. I), or by indifference; or they arouse sudden fright or unnoticeable pain reactions in breathing and pulse. We see this tendency slowly overcome by pleasure in seeing, by sexual pleasure, and finally by the gain from auditory pleasure. This reaction is again reflected in the motor complex of laughing. In a sudden outbreak it is reproduced, as it were, in a condensed form, and indicates the newly-acquired attitude to the outer world, which is no longer wholly hostile, but which contains a complex of the familiar and the loved, which are no longer repudiated and no longer frightening, but are sought for and enjoyed. The R.-instinct reaction is released from the libidinal.

This consideration places laughing in a certain relation to fright; they are diametrically opposite discharge-phenomena, which are neither directly contrary nor actually fused in their motor relations. Their relationship is more complicated than it would seem at first glance. The breathing reaction is different: fright is the paralysis, the reduction of the breathing activity to the lowest level; laughing is not simply increased normal breathing, but also increased breathing activity.

The same holds true for the distention of the bloodvessels in laughing, and for their contraction during fright. Fright goes further back than laughing. It reproduces, in a certain sense, at the moment of its inception, the state of apnœa of prenatal life (Eisler). But the most conspicuous difference is that fright produces a diffuse discharge, general shock, and weakness, shivering, twitching, etc., whereas the discharge through laughing is an organized motor phenomenon. The very rhythm of inspiration reveals the organization. But it can be seen still more clearly in the easily analyzed co-ordinated movement-complexes of the facial expressions, which are concentrated on a few muscles, even when, as in the case of violent and sustained laughter, other parts of the body participate. These complexes are centred characteristically on the head, to which we previously have called attention, on the place of all organized discharge- and movement-phenomena, of all the activities of the new-born and the three-months-old child. Perhaps the overcoming of fright, of anxiety—which for the present we need not distinguish from each other—means that the general (traumatic) discharge has found paths, has organized itself. And, indeed, the discharge movements, each of which has a significance as an activity in itself, are used for sudden

8

excitation-discharge, independent of its significance as an activity. Thus laughter would comprise a number of R.-instinct activities and sexual instinct activities, not to perform a complicated act which is inherent in one of these instincts, but to discharge an excess of excitation which is released by a stimulus. And this phenomenon would secondarily fulfil a psycho-social function, and through it would finally produce a new gratification of the sexual instinct, if we do not wish completely to disregard the discussions concerning laughter as a love activity.

But with this we have arrived at the limits of the economic consideration and must ask: what energy is discharged by laughing, what energy by fright, and what do the dynamic indications, such as overcoming anxiety, disposing of ' pain,' mean from the economic viewpoint ? And we expect especially at this point a more precise formulation of the expression " trauma of birth," a phrase used continuously as a substitute and to cover embarrassment.

Some factors of this question can easily be answered in accordance with the foregoing statements and assumptions. First of all, the energy which is released by laughing as well as by fright is obviously free energy. This conclusion results *per definitionem*, since by way of experiment we are proceeding on the basis of the Freudian theory of energy—recognizably influenced by Fechner. It is more difficult to decide what conception we are to adopt concerning the origin of this quantity of free energy. There are two possibilities: first, it may be energy which is free at birth, which is perhaps being kept free for the purpose of discharge when necessary; second, the stimulus—or any other circumstance—which released the laughter or fright, may also have freed the " bound " energy. According to the Spencerian and Freudian conception, the second possibility is to be assumed with regard to laughter; the ridiculous removes an existing binding of energy (Freud's repressive force, the expenditure in preparation) which is then discharged in laughter without utilization. This complicated psychic mechanism does not exist in the infant, it cannot expend any energy in repression, and therefore does not need to economize it; but, nevertheless, the Freudian conception seems to apply particularly well to the child. For it does expend in anxiety energy which it economizes in the case of laughter. We can easily demonstrate this process in the

auditory reactions. An auditory stimulus occurs, the phenomenon of attention follows it; the stimulus continues, the child
laughs aloud and creates for itself new rhythmic auditory
stimuli. Attention as a cathectic phenomenon is already
known to us; to some extent, as protection against the threatening increase of the level of energy; energy as counter-cathexis
is added which immediately shows that the stimulus is not
dangerous, the cathectic energy proves to be superfluous in
this place and is discharged. The energy situation that existed
before the stimulus is re-established, and a feeling of pleasure
has been experienced.

The situation during fright is completely different. Here
no cathexis of the danger zone took place; the stimulus brought
a sudden strong increase of the level of energy from the outside,
the entire energy situation is resolved, bindings are resolved
in various places and discharged diffusely; the individual needs
after this discharge a certain time to recover—that is, to reinstate the interrupted situation after the discharged stimulus
—in order to restore the released bindings again. Even in
this case the expenditure was unnecessary; but this is realized
only after it has been spent. Fright, viewed in this light, thus
appears senseless. It is, therefore, in both instances " bound "
energy which is freed and discharged. But it seems as if there
existed a quantum of energy which finds itself relatively free,
which is used for certain more transitory cathexes, more mobile,
more displaceable than the rest; Freud (1) calls this quantum
" cathectic energy " (Besetzungsenergie).[1] It is with this we
obviously deal in the case of laughter, with the bound energy
in the case of fright in general.

From what source is the cathectic energy derived? We
need not give a final answer, but the origin of one part of it
seems easily understood. It serves to prevent attacks of
fright; it serves as protection against such undesired surprises.
Perhaps in the many shocks which the child experiences in the
first weeks a quantum of energy remains free during the new
organization which is necessary after each spasm, and thus
creates for itself a supply of reserve energy which is at the
disposal of all kinds of cathectic phenomena. If this were so,
it would at least indicate an effect of fright, which had some
meaning, certainly an affectively satisfying construction.
What applies to the repetition is no less valid for the first shock,

[1] Investment energy.—*Translator*.

birth. But this reference in particular brings before us the reverse possibilities. By birth, in any case, the energy situation of the fœtus is suddenly and radically disturbed. These freed quantities of energy are discharged in the new physiological movements: breathing, blood circulation, crying and movement of the limbs.

The first sleep temporarily reinstates the prenatal situation, but obviously the binding is no longer completely successful, the quantity of energy (cathectic energy) remaining free causes a *labile* situation. A stimulus originating from the syndrome of birth stimuli gives this quantum opportunity for discharge: the birth situation is reproduced.

The repetition of shocks lessens the quantum, because it is consumed by the frequent discharges up to the limits of the residue which is reserved throughout life for the actual passing cathexes. The diminution of the quantum of cathectic energy occurs undoubtedly through the new bindings of energy which happen during the first months of life. Which of these two conceptions is preferable could hardly be decided without establishing the exact meaning of the expressions " strong " and " weak " binding, and a definite attitude concerning the " consumption " of energy by discharge. I do not feel justified in pursuing these ideas in this connection, so the problem is left open; perhaps the nearest approach to reality lies in the supposition that both conceptions merge into each other and unite.

If it were not the object of this book to attempt a comprehensive presentation which may fill in the gaps in our knowledge by hypotheses and conjectures, by putting forward transitory views, so that the gaps may become the more obvious and intolerable, a discussion such as that of cathectic energy would hardly be justified. I fear that the suggestions which are now current concerning pleasure and its relation to the discharge phenomena will even in this book appear too bold. Nevertheless I do not wish to omit them; but I will again emphasize the fact that I am aware that such theoretic discussions in connection with child-psychology are suspect so long as psychology has not achieved an independent solution of those of its branches which are concerned with psychic energy, its origin and source, its changes, its qualitative and quantitative relations. This group of questions could very well constitute a theoretic psychology. So long as this does not exist, save in the scattered comments, more or less responsible, of various authors, it is of course impossible to apply it to child-psychology. And the presumptuous attempt to build up a psychology of energy casually and incidentally, in a psychology of the infant, would promise very little. If, in spite of this, I go beyond the limits of what can justly be expected today of child-psychology, I do so in order to call attention particularly to the necessity, and I hope also to the fruitfulness of theoretical assumptions and considerations. The ideas which these chapters of my book contain scarcely need in themselves any justification. In almost all instances they are conceptions which have already found advocates and defenders in psychological literature; they are in essence Freud's well-considered and studied theories. But the reason for allying myself with these opinions, for dispersing the objections which are, or might be, raised against them, and, above all, the basis for such obscure defences of theoretical assumptions, I must continue to owe the reader, who might otherwise be disappointed in his expectation of finding a comprehensive psychology of the infant, and would not be satisfied with finding instead the beginnings of a theoretical psychology.

With this apology we ask: what is the dynamic presentation, from the economic point of view ?[1] Why is discharge of cathectic energy pleasurable, why is the discharge of freed energy painful—at least in the case of fright ? Fundamentally two conceptions of pleasure have been expressed: pleasure as an indication of utility, and pleasure as perception of a definite state of energy. These two points of view are not incompatible, as, *e.g.*, G. Heilig's book on the perceptual sensations shows; starting from the principle of utility, it reaches conclusions which agree well with ours. We follow up the Freudian conception of pleasure as perception varying in the amount of energy. And indeed it is assumed that perception carrying a high amount of excitability yields ' pain,' and carrying a small amount yields pleasure. This idea leads to various difficulties, even though it is well substantiated. In the first place, according to this idea of energy, any discharge must be pleasurable; for discharge obviously means utilization of energy: and further, every stimulus must be painful, for stimulation obviously means an increase in the amount of excitation. To a certain degree both apply, and the correct-

[1] Freud's metapsychological classification.—*Translator.*

ness of this viewpoint is thus proved; nevertheless, it is not valid for the more differentiated relationships. Undoubtedly there is a pleasure in increased excitation, stimulus-pleasure, and it is indeed the greatest pleasure we know. Stimulus-pleasure can probably be traced back to pleasure in the reduction of excitation, but this is not our task. We can be content with stressing, in agreement with much that has been said earlier, the difference between both kinds of pleasure. If the infant obtains pleasure from light and auditory stimuli, from the rhythmic stimulation of sucking, we can contrast this, as the stimulus-pleasure in gratification-pleasure, with the rest-pleasure which it may have when, satiated and satisfied, it falls asleep. We might classify the stimulus-pleasure as the aim of the sexual instincts, and the rest-pleasure as the aim of the R.-instincts. In concluding the investigations which we presented, if one were willing to overlook the fact that the stimulus-pleasure in seeing and sucking is indicated from birth, one might further say that the stimulus-pleasure is acquired, while rest-pleasure is primary.

It is difficult to understand the economic situation in stimulus pleasure, but one condition for its realization can be made evident to a certain degree. It is noticeable that many of the stimuli which apparently produce pleasure in the infant possess rhythm as a common and characteristic property. Of course we must not use the word rhythm in its strictest sense, but must always keep in mind the simple form of some kind of alternation of stimulus and rest in which the rest has a duration equal to that of the stimulus; but this duration must not be so long that the next stimulus will be conceived as a completely new one, but must be short enough to be connected with the first. That rhythms are pleasant, that every rhythm as such is agreeable (even if there be other factors which spoil and conceal the pleasure), and that the children of the earliest age are particularly sensitive to it— these are facts from which it follows that we can, on the whole, perceive as pleasure the repetitions and gradual descents of energy in quick succession, ascents during stimulation, descent during pause. And it appears that this occurs regularly in the infant. We see nothing like it in the new-born; this reaction is clearly noticeable only after several weeks of life. In this period the cathectic energy begins to function. It is prepared for the counter-cathexis if the stimulus follows. The reduction of confined energy is consummated in counter-cathexis when the stimulus occurs rhythmically. We have reason to believe, as we shall explain in the chapter on "Perceptions," that during the waking state a quantity of energy is at the disposal of the sense organs even before they have met stimuli, that an increase of the level of energy of the sense organs begins with awaking, which makes intelligible the paradoxical facts of hunger for stimuli even without this assumption. This relative duration-cathexis of the sense organs is evidently consummated in the first weeks of life, and creates the basis for possibilities of prolonged stimulus-pleasure in the sense organs. If this is accepted, it would appear that the stimulus pleasure consisted in the countless repetitions of the birth situation and the "overcoming" of it in the first sleep, *i.e.*, absence of stimulus—stimulus—absence of stimulus, in rapid succession. It would seem that the energy thus frequently released and bound is not the whole quantity of energy of the psychic apparatus, but only a small quantity—the cathectic energy; it is not the energy that is difficult to release and difficult to bind, but the relatively free, easily mobile cathectic energy. One might directly say: the stimulus-pleasure occurs instead of ' pain ' because the same process—which, if it took place on the whole mass of energy, would result in ' pain '—is enacted on a suitably small scale, because it is not in earnest but in play.

Speaking of " in play " and " in earnest " is no stylistic phrase; it is more probably an analogy. If we would explain play we should have to begin at the "playful" repetition of birth which manifests itself at every rhythmic stimulus. But since we reflect on the energy relationships of stimulus-pleasure, we can only make them intelligible in processes identical with those which we have directly experienced. It is a game of energy, a game of fright, a game of being born, which we experience as stimulus pleasure. All these are co-existent, and it is immaterial what causes, content, and forms pleasure may have. It should not be forgotten that we neither explain pleasure thereby nor completely understand it; we have merely, in one instance, clarified its possibilities within the realm of the Freudian-Fechnerian conception of pleasure-pain phenomena. (The expectation expressed at the beginning of this discussion, that the idea of the birth trauma would find a precise formulation through it, has remained of course unfulfilled; and the relation to birth, so frequently mentioned, and its " repetition " and " overcoming " (*Über-windungen*) must be understood as merely a figurative expression.)

One fact which is relevant in this connection, and which is occasionally noticed, deserves mention. Laughing is an outcome of tickling. In adults and in children this follows so frequently, indeed to such a degree regardless of whether tickling is perceived first as pleasurable or as painful, that one speaks of laughing as a reflex. But in the infant a noteworthy reaction should be recorded. At the beginning, laughing cannot be produced by tickling. Different times have been cited for the first appearance of laughter after tickling, but Sully's (2) evidence that the first laughter occurs when the child has already laughed for some time from other causes seems to fit; but the beginnings of both do not seem to be far from each other. Tickling stimulates laughter in the child only when it is done by a familiar person, and when the child is not suddenly surprised by the stimulation. In the case of tickling, the way in which laughing is substituted for fright is so conspicuous that Sully—as well as other authors—builds up his explanation of its appearance on this antithesis. And indeed Sully sees an intellectual factor operative here, the understanding that this stimulus produced by this person, in spite of the surprising aggressive character which tends to release instinctive fright, is not dangerous, but only a game. This understanding, which in itself is by no means pleasurable, is made possible by the pleasurable nature of the process. Sully consistently reckons pleasure derived from tickling as a game. The fusion of painful movements (defence) and pleasurable movements during tickling is stressed by Sully in his treatment of this complicated phenomenon, just as we attempted to do in the case of laughter. Sully is not successful in making this intelligible as a result of tickling, nor even as the result of the pleasure of the process as a whole. He had to make daring and uncontrolled leaps into the phylogenetic realms: he had to refer to the pleasure which the young animal may feel when it is freed from fleas by its solicitous mother, and, on the other hand, he had to call in specific situations which may arise in the fights of older children, but which do not exist for the infant. Laughter is the most evident indication of the playmate; it has comprehended the nature of aggression as play and wishes to continue it as such. In our construction, the facts mentioned, as well as their play character, dovetail well without our having to assume such remote ideas, and without having to expect that the child in the first months of its life controls intellectual processes of such a complicated kind. Tickling as rhythmic stimulation is quite capable of calling forth that special course of the discharge of the cathectic energy which expresses itself as pleasure, play, or laughter. And one point which we left completely unclarified in visual pleasure, and which we did not consider carefully in auditory pleasure, can here be decided beyond a doubt. The tickling pleasure is tactual pleasure, the energy at its disposal is libido; laughing is here clearly sexual pleasure, and the tendency to permit tickling, the preparation for it, is in the service of the sexual instinct. We shall here be able to speak of libido without discussing whether it always applies in cases of stimulus-pleasure, and regardless of what the complicated relation between energy and libido and their quantities may be when it is not relevant.

PERCEPTIONS

Of all the advances in development during the first quarter of the first year, the advances in perception seem the most remarkable and almost improbable. For as far removed in a thousand details as the world of the three-months-old child may be from ours, the world, as the child perceives it, is not only incomparably far advanced quantitatively, but it is fundamentally separated from the condition which we consider primitive and which the new-born represents. For the three-months-old child the world is most assuredly not a chaos of light and darkness, of numberless inextricable spots of colour, of tones and noises. On the contrary, it sees its mother, the milk bottle, its toys; it hears combinations of tones and voices; it recognizes familiar and unfamiliar faces, friendly and unfriendly voices: thus it sees the world fundamentally as we see it, even if the number of objects be very much smaller. But not only this holds good; the agreement with adult perceptions is even greater. The bare breasts of the mother are not spots of colour, but something which the child takes as a whole, from other units or mere spots of colour, as structure or "*Gestalt*," as the psychologists Köhler and Wertheimer (Koffka) say, something differentiated. The child really sees the mother's breasts, but it does not see them as the naturalist contemplates an object in order to fix its contour, its form (*Gestalt*) and properties; but it sees this whole simultaneously in relation to itself: it knows the breast as something which should be taken into the mouth, something to be suckled; it prepares itself immediately for suckling, and anticipates what is coming. Fitting examples of the clearness of such expectations of its fulfilment, as it were, are seen in the following instances:

Scupin, sixth week: "Before imbibing, a bib is tied under the child's chin. The boy for some time now associates with the bib the idea of a coming delight; for the eyes immediately become greedy, the mouth seeks, the hands are joyously flung about; if the child thinks his expectation is going to be thwarted, or if the breast is not reached quickly enough, he breaks out into a vigorous, angry, resounding scream." Scupin, twelfth week: "Today we noticed for the first time that the child recognized the breast. As soon as he caught sight of it, he opened his eyes wide, and followed it with all the signs of greed. Hitherto, it was only after the preparatory operations of being placed at the breast that he realized that he was to be suckled, and indeed on seeing the nude breast he turned elsewhere and clumsily panted in the air." Queck: "On the sixty-seventh day he takes three spoonfuls of honey with great relish. He licks the spoon till it is clean. . . . Several days later, when he was about to receive fruit juice . . . he at first smiled at his father who extended the bottle to him, pouted his mouth, and then opened it as if begging for a drink."

This is quite obviously adult perception; here a thing is seen and is not a chaos of sensations; simultaneously there occurs a relation of the object to himself on the basis of expectation, which his own experience and knowledge up to this point makes possible. The perception of the three-months-old child, accordingly, refers to things, *Strukturen, Gestalten*, and it occurs influenced by memory, or at any rate is accompanied by memory. This, of course, can be asserted with certainty only of visual and auditory perceptions, but probably only because observations in the fields of the other senses are insufficient, and because *Gestalt* psychology is scarcely advanced enough in these fields. For it is highly improbable that the child, at the time when it recognizes the breast, does not yet know milk, and indeed it has not a perception of a chaos of coloured spots; but it has rather perceptions of sweetness, moisture, warmth, instead of the " taste-pattern " (*Geschmacksgestalt*) milk.

The difficulty for our explanation which results from these facts is still further aggravated because unfortunately no development of perception can be established—that is, none of its essential characteristics, none which go beyond quantitative elaborations. As soon as the reactions of children to perceptions become so varied and unambiguous that they permit of only one inference from a perceptive act, only one possible conception of it presents itself: the child has perceived structures and their relation to itself, modified by memories of its personal experiences. One may doubt whether the observation of Preyer which we examined (p. 57) was correct, whether this reaction of the new-born actually occurs; one may consider whether it was not the accidental result of other causes; if it were established beyond a doubt, the only rational conclusion would be that the new-born already recalls a certain taste pattern (*Gestalt*), has therefore perceived it before, compares it with the original one, and repudiates it. The time given to the psychic apparatus to develop from the accepted primitive initial stage to the adult stage is not even three months, but at most two months, perhaps only one; for already at this time activities are noticeable from which the assumed inference must be drawn.

The same problem exists here as in the question of consciousness. That this is present in the three-months-old child cannot be doubted; it may be possible to discover when and how it has developed. Furthermore, both questions seem to stand in a certain relationship to each other, for those instances in which we must assume a perceptual act in essentials similar to the adult's act are those which give the strongest impression of the existence of *consciousness*.

There is a simple way to dispose of these difficulties. But one must abandon presuppositions about the primitive states and substitute new ones which agree more closely with the facts. Among child psychologists Bühler and, more definitely, Koffka take this step; they apply a new conception of psychology in interpreting the developmental phases, making this interpretation more understandable and substantially supporting the new conception. It is a question of the ideas of the so-called *Gestalt* psychologists. These ideas need not concern us, since attempts are already being made to apply them to the fields of our facts. One must only assume that friendliness, for example, is a simple phenomenon, more simple than the so-called simple sense impression (Koffka). And the facts of infant-psychology indicate precisely this. We cannot determine exactly when the child has a perception for the first time; the error in estimating the time, however, is probably the less the earlier this point is placed; in any case, it occurs during the first weeks; perhaps even in the first days. But these earliest perceptions are really perceptions and not isolated sensations. There are a collection of sensations which come from a " neutral cause," which are emotionally toned, and which, finally, have also some relation to expectations resulting from the previous experiences of the individual. This must be our assumption, according to the findings which observations offer us. Whether this is phylogenetically the primitive stage of perception we need not decide, although there may be much in favour of such a decision. There are no ontogenetic reasons to assume earlier stages out of which it could develop; indeed, whatever earlier stage we might conceive, the path from it to the empirical-primitive stage is so complicated that it would be extremely difficult to believe it was passed through in a few days, when we also consider that the first weeks and days are spent to so great an extent in a sleep state—in absence of perception.

This conception will not be received in the literature without objections; I, too, shall have to suggest further limitations, for some arising from affective causes are too apparent to be delayed. One is so accustomed to consider sensations as the elementary component of our perceptual world that it is easy to understand that they are fictions which may appropriately serve general psychology, but are certainly not useful in making intelligible the development of the phenomena (Krüger). Developmental psychology does not try to reduce the " composite " manifestations to the " simple," but the developed to the undeveloped, the complicated to the primitive. A " primitive " phenomenon can also be a " simple " one; but need not be. But the primitive phenomena must by no means be construed in analogy with physics or geometry. The conception of " simple " sensations of which our perceptual world is " composed " refers to the perceptual content, and not to the perceptual process or act. I can separate this room before me (physically and geometrically) actually into simple forms, spots of colour, light and darkness, and can think of it as built up out of these. This simplicity and composition has nothing to do with the simplicity of mental processes or their complexity. Why should it be simpler—more primitive—to perceive a red spot than a red circle on a blue background, for what other reason than that one is a simple figure, the other a composite geometric figure? We are so proud of our consciousness, of its intellectual function, its power of comparison, conclusion, and judgment that we would like to reserve all these as our higher function, and allow the infant only the earlier stages, only, as it were, perception. But in truth every perception is already an intellectual process, it is already comparison, it has relationship, and it is part of the most primitive process, as well as of the complicated process. It is like " talking " horses. One does not wish to believe that a horse can count, because if one did the horse would have to be placed on a much higher level. But the worst is yet to come. I do not believe that horses can count. But should it prove true that animals can perform counting operations, it would follow that counting is a much more primitive accomplishment than we think. We are brought down a step, which is even worse than exalting the animals.

We must not be satisfied with emphasizing the principal similarity between the perceptions of infants and those of adults; we may try to imagine the differences. For after it is proved that the primitiveness of perceptions does not lie in their simplicity, we can try to give a more precise definition of primitiveness. The observations here are too scattered and ambiguous for an inductive method: but they support an attitude which results from reflection. The use of perceptions for the individual is that they offer proofs of the outer-world (Freud, 9) in accordance with which the individual orients himself in his behaviour. The most rationalized process runs its course, so that the individual reflecting on the perceptions interprets and acts accordingly; the evaluation of perceptions—the insight made possible by them into the situation World—Ego—follows from the exclusion of every affective colouring. But in general rationalization is not so unalloyed. The evaluation is more probably found through reflection accompanied and influenced by affects of joy or fright, for example. This is not the empirical, most common, reaction, but in this reaction thought is more or less pushed into the background and the evaluation of perceptions results first of all affectively. That is, there are two series of perceptions at the same time: the optical, for instance, mediates toward an insight into the situation: fright, which is connected with it, gives us an insight into the reaction of our psyche to the situation. The inner and outer perceptions occur together; our conscious is in this case, so to speak, not an observer of this process, which is consummated without it and its reflection. One does not really understand why both series of perceptions should be necessary; it is advisable not to state this question as a scientific problem, but to be content with the assertion that as far as consciousness comes into the question all indications point to calling the inner perceptions the more primitive.[1]

We therefore assume that in the outer perceptions of infants the affective element greatly predominates. Of course, what the infant perceives are structures, but optically-affective, acoustically-affective, etc., and not only optical, etc. More concrete formulations are not possible here, but one can express oneself for example thus: from the dark background not a milk-bottle is taken away, but a beloved milk-bottle. Thus we do not know which element constitutes the concept milk-bottle, but we can be sure that the combining, form-creating element is the awakening of a desire for oral pleasure or gratification. Experiments, Bühler thinks, will, perhaps, be able to accord us an insight into what changes of form and colour are sufficient to change the loved milk-bottle into an unfamiliar feared one. But there is little hope that we shall be able to comprehend precisely the whole range of the affective factor. It were well, then, not to underestimate its importance, but to remember that we can notice in the infant almost from birth a certain interest in stimuli whose affective significance is insufficiently understood. It is, therefore, probable that the early perceptions already contain obvious optical elements in the optical affective relation.

Perhaps, too, there are also perceptions of the outer world in which the affective element absolutely predominates, in which the sensory element is perhaps entirely lacking. The adult mental life also knows such perceptual experiences bordering, as we may say, on the threshold of the primitive.

[1] There is much evidence in support of this conception in Heilig.

A sudden, violent pain gives us almost no insight into the environmental situation; we have not recognized that we felt the source of the stimulus, but we know it only—as intense pain—from our own reaction to this interference. Some psychologists endeavour, of course, to interpret even pain as the sum of certain tactual perceptions: the question is disputable, and therefore we select another instance of a similar nature: even during vehement fright the sensory element of perception, in contrast to the affective element, recedes considerably into the background; if I am startled, I know much less about the situation which frightened me than about my behaviour; I only know my timidity or momentary fright. It is easy to assume the same in infants, only in a more intensified form. The shrill whistle which frightened the infant recedes sensorially so completely into the background of perception that one can say paradoxically that the infant has not heard it at all. This is probably valid to a certain degree for painful reactions in general. They consist in great part—as our Reaction Type I—in this: that the sense organs are protected from further stimulation; and if the sensory element in perception is to gain in significance, it needs some time for development, which is only given when the individual turns his attention to it and offers his sense organs to it. The development of sensory perceptions will, therefore, unfold and open up channels for such things of the outer-world as are connected with pleasure. One could at once predict from the above the results of observations. Fortunately the observations exist, so we must obtain the confirmation of this statement from them. The three-months-old child knows most of the things, and all of the people who create the means of satisfying its nutritional instinct; it knows the comforter, the finger, and similar dispensers of oral pleasures; it knows the preparations for the bath, and ablution, articles of clothing, which are connected with its pleasure from skin excitation; and in conclusion it knows a number of those things which help it really to create sensory stimulus-pleasure, the relation of the quantity of cathectic libido: the celluloid ball, the rattle, and similar toys.

Primitive perception is dominated more by the affective element than developed perception—this would be the first assumption which we could enlist for the recognition of the characteristics of the infant's perceptions. As the second assumption we can observe more exactly the relation between the reproductive and the perceptive element. We need not investigate whether a perception is possible without a reproductive process, whether it has any meaning without memory.[1] For something definite can be said about infant perception when we observe effects of memory. Only when the child recognizes an object, recognizes it beyond a doubt, does it have a primitive perception. But even if we wish to make some interpretation of its earlier perceptions, we would sooner attribute perception to those cases in which the infant shows apparent interest for changes, movements, rhythms; and to perceive these surely implies in some way the recall, during moment B, of the moment A which has just passed. It is remarkable that the perception of changes, which does not appear simple to us but very complicated, belongs particularly to the earliest perceptions. It is very primitive; it falls completely within the relationship already discussed. But in any case, memory and perception are two processes which appear very early in the development of the child, certainly before the end of the third month, probably considerably earlier, perhaps already in the first days or perhaps immediately after birth; and their relation to each other is so close that we must assume memory to be already operative where any signs of the existence of perception can be surmised. Max Offner has written: " We know that small children in the first few months of their life show no signs of memory; only after the third or fourth month are the first indications observed"; though such formulations as this are frequently found in the literature they are nevertheless insufficient if they presuppose too narrow an idea of " memory," and otherwise they are absolutely wrong. On the other hand, in order to grasp our conception, one need not assume memory as an organic phenomenon; the manifestation of which we speak here means only the individual memory; reproduction wholly within the realm of individual sensory experience. Only one amplification—if it is not obviously implicit—has to be undertaken. One must not think that a long latency period elapses between perception and the reproductive process, the actualization of perceptual traces. When the clapper of a bell strikes against one side the perception of the noise becomes a memory trace in the brain, and

[1] See, *e.g.*, Bleuler's interesting arguments, which deny this emphatically.

if the clapper reaches the other side of the bell, and if the perceived sound is not experienced as an isolated first tone but in some relation to the first tone, it is, then, the effect of reproduction, in spite of the fact that the interval between the formation of the memory trace and its first reawakening may be only a fraction of a second. In this sense, perception without memory, as far as we can empirically determine, does not exist.

From two angles it is easy to make an assumption, of course not capable of proof, about primitive reproduction. Dream and hallucination can be easily understood if they are conceived as the regression of the mental apparatus to a primitive state. Thus Freud (4) evolved this idea of the most primitive course of the mental life: " the state of mental equilibrium was originally disturbed by the peremptory demands of inner needs. In the situation I am considering, whatever was thought of (desired) was simply imagined in an hallucinatory form. . . . This attempt at satisfaction by means of hallucination was abandoned only in consequence of the absence of the expected gratification, because of the disappointment experienced."

This means that reproduction occurs in primitive stages with much greater animation than in more developed stages. The reproduction has the sensuous vivacity of reality. . . . This does not apply to the adult. Indeed, there are types varying greatly in reaction, and one may justly seek the nature of reproduction in characteristics other than its lesser intensity. This, therefore, remains the rule. In the case of vision and hallucination (and inspiration, one might add) the rule finds exceptions in that the primitive stage, the stage of the infant, is attained. The hallucinatory character of reproduction need not be the usual one, it can be reduced to wish fulfilment; thus one idea still remains which does not seem to offer fewer difficulties, but it does not seem worth while to reject it outright, because it is, though by no means an indispensable, a very convenient stone in the structure of Freudian psychology. However, investigations undertaken from an entirely different angle, by Jaensch and his pupil (Kroh), gave the very noteworthy result that the hallucinatory clarity in reproduction obviously decreases with age; that childhood is distinguished by its more frequent hallucinatory images. And although the experiments have not been traced back to early childhood, and their general meaning is not yet accepted beyond a doubt, yet we

9

have every reason to expect that they can be seen also in early childhood and especially then. For the plausibility of the Freudian construction (the usual adult manifestation of reproduction is the result of a repressive-depreciation process), which in itself is so well built up, is extraordinarily increased if it is confirmed from wholly different points of view which apply completely different methods, and if the results found allow similar interpretations.

To all this can be added that the three-months-old child cannot possibly have any cognizance of the outer-world, any insight into the difference between reality and its subjective ideas. And this will perhaps help as much as anything else to obliterate the difference between perception and reproduction. Here it remains relatively immaterial whether one ascribes any subjective attributes to reproduction from the beginning, or whether one wishes to make its origin dependent upon an experience already in progress; for this certainly defines those attributes, and since such experience is lacking the difference is less.

Having summarized this, we are led to a construction which is not without difficulties. The infant is hungry; at first hallucinations of oft-experienced gratification-situations set in. As soon as the mother steps near his bed, he will have a perception simultaneously with the hallucination (reproduction), and both, although of similar intensity, will be slightly different in structure and attributes. One must admit that this simultaneity of reproduction and perception is not easy to conceive and appears somewhat strange. But if we substitute rapid succession for simultaneity, we see very fruitful prospects. The substitution is justifiable. Indeed, the hallucination of an adult is usually stronger than the perception and obliterates it; but this is a pathological case. Although we have ascribed to infant reproduction the vitality of hallucination, and the similarity of hallucination to perception, we must not think of it with its other characteristics too. The reproduction of the infant remains reproduction—*i.e.*, the influx of stimuli from the outer-world withdraws the energy from reproduction which is used for the process of perception; reproduction becomes weak or completely disappears; the memory paths (*Ekphorierung des Engramms*) are not retraced. Apparently the infant learns very soon, especially from the nutritional instinct, to distinguish between reproduction and perception, because he soon makes the disagreeable discovery that reproduction does not lead to gratification, but that it also needs the occurrence of those images which differ from reproduction in certain characteristics. He presumably learns from the hallucinatory reproductions, which are connected with hunger and its gratification, to recognize the ideational properties, regardless of whether these adhere to the idea from the beginning, or whether they develop only with the process. We should not be surprised if further investigations show the early application of the best possible means for preventing continual disappointment over the reproduction, namely, prevention of too strong a flow of energy to them, their relative paleness and unreal attitude. The progressive dimming of reproductions would accordingly start from conceptions which are connected with the nutritional instinct, and lead, in one type, to total absence of visualization, and in other types to relative absence of visualization. That it may be a question of real processes, and not merely of fiction, is proved by hunger-visions, in which, after exhausting all normal means of instinctual gratification, and perhaps also after injury to the mental apparatus, the primal process of hallucination—abandoned as useless long ago—is reverted to in desperation. This withdrawal of energy which occurs in the memory path, hunger-gratification, would be the primal predisposition, the prototype of real repression; the memory traces are shut off from the supply of energy which would stimulate them to reproduction—in this case only to a certain degree.

The great similarity, the close connection between reproduction and perception, revises for us a little the idea of intellectual functioning, which one perhaps might have built up from what has been said before. If we agree that comparison, expectation, and even reasoning, to say nothing of remembering, are more primitive processes than they are frequently believed to be, it can then be further recognized that these primitive processes in the three-months-old child are carried out in more primitive forms than is the case in older children or adults. It is really the quantitative factor, the interval between the parts compared, which plays a rôle here. It is not easy to believe that a child of eight or ten weeks " recalls " when it is laid into the cradle how it was done yesterday, and now " knows " what will follow. And yet the infant's conduct is completely and correctly described thus (there are even more surprising instances, only this process of remembering, and indeed, this knowing, is quite different from ours): it consists—in everything that is important to the child—of an affective-sensory reproduction of yesterday's (and probably even earlier) experience, faithful and similar to reality, because hallucinatory. The child can, so to speak, do nothing but correlate both the images of memory and actuality, appearing almost simultaneously. If it succeeds, it then has the feeling of familiarity, and expects something, since the one picture already conveys what the other will show in a second or in a minute. Nevertheless, to speak of a feeling of familiarity is not quite accurate. For one must imagine that in the case of essential superimposition, both images are experienced only as an affective evaluation of them, as a single one; a situation of gratification (or one offering stimulus-pleasure) occurred. But since the increasing difference between reproduction, perception, and the disappointments frequently experienced may set in, and also a certain recognition of the familiar, which is always positively perceived, the abbreviated evaluation, the feeling of familiarity, suffices. The coincident occurrence of reproduction and perception is in most cases pleasurable; since certainly only pleasant stages in general lead to real perception. It obviously takes a long time—certainly far into the second or even third quarter of the first year—before the sensory element of perception during a state of ' pain ' attains formation and relative dominance in the child. But the reproduction of unpleasant situations is certainly very infrequent. As far as I can see, the facts do not literally contradict a generalization, but neither can it be proved. For the present the reasons which induce me to generalize are still theoretical ones: in the first month of life no hallucinatory reproduction of an unpleasant experience occurs. In any case it seems to me that this assumption has been ventured even less frequently than the assumption that no sensory perception exists in an unpleasant (' pain ') situation. And yet this is obviously true, to a certain degree—as we have explained above—in so far as the sensory element recedes very far into the background compared with the affective element. Even if this were absolutely true, reproduction, which nevertheless applies to a previous perception, could at best contain only a very meagre sensory part. But even this part is highly improbable, since it contradicts the pleasure-principle so fundamentally that it would hardly be possible to discover its dominance at all. But if the validity of such deductions is not admitted, I gladly yield and offer the following for consideration: After the infant has finally come to terms with the existence of stimuli alien to the embryo (which occurs very soon for the eye, and for the ear last), it generally knows no sensory elements painful in themselves; but knows only such as are connected with a situation of gratification (or stimulus-pleasure) with the exception of fright, of which we will soon speak. And it cannot know them, for all its perceptions have been bound up with pleasure- as well as with ' pain '-situations. The milk-bottle is part of the hunger-situation, during which it first appears, as well as of the gratification-situation, when the infant sucks it. The mother's face belongs to all (or most) ' pain '-situations, as well as to many gratifying situations. If it were really possible easily to reproduce the pleasure- and ' pain '-situation from the sensory perceptions, it would be impossible to understand how an endurable attitude to the outer-world, which the three-months-old child has beyond doubt attained, came about. This result is only possible if the ' pain '-situation is very difficult to reproduce, possibly incapable of reproduction. And this can be attained best in this way: (1) perception in the ' pain '-situation was generally inconsiderable; (2) memory paths, which were formed exclusively in the ' pain '-situation, are in great part cut off from energy-cathexis. Both possibilities may be plausible; the first alone would suffice for the understanding of most cases, the second needs some additional assumptions which are none too simple.

In the beginning perceptions are not in themselves reproductive of ' pain,' on the contrary they embrace—as it seems, at least—a fair quantum of potential pleasure. If we reach this conclusion from the assumption which we made concerning stimulus-pleasure of a sensory nature—according to which also those perceptions which are not necessarily connected with instinctual gratification situations are enjoyed numberless times in the games of overcoming fright—it would certainly be a conclusive proof, if the assumption of the hallucinatory reproduction as an attempt at instinctual gratification were confirmed. For here it is clear how the cathexis of an idea, which is related to ' pain ' as well as to pleasure, comes into contrast with the actual affective situation: the pain of dissatisfaction changes gratification into pleasure. As I see it, one can set aside these arguments as worthless only when one decides to ascribe understanding of causal relations to the infant, and even then only as partially worthless. If this is agreed to, then it can scarcely be dismissed *a priori*, although it will interest us in a later connection.

Of course, there is, too, a kind of reproduction, a kind of memory of ' pain ' in this early period of life, only it is not of a sensory, but of a motor, nature. We often come upon phenomena which we do not know how to organize in any other way than by saying, here the birth situation is being produced —that is, by motor repetition. First, fright is involved. A stimulus " recalls " birth, as we say, which, considering the figurative expression, is obvious enough. But the memory consists solely of a motor action whose meaning we knew how to formulate only from the point of view of energy. It must be stressed that such stimuli release memory, although not on the strength of the content of its perceptions (its sensory value), but according to its formal quality (suddennesss, intensity, etc.). We ourselves know anxiety (fear, fright) as an " expression " of this reaction; we may ascribe it also to the infant and the new-born. But it is fundamentally independent of all sensory elements, it releases them, accompanies them, but in optional variability. One might say that anxiety is the recollection of birth, but this means something different from recollection as the word has been used hitherto. It would be more correct to say: instead of the memory of birth, instead of sensory reproduction of all perceptions, we have anxiety. No one can have a sensory recollection of birth; even hypnosis and psycho-analysis, which can drive memory back into the depths of early childhood, have not the power to recall birth. That is in general impossible, because the individual sensory memory—at least, we must for the present assume so— begins first with the overcoming of the trauma of birth. The preceding sentence is reversible: sensory reproduction stands in the place of anxiety. The individual sensory memory originates in a struggle to overcome the anxiety of birth, which tends to reproduce itself in response to every post-natal stimulus.[1] At present these last conceptions are only gropings in the dark. To me personally they are nothing but tentative conjectures for thrusting back the boundaries of psychological knowledge by starting new hypotheses. Later an attempt

[1] This seems to be Rank's opinion too.

will be made to formulate what in general can be said about this today. Here the apperceptive connection must suffice. An observation frequently made " which is insufficiently understood " (Bühler) finds a simple explanation in our conception. A relatively small change in the object will often be enough to awaken fright in the infant instead of a feeling of familiarity. Thus it is sufficient that the mother put on a black hat unfamiliar to the child, to make it recoil anxiously from her instead of greeting her with joy; it obviously oscillates between recognition and anxiety. In this example, perception and reproduction do not coincide at one point essential for the child. It expects to see mother and is disappointed because it sees mother in a black hat. It cannot be the unfamiliarity of the impression which creates anxiety in the child, for it clearly has a perceptive interest in new impressions (Claparède, 2). This interest of the infant in seeing and hearing is already very strongly developed at this age, and does not break down in relation to any thing or any noise which does not call forth shock reactions by the suddenness or intensity of its occurrence. The child at this age does not yet fear at all. As far as I gather from the literature and the impression I gained from my own observations, it does not even fear things with which it has had unfortunate experiences.

The perceptive interest changes into ' pain ' only in two instances: (1) When an urgent need demands appeasement—sleep, hunger, pleasure-sucking; but even then there is still sufficient capacity for diversion, at least for a short time, and indeed to completely new stimuli. (2) When an otherwise familiar loved object, may we say, is changed. The first case is simple. The necessity. has produced a vivid reproduction of a gratifying situation. What does not coincide with this reproduction is sometimes accepted, sometimes rejected, according to the circumstances. The second is more complicated. It calls forth not repudiation, but anxiety. In this case a gratification-situation has set in. The mother is here, but she does not coincide completely with the reproduced image. The child has no fear, but a feeling of unfamiliarity, as Stern says, or as we would say, anxiety, because even unfamiliarity requires too much reflection and experience. Fear and anxiety deserve to be kept distinctly separated, as Lehmann and Freud (11) separate them. Fear is justified fear of an object. Anxiety is objectless, unfounded fear. Infants of this early age know no fear, but experience pure anxiety. Only a confusion of both of these ideas could lead to so impossible an assumption as that of the inherent fear of certain animals. In the case of the mother's black hat real anxiety occurs, not fright, which is an instantaneous motor discharge of anxiety, but this as a phenomenon continues for some time. Reproduction (hallucination) promises stimulus-pleasure, perception hinders it; libido, in the process of development, is inhibited, and must change into anxiety; this, according to Freud's fundamental discovery, is the general formula for anxiety.

Originally the world of stimulation released only the reaction to the primal stimulus: starting from birth: fright (anxiety); the *R.*-instincts seek to hinder the possibility of such continuous repetitions by continual reinstatement of the fœtal situation; they respond to stimuli with Reaction Type I. In exercising the nutritional instinct, which serves to re-establish the disturbed fœtal situation, the individual experiences the stimulus-pleasure of perception, which the "playful repetition" of the trauma of birth overcomes. The sexual instincts react to the stimuli with Reaction Type II; the stimulus-pleasure is vigorously sought at the expense of the fœtal situation. Gratifying situations also become more and more the agents of perceptual-pleasure-experiences. Thus the perceptual world and especially certain preferred things (*e.g.*, the mother) become strongly cathexed with libido. Where its development, initiated by perception or reproduction, is inhibited, anxiety (fright) again sets in as the regression to the original state.

Some may perhaps think that a brief justification for speaking of libido in connection with perception is necessary. Admittedly, the statement that processes of energy which play a part in perception and reproduction are fundamentally libidinal is convenient, and good sense, but in the present state of our knowledge the assertion cannot be represented as indisputable. Of course, we must ascribe a good part of all these processes to libido, for stimulus-pleasure is, according to the definition, the aim of the sexual instincts, and the energy which is at their disposal we call, with Freud, libido. In the same way, anxiety, the negative of stimulus-pleasure, is always libidinal. In any case, a greater quantity of libido is given to the perceptual processes than one might without question admit, for undoubtedly a great number of perceptual acts are in the service of the sexual instincts. This is not, of course, decisive, because occasionally the same processes are in the service of the R.-instincts too. But the apparent stimulus-pleasure and the facts that the perceptual life, as a whole, promotes the progressive tendency, that it is in strong contrast to the fœtus situation, that it is generally only possible after, and in so far as, the effects of the R.-instincts are overcome, all speak for the conception of energy as libido.

The relations of perceptions (and reproductions) are not entirely simple. First of all, they are different from what one might expect without careful consideration. We understand perception as a test of the outer-world stimulus-situation, if it leads to action. One must have observed the harmful influences in order to escape them, one must observe food in order to seize it. The psychological and social situation of the infant by no means assumes this necessity. It may be blind and dumb, and will be fed in spite of it; on the other hand, that it is neither blind nor dumb is of little or no use to it, for it cannot flee from perceived danger, cannot take possession of (master) perceived things, in the first quarter of the first year of its life. The possessive (mastery) apparatus—hands, legs, body—begins to develop only in the second quarter of the first year, and completes its development in the fifth quarter, while the perceptual apparatus has already attained a considerable degree of development before the beginning of the ability to grasp (which is only the most primitive expression of the possessive apparatus), and, as we shall later see, is almost completely developed before the child has really learned to walk. We do not know what causes have produced this division between the development of the perceptual apparatus and the mastery apparatus, which is specific in humans, and as far as I see does not exist in animals; nor is this a problem for child-psychology. The results of this speeding up of the intellectual development are obvious. This fact is possible because pleasure is created from perception, because libido is the motive power of this development. Pleasure is gained from perception itself, at first independent of its content, and further independent of the gratification of the R.-instincts and the remaining sexual instincts. Thereby a part of the world is libidinally charged (cathexed) even before the individual can take possession of it, and before it has comprehended this world as Not-I. This deep, matter-of-fact confidence in the outer-world which we normally have is the result of this primal cathexis, which occurs even before the separation between the ego and the outer-world, even before the mastery impulses aim—as we shall see—to destroy this world.

Here the Schopenhauerian " World as Idea " is realized; and, indeed, the infant loves this world as it loves every part of itself, for there is no difference between reproduction and perception, in any case no difference in libidinal cathexis, but there is also none between pleasure-dispensing parts of the body (e.g., the mouth), and pleasure-dispensing reproductions and perceptions. The significance of the fact that by the remarkable prematurity of the sensory processes themselves the mental functions of perception, attention, and reproduction have at their disposal and retain forever, presupposing a normal development, a considerable quantity of energy, is not to be underestimated for the whole future development. The powerful significance of the intellectual processes—perception, phantasy, thinking, and their social results in science, art, and philosophy in the human being—have their first roots in this specifically human mental structure of the three-months-old child.

THE STRUCTURE OF THE THREE-MONTHS-OLD CHILD

I should like to combine in this chapter a cross-section of the mental structure of the three-months-old child, with clear and summarized presentation of the fundamental ideas and developmental principles, which I fear are obscured by the factual material and the special discussions.

We found the new-born governed by the R.-instincts; long sleep periods, short waking periods which are dedicated almost exclusively to feeding; indifference or repudiation of all stimuli from the outer-world greatly predominating; expressing itself pleasurably in situations which recall the fœtal situation, in its bodily attitude—and in great part, too, through the customs of child rearing—continuing the fœtal-situation. It has not taken cognizance of birth; it strives to continue, and when disturbed to reinstate as quickly as possible, the environmental situation and the life processes existing before birth. Thus the new-born presents a psychic system at rest which reacts to stimuli in so far as they penetrate beyond its indifference—reacts only so far as is necessary in order to dispose of them, in order to re-establish its state of equilibrium. It is extremely narcissistic in relation to the outer-world. In general there are only two groups of manifestations which do not fit in with this picture: (1) discharge phenomena of a surprising nature, whose significance we do not yet understand, but which we suppose to be connected with the traumatic consequences of birth; (2) the beginning of a new distribution of libido indicated only in visual pleasure, and perhaps also in sucking-pleasure, which is really independent of the gratification of the nutritional instinct. Both groups are of almost unlimited scope.

The first quarter of the first year is dedicated to the intensive achievement of this new division of libido. This means that the new organization is already completely developed, in the normal case, at the end of the third month. We find a considerable concentration of energy on the head, which offers strong possibilities of stimulus-pleasure. Three well-characterized zones result from libido cathexis: eyes, oral zone (mouth), ears. The zone around the mouth is obviously erotogenetic; it offers sexual pleasure (tactual pleasure) in its restricted sense; the ears and eyes offer stimulus-pleasure; this pleasure from the ear is even more closely related to sexual pleasure than that from the eyes. The sexual instincts strive unceasingly and energetically during the waking periods to gain pleasure from these three zones.

Most activities are likewise dependent on the head as the motor apparatus. We can differentiate a specially mobile and easily displaceable quantity of the energy (libido) which is presumably concentrated on the head; this quantity is cathectic energy, which is changed during the act of attention into perceptual and reproductive energy and offers pleasure. Secondary to this is the possibility for pleasure which the rest of the body, the skin, offers, and for the kinæsthetic pleasure of moving the limbs. But even this pleasure is invested with libido, giving pleasure. The waking periods have become considerably longer, and are almost filled with expressions (in part real activities) of the sexual instincts which, in part, actively seek that varied pleasure; but first the infant must wait passively until, through changes in the outer-world, suitable stimuli release the pleasure. The infant's activity can operate first in sound utterances, so that the auditory pleasure can to a great extent be gratified; secondly, putting the hand into the mouth or movements of the head produce sucking-pleasure; expressions of pleasure are at the same time further excitation of the oral zone and the auditory zone; finally, by moving the arms and legs it also produces independent kinæsthetic pleasure.

And yet at least three-quarters of its activity belongs to sleep, to the continuation of the fœtus life, the daily return to the pre-natal energy situation. Many activities of the child aim to prevent stimuli, to reinstate situations which existed before birth, to attain rest-pleasure. In the strictest sense of the word, the nutritional instinctual activities belong to these. These activities clearly show how, in the exercise of such R.-instinct activities, the possibility of stimulus-pleasure-gain is increased, or how the sexual instincts dependent upon such activities are differentiated and developed. So that from this point also the initial narcissistic organization is broken through more and more.

The possessive apparatus makes no very important advances in its development in the first quarter of the first year. It belongs completely, in so far as the waking life is concerned, to the development of stimulus-pleasure, which is closely related to the overcoming of anxiety. This late development of the possessive apparatus results in a strong libidinal cathexis of perceptual and reproductive processes; the formation of a very mobile quantity of energy, and the binding of libido to a number of perceptions (and reproductions). A part of the world-image invested with libido consists of a series of forms (things) on an indifferent background. The development of this perceived world is bound up with pleasure-situations; even its appearance is pleasure, and brings the expectations of further pleasure. The 'pain' situation calls forth hallucinations as primitive mechanisms of the gratification of every wish. Perception and reproduction are not differentiated as inner- and outer-world, and indeed have libido bound in the same way; a portion of primitive love belongs to these things—regardless of whether they are endopsychic pictures or perceptions—exactly like the erotogenic zones themselves. Recognition, recognizing again, the joy in the identical (the pleasure in the overlapping of reproduction and perception), anxiety at the foreign-familiar (partly overlapping), expectation, and perhaps a primitive comparing and reasoning, are the functions which belong to the intellectual sphere, and are more or less clearly developed in the three-months-old child. The delay of the motor development, the prematurity of the sensory development, appears of the greatest importance for the future configuration of specifically human phenomena. The first period of life is far from being the "dumb quarter" (Sigismund). It is, on the contrary, the foundation of the development of all intelligence.

On the long road from the structure of the new-born to the organization of the adult, the first important step is made toward the end of the first quarter of the first year. Neglecting what is unimportant for us in this connection, the development must progress from that extreme narcissistic state—still possible in the world of given stimuli—to a coherent personality, which possesses as the object (objects) of its instincts a coherent, varied, articulate, world of judgments and values. The stage earliest attained shows us the first unfolding of the instincts, which are directed at objects, and the formation of such objects. The three zones, eyes, ears, and mouth (and in a certain sense the whole skin surface as a fourth) are seats of strivings, which aim at objects outside themselves. Now whether the object is the mother's breast or the infant's own finger; whether it is a rhythmic rattling of a celluloid ball or the swinging to and fro of a coloured cloth, in any case it releases pleasure-experiences in one of the zones, and is desired as a dispenser of pleasure. To perception they are things, to pleasure strivings (the sexual instincts) they are objects. A certain amount of libido is bound to them, and the oral zone certainly leads in this respect. We need not characterize the differences from the adult structure. They are present in every other relation. But in one respect, the decisive progress is built up from the previous state, that of the new-born, almost completely on narcissism. A primal world is, so to say, constructed; instincts become evident which are directed toward the primal world as objects, and which no longer oppose that world, nor turn completely away from it, nor shut it out.

The following can be said of the way in which this progress is attained: (1) The conversion of anxiety into pleasure. We have already studied this in the case of hearing. The fright reaction of auditory stimuli gives way first to sustained attention, and finally to joyous pleasure. Although at this point it does not appear completely justifiable, fright and sustained attention are listed under the anxiety phenomena. Thus the development of the auditory zone can be formulated as the conversion of fear of stimuli into pleasure in stimuli. Laughing is to a certain degree the general expression of the consummation of this conversion. (2) The differentiation of the instinctual aims. We studied them in detail as an instance of the functions of the oral zone, and saw how, out of undifferentiated sucking, hunger-sucking as an R.-instinct activity is differentiated from pleasure-sucking (*Wonnesaugen*) as an activity of the sexual instincts, because the oral zone, in exercising its nutritional function, becomes eroticized, gives taste-pleasure; in order to attain this in isolation, a complex of actions must be singled out from the nutritional instinct. (3) The organization of movements. We saw this (*a*) in the increasing control of various discharge and reflex movements of the eye muscles emanating from " seeing-pleasure " or an ego-kernel; in any case from an organizing factor in the service of a need, namely, gaining pleasure; or (*b*) as the organizing of manifold discharge phenomena, reflexes and activities, into a unit of complete discharge, which is bound to a definite affect: laughing when anxiety is changed into pleasure.

Thus the profusion of facts can be organized by assuming two opposing groups of instincts, which alternately take possession of the psychic energy and control its distribution, binding, discharge, and release. They can be classified in relation to the dominance of the instincts and in relation to the moment of birth and its physical and mental qualities. Accordingly, in my opinion, it seems that the one instinct group strives to undo birth again in order to resume the fœtal life; the other is able to get pleasure out of the new situation, and apparently strives to make use of this capacity. One can picture the relationship of these two groups as analogous to a battle; the sexual instincts, in the first quarter of the first year, snatch a third of the day from the rest-instincts, and fill it with pleasure-gain, which consists to a great extent of triumph over the R.-instincts; but one can say the R.-instincts are the victors and drown in sleep every stimulus-pleasure almost before it is enjoyed, even the pleasure-gain of the sexual instinct itself, and through the continual " recollection " of birth and the obvious admixture of ' pain,' set their stamp—by the tension in every stimulus-pleasure—during the whole waking life.

But instead of comparing it with war one can choose the English parliamentary procedure, and say that the Tory-R.-instincts and Whig-sexual-instincts follow each other in ruling the mental apparatus at short intervals, but that both parties are clever enough during their reign of power to consider, as far as possible, the strong opposition which is waiting for the moment when it will take over the reins, so that, finally, every Tory decree contains Whig ideas, and every Whig act contains Tory restrictions. But one can renounce this comparison and say: the libidinal unwindings join the katergy[1] (the R.-instincts), whereas their new libidinal accumulations mature to libidinal processes, and every libidinal process represents at the same time a compromise with the katergic forces; probably this is also reversely true. And if we speak figuratively or abstractly, it must not be forgotten that in the last analysis the libidinal processes also strive toward the same final goal as the katergic: for " the goal of all life is death " (Freud).

A certain difficulty with the nomenclature continuously presented itself as soon as the economic question—such as the question of psychic energy—was touched upon. We need not be ashamed of this difficulty, nor of the uncertainties and ambiguities which it produces or which result from it. For in this field of psychology we are dealing with a question which is seldom touched upon by experimenters, and which they all are glad to desert quickly. Besides this, it is the outer boundary of psychology, that strip which touches biology; and the frontier-line is but vaguely defined. Freud, our reliable leader in psychology, is more than careful in stepping over the boundary. I am finding a way out of the difficulty by attempting to draw a sharper line of demarcation; this is by no means a virtue, but frankly a substitute which may perhaps serve only for this book, which does not aim to be a psychology, but only offers a Psychology of the Infant, in dangerous proximity to the alluring fields of biology—bio-analysis as Ferenczi (2) calls it.

I agree with Ferenczi completely in this—and cannot believe that anyone who has an understanding of Freud's theories could oppose them—that it is permissible and desirable to operate in biology with the suppositions and conceptions, of course

---

[1] Katergy and katergic are words coined by Dr. Bernfeld to designate the opposite of " energy."—*Translator*.

also with the terminology of analytical psychology (psycho-analysis). Nor can a book which in its province, that of child-psychology, deals so much with what is unspoken and unseen, venture to depart from its special province; especially since all this new theory, or far the greater part of it, is not new in itself, but is only new in the special branch of child-psychology. Biology, therefore, remains an untouched field. Disappointed as the reader may be, the author gives up these prospects with equal reluctance.

We therefore omit all discussion as to whether psychic energy is identical with nerve energy, with organ energy, vital energy, etc., or as to what its relation to these is; nor have we entered upon the question as to whether the embryo possesses psychic energy and what its nature may be. But this deficiency with reference to the conclusion inevitably demands a certain precision of terminology and of the fundamental general viewpoints. Both instinct groups share the psychic energy: when it is a sexual instinct force we call it libido; if on occasion we find the need to characterize the R.-instinct force, we call the psychic energy which it provides katergy. The relationship need not interest us; both names are abstract designations for psychic energy, depending upon the stand-point from which we view it; what they actually represent, whether a difference of direction, of quantity, of forms of energy, or whether a difference exists at all, we need not decide. Libido will be put on an equal footing with psychic energy from another viewpoint—*i.e.*, the biological. When we wish to speak of organic force, we call it libido or " organ-libido," bearing in mind the terminology of psycho-analysis, but organ-libido is not libido (in our limited sense) of the organs, but something else, whose relation to libido and psychic energy we need not investigate—that is, organ-libido may also be the same as libido. We do not know, nor do we need to know in this connection.

One can speak only very cautiously and tentatively of the quantities of energy; I should, therefore, like to bring into prominence a somewhat more comprehensible difference, although it does not offer any very striking illumination of the question. We can graphically organize the various forms of energy, or the nature of the manifestations of psychic energy, according to their mobility. We can suppose, next to the usual degree of binding, a degree of especially close binding difficult to release, and a degree of especially transitory and easily releasable binding, whereby the most closely bound energy, which is finally freed, is difficult to discharge and difficult to bind again. It strives to attain the old binding again, and when this is not possible needs intensive and frequent discharges, whereas the lightly bound energy, having become free, tends to assume new bindings easily or to use itself up in moderate discharges. The most closely bound energy is nearly related to organ-libido, is perhaps identical with it; it participates in those processes which are of an organic nature—in growth, for example; the easily bound energy belongs to the process of consciousness, perhaps especially to the cathectic energy of the system (perception-consciousness). One must finally suppose that the transitory nature is attainable up to a certain degree, at least for a certain mass, by the organ-libido being repeatedly forced to deep and frequent release.

Collecting scattered observations into a comprehensive formula, we describe the path of development thus: the embryo may have closely bound all its psychic energy as organ-libido; in the inner part of the body, for example, the violent shock of birth releases an important part of it. The residue continues to remain within the organ indistinguishable from organ-libido. The energy so freed will have, to a great extent, to undertake new bindings to some organ; these, as libido, now change into sources of pleasure; and, in fact, it is on the head that this new binding is accumulated; the constant shocks of the first weeks force new releases and new bindings, in which considerable quantities may participate. Thereby the libido-binding attains that moderate degree of density which is the optimum for all tactual pleasure, for all sexual pleasure in the restricted sense. But a certain quantity may be forced to more transitory bindings, which are necessary for cathectic energy, and may perhaps bind itself with a residue freed at the birth-trauma. These are processes which continue perhaps throughout life to a certain degree, and probably can also become retroactive through katergic influence. But katergy can at least displace libido into a state of latency. A good illustration of the above statement is the increase of the growth-energy in the fœtal state, its decrease after birth, and the periodic increases during sleep and decreases during the waking state (Friedenthal). Here we see clearly how the libidinal processes (during the waking state) and the katergic processes (during sleep) are correlative.

The difference between the organization of the three-months-old child and that of the fœtus in comparison with the adult can be expressed in one sentence: the head has consummated its adaptation to the new biosphere; the rest of the body has remained almost completely in the libido-situation of the fœtus. Its body, therefore, repeatedly experiences birth (in response to every shock): diffuse shock reactions of the extremities and musculature; in breathing, heart beat, musculature, anxiety reaction of the digestion-apparatus; whereas mechanisms organized in the head (laughing) have overcome fright, anxiety. A common symptom of this change is that the head does not need the fœtal warmth any more, whereas the body needs it just as much as the new-born. This renunciation of the fœtus situation takes place in the head—if we wish to speak in an abbreviated manner—as compensation: the strong libido-cathexis which assures it great possibilities of pleasure. The difference from the adult might be formulated in these two tasks that (1) the body must catch up with the lead of the head (though this never happens completely); (2) the head must become de-erotized in its functions, the oral zone, ears, eyes, must renounce[1] the lively stimulus-pleasure (this, too, is not completely accomplished during life) in order to become capable of purposive action.

If we are to make a thorough study of matters important in further development, mention must be made of one bodily zone, as yet not discussed; one in which, for reasons which I shall indicate, a similar adaptation to the new situation must be effected at this time—namely, the anal zone. Little further, mention of it will be made. The prudery of observers and experimenters has caused them to omit to make even the most timid comment on this phase of the infant's existence. There remains nothing for us to do but to disclose this prudery and show how regrettable it is. Defæcation is a process which is alien to fœtal life. It offers new stimulation to the new-born, and most certainly to the infant. How does it react? There is no doubt that the infant does not reject it, at least not for any length of time, for these stimulations are not to be prevented; perhaps the child controls the mechanisms of inhibition very early; as a consequence of the prudish attitude

[1] See Ferenczi (2).

we do not know approximately when. But if the inhibition existed from the very beginning, then it can have only a postponing effect, for the new-born apparently defæcates and urinates regularly. Does he react pleasurably to the tactual stimulation of the outer anal zone and intestinal mucous membrane as soon as to light-stimuli? I will not make any assumption. But some kind of adjustment to these stimuli—and, indeed, not a very simple one—must arise in the first three months. For it is certain that the child's acts of urination and defæcation are not accompanied by cries of 'pain,' nor by any expressions of displeasure. On the contrary, the experienced mother most likely concludes from the sudden, snug quiet that the " accident " has happened. It is certain, too, that the child does not give notice immediately, and often does not indicate what has happened at all. In other instances it gives the impression that the wetness and skin irritation are disagreeable. But since here a stimulus foreign to the fœtus-situation exists, and since defæcation and urination are not undoubtedly answered by 'pain,' fright, and anxiety, an adjustment to the excretion stimulations must have taken place, perhaps similar to the adjustment to auditory stimuli. Or is there another way which is not found in the rest of the body? One should be ashamed of the unscientific prudery which has no data of any kind ready in answer to these questions.

Biologically the three-months-old child is like the new-born, an "*ectoparasite*, which eats its mother" (Ferenczi, 2), except that it has become energetic and greedy. Nothing, therefore, in its social structure changes, at least nothing essential. Yet two details show accurately how the behaviour of society (the mother) and the mental development correlate.

The artificial womb in which the one main type of child rearing, the fœtusphile type, allows the new-born to grow up, opens itself, allows the head freedom, and enfolds protectively and conservatively the rest of the body only. This is especially obvious in those countries where the child is carried in a basket on the back out of which only its head and hands project. With this in mind one might speak of the kangaroo phase of child-rearing, which represents the adaptation of the head to the stimulus world of adults.

The child receives its first toy. It is not only in Scupin and Preyer that the child receives a rattle, for the purpose of giving stimulation-pleasure to the eyes and ears, for objects have always been used exclusively for this purpose. The rattle, toys, and varieties of small bells are widely used; by the Dayaks, in India, as well as among European peoples, these are specifically used as toys for infants (Ploss). The old Egyptians knew them as well as the Romans and Greeks (Claretie). To them the child's rattle seemed to be a specially interesting and important instrument; their legends ascribe its discovery to no less a person than the wise Archytas. Of course this is incorrect as far as the name is concerned, for the discovery was made in the antiquity of human culture: neolithic child rattles have been found, made in primitive fashion, of reindeer bones (L'Allemagne).

C. THE INSTINCT OF MASTERY

THE chief cause of the infant's helplessness lies in the undeveloped state of its locomotor apparatus. It cannot withdraw from disagreeable situations by means of its own body; it cannot seek agreeable situations. As far as its whole body is concerned, the infant is passively exposed to the stimulus world. The infant cannot exercise actively to any considerable extent, and, above all, not completely; an action of the entire body cannot be accomplished; but each organ acts independently. The child attains some degree of co-ordination in the third month, when the head turns toward the source of the sound, so that it can also be seen; but even this action, combining three different organs, is limited to the head. The second quarter of the first year brings with it considerable progress, in that the arms, and hands, later the upper part of the body, and finally the legs, are called into the unified act. To present this stage of the infant's development will be my next task. I refer in some phases to the first quarter of the first year, for all demarcations, and especially temporal demarcations, are flexible. Thus there will be an opportunity to follow up some manifestations which were not mentioned, or barely mentioned, in the preceding chapters.

The arms are from birth organs of vigorous discharge-phenomena. They discharge " impulsive movements," during fright, during sucking, crying, and for " inner reasons " which cannot be determined more exactly; which cannot be stated more concretely even when they are considered as discharge-manifestations; we do not know in detail what causes for the unbinding of energy are to be assumed in this instance. In any case, moving the arms—unless an understandable stimulus-state can be observed—is infrequent. Watson gives graphic records of arm movements of a child less than a day old, which clearly show jerk reactions to stimuli, such as tearing a paper, saying the word " Boo " loudly, and applications of ammonia. If these experiences are confirmed, the interpretation of all arm movements in the first days as discharge-manifestations is quite certain.

Closing the hand when the palm is stimulated is likewise to be observed from birth (Dix). One therefore speaks correctly of a grasping reflex. Of course one must not be led by this name, which applies to the earliest beginnings of hand activity, to a false conception of the later grasping processes. The weight which the new-born is able to hold with the grasping reflex is considerable. According to Watson, it is almost equal to the infant's own weight; this bodily power scarcely increases at all in the first three weeks. This original Stage I of arm and hand movement remains, from birth for the rest of life, behind all the changes and developments; strong effects also affect the movements of the arms in specific ways, and in case of danger (above all the danger of losing balance, but symbolically also in other dangers too), or in intense anxiety, our hand grasps convulsively at the air.

But the movements of arms and hands soon become inde-pendent of discharge processes. The child begins to "fidget" with the arms, and moves them back and forth without any apparent aim. Since the common resting position of the hands continues, far into the infant period, to be that of the embryonic position (pushing the hands on each other in front of the mouth), in the same way the child moves them about in front of the mouth and eyes. · Thus often enough the hand, coming within the grasping region of the mouth, is caught there and sucked, or is noticed in gesticulations and is followed attentively with the eyes. Exact data for the occurrence and duration of this Stage II cannot, of course, be given. Observers disagree with each other, for their conceptions are by no means uniform, and the development itself seems to be dependent upon individual characteristics. Certainly this stage is completely developed in the second week (mouth and eyes are even at that time—or so it would appear—the preferred goal of the arm movements, if they do not take their start from the embryonic position). Dix writes: "I frequently observe the *upward movement* of the arms toward the head," and it continues until the end of the first quarter of the first year. The hands behave peculiarly: that "objects put into the hand are held fast for some time, *but the child does not look at them*, and he then drops them again," is reported of the second month. Whatever comes within the child's reach, whatever comes within its "near-space" (Stern), is whenever possible grasped and touched; it is often beaten with the fists; its own body and hand fare no better. There is no doubt that touching and gesticulating are pleasurable. They are obviously pleasurable in themselves, regardless of whether they are or are not means to seeing-pleasure, or sucking-pleasure. Whether this is also true for the grasping act can scarcely be decided. It will not be difficult to determine what kind of pleasure this is; the observation I made above about the spontaneous fidgeting movements in general certainly applies to these movements: they interpose stimulus-pleasure of a tactual nature; they are activities of the sexual instinct.

The sexual-instinctual function of arm movement does not continue for long, at least not as a phase in itself. Their case is different from that of the kicking movements of the legs, which not only become more lively, and seem more obvious stimulus-pleasure, but can have for months no other function than that of gaining pleasure; this very soon blends—strictly speaking in the very first days—with another factor in gesticulating and touching which designates Stage III, in which the arm movements are means to a further purpose. Already in the second week the infant frequently gives the impression that its arm and hand movements are not or no longer merely ends in themselves, but that the ever-existing relation between mouth and hand has been intensified. It is as if the infant were trying to put its hand into its mouth. It is often successful, but not always; at times the finger happens to be put on the nose, not infrequently into the eyes. An experiment can easily show that a striving toward a goal really exists here: " I drew his hand out of his mouth and held the outstretched arm fast; as soon as I released the hand he directed it again to his mouth; this attempt was ' successful,' not only on this day, but on the following days " (Dix). The child obviously has already learned to retain the direction for a while, once it has been found, but is not yet sure to find it if the hand comes into the mouth from another direction. This interpretation is not positive; perhaps the infant does not " want " to reach the mouth, but really the eyes. But whether the fingers are put into the mouth or into the eyes, we have before us a movement which is not a pleasure-movement. For not kinæsthetic pleasure is sought, but sucking-pleasure, to be obtained by a purposive hand movement. Kinæsthetic pleasure may be a desirable by-product, but it may be completely omitted without discontinuing the movement, whereas in Stage II a movement which did not bring stimulus-pleasure could not take place. We know too little about the conditions of this pleasure to be able to say which form of movement is the best for gaining kinæsthetic pleasure. By analogy with similar manifestations one may assume that rhythmic movements to and fro of a certain amplitude, not too small but also not too great, will be favourable for gaining pleasure. From the standpoint of the rational intention of a hand movement just this kind of movement would be rejected as too circuitous, too slow in leading toward its aim, too " luxurious," clumsy, and uncertain. But is not this exactly what we observe in a child at this stage ? The hand should go to the mouth; it does not find its way there, but moves back and forth a while around the nose, the cheeks, the eyes, and mouth, a little to the right, a little to the left. This observation almost gives one the courage to say that the hand does not want to go by the shortest route straight into the mouth, as it should, but enjoys itself a while, plays before it fulfils its commission. The possessor of the hand will behave in just this way in a few years: ordered to leave the room of the " adults " and go to bed, he will turn here and there, will walk around every chair, will step only in the red spots of the rug pattern, will go toward the door zigzag, concluding a compromise between his own wish and the request. We will discuss later how far this comparison is more than a casual notion. Whatever the reasons for this vacillation may be, the child controls the path of the hand to the mouth in the second month at the latest, and directs into or to its mouth, with very few false movements, almost every object which its pleasure-seeking hand accidentally gets hold of.

But an important factor is still lacking to make this putting into the mouth of accidentally grasped objects, actual grasping in its real sense. This happens in Stage IV when the eye also is drawn into the mouth-hand-relation. Henceforth the hand grasps under the guidance of the eyes. At first the eye focuses on the object already grasped, it also attentively observes the finger play, the grasping hand, the hand with the grasped object, and follows the hand on its way to the mouth (Dix's son in the twelfth week). The final step does not occur until a short while later. Dix notes it on the one hundred and seventh day (three and a half months): "Heinz locates his rubber dog, his eyes widen and sparkle (pleasure feeling !), the fingers spread apart; the typical indication of attention, open and pouted mouth, was to be observed. A tendency to touch appeared, and he grasped it, clutching it with thumb and fingers, and hastily drew it to his mouth and his eyes." After this the process which in the adult also constitutes "grasping" is practically complete; it signifies an advance upon the earlier stage in two relations. First, the motive of the act has changed; it is no longer kinæsthetic pleasure; second, the act itself is not released by a tactual stimulus on the hand, but by an optical stimulus in relation to an erotogenetic zone (mouth), by a wish, we may say succinctly. The kinæsthetic pleasure is subordinated to the gratification of a wish; it is shortened and decreased at its own expense. But one must not imagine that this happens all at once. Just as the discharge-function of the hand movements (Stage I) remains in existence to a certain degree throughout life, so does the pleasure-function (Stage II). Yet we see also for a long time a considerable insecurity in the fulfilment of the wish-function (Stage IV), which probably is not yet quite dependent on the little practice and experience, but in part, too, upon the "passive resistance," of the arms and hands, which will not entirely give up their pleasure. The fact is that there are always relapses to a state of uncertainty in grasping, which has already been practically overcome. In conclusion the development of the capacity to grasp may be described briefly, very much like that of the eye movements, as a progressive control of the motor apparatus by a need, a wish to grasp, as we shall express it for the present.

The development of the hand is not actually completed during childhood; the highest degree of speed, precision, assurance, and fineness of hand movements is only attained by the adult. Yet a good part of this development falls within the first year of life. It would be most fascinating to describe it in detail, but unfortunately the observations do not extend far enough for us to recognize to any considerable extent the typical steps, and certainly not far enough for us to deduce general rules from this process of development. We must therefore be content with a few hints. In the fourth month, the accuracy with which objects seen are grasped grows very quickly; soon the child also grasps objects which are out of its reach, to the side, at times even those which are behind it and hanging above it. Every improvement in the trunk movements is used in grasping. Many more complicated movements of the upper part of the body are performed for the first time to aid grasping; creeping retains even later its auxiliary function during grasping (Dix). According to Dix the child grasps at first with both hands at the same time, and later uses one hand alone, and, according to Baldwin, he uses from the first (fifth month) preferably the right hand, whereas Watson could not establish any difference between the use and strength of the right and of the left hand in the first weeks of life. It is also worthy of note that the original grasping process occurs with outstretched arms (elbows slightly bent), so that the child must lean back in order to grasp objects that are too near. Dix's son abandoned this stiff posture only in the seventh month. Grasping very small objects, such as paper-shavings, did not occur for a long while. Shinn's niece showed great awkwardness in this even in the eighth month, and made efforts even in the fifteenth month to get hold of lead shot. The infant's hand, one can say, has at first only two fingers, the thumb, and the other four opposed to it. Their co-ordinated movement develops only gradually. Until far into the seventh month Shinn's observation is valid: " How many and which fingers are used in grasping up to this point depends much more on the position and form of the object and on the accidental placing of the hand than on intention."

What does the child do with the object which he grasps with increasing accuracy ? He directs it with equally increasing speed and certainty to the mouth. This answer is absolutely valid until far into the third quarter. The child seizes the object almost exclusively in order to put it into his mouth as soon as possible. Toward the end of the first year of life this behaviour changes considerably. What formerly happened intermittently now becomes the principal use of the grasped object: it serves for the creation of noise, or is discarded.

SITTING, CRAWLING, CLIMBING

The ability of the hand to grasp objects seen and to put them into the mouth is greatly increased as soon as the child learns to change, without assistance, a given position of its whole body into a more satisfactory one. When the child can raise itself, the hand has a larger field of reach; when it can crawl, the active range of the hand increases greatly. The first stages on this path are sitting and crawling. Sitting extends the reaching power of the hand considerably beyond that of the child lying on its back; crawling is the natural enlargement of the grasping sphere of the child lying on its stomach. To the child-rearing customs of modern Europe, the natural position of the infant when awake appears to be on the back; it lies on its stomach only for definite rearing measures. Accordingly, sitting is encouraged by the environment; crawling is sometimes even suppressed. This naïve procedure in child-rearing has attracted the attention of doctors, child-psychologists, and pedagogues to such an extent that they have at times been provoked to pointing out the importance of crawling for the natural development of the child (Preyer, Dix). Uninfluenced and unconfined by the measures of the environment, the infant appears to prefer a side position (according to Dix, the right side), which somewhat approximates to a stomach position. This position is obviously better suited to the child's way of holding its arms and legs than the position on the back, which at times makes the onlooker wish to give these raised knees and hands something to rest on, to turn the child around, an action which in many instances is greeted by the child with expressions of pleasure. Touching the whole chest and parts of the stomach seems to be pleasant enough to the child; indeed, when in its mother's arms, it loves to press its chest and belly actively to her body. This situation, often realized for the infant, but only as an exceptional situation, is the usual one among forms of child-rearing outside of Europe—namely, when the usual carrying place for the child is at the breast, on the hip or the back of the mother, and when its usual nightly sleeping place is at her breast. In the next chapter I shall bring forward a conjecture as to the possible reasons for this difference in child-rearing, in spite of the fact that the question has as yet been given no attention, and although facts concerning it are not at our disposal. It will suffice here to observe that the methods of child-rearing which favour the position of the child on its belly offer stronger provocation to crawling and climbing, and that the other forms offer provocation to sitting.

The child seemingly learns more easily to sit than to grasp; it is to a certain degree a purely purposive activity. Observers have noted in the third month attempts on the part of the child to raise itself from the right side (Dix); these efforts were preceded by lifting the head forward a little. Then follows supported sitting produced by the environment until the child can sit erect in the lap or in the carriage, etc., without support in the fifth month. The earlier attempts to sit up from a position of lying on its back become more frequent and more successful. They have the character of work. They occur in order "to see better," "to reach the rattle," etc. Dix records that on the two hundredth day (sixth month): "He pulls himself up, holding fast to the side of the carriage with his right hand; becomes purple from exertion, the eyes become moist with tears, the corners of the mouth drop—and it is accomplished: he sits alone without a back-rest." Very soon the child masters sitting up and sits completely alone, whereas lying down from a sitting position is still awkward for a long time, and sitting down from a standing position is learned only in the second year.

The description of this development given by Dix is similar to the descriptions of other observers, if their records are correctly understood; but children vary considerably with regard to time; for instance, Preyer's son raised himself to a sitting position in the fifth month, but could not maintain it until the ninth month, could not sit without a back-rest. Of course, Preyer is right when he says the variation in time is explained "by the premature attempts of relatives to produce sitting artificially, by imitation of sisters and brothers growing up with it, by negligence and inattention."

Setting aside the question of the variation in time (and the details in general), the important fact for our argument is certain—namely, sitting up and sitting are not pleasure-activities, but purposive activities which are primarily in the service of grasping: to increase the reach of the arms. Next comes into consideration the wish to see better, and finally the pain with which lying on the back may occasionally be connected. No discharge-movements, no pleasure-activities precede the efforts to sit up. The process itself offers no pleasure, just as little as sitting itself is able to offer. But in the efforts made during these earliest experiences, the child comes to know the pleasure of overcoming difficulties, which at times is so great that it causes the child to forget for a time that the exertion was undertaken in order to reach the rattle, for example.

In contrast to the development of sitting, the development of crawling gives us again an indistinct picture of the eye movements and a clear one of grasping. A purposeless, unalloyed pleasure phase is very well characterized here. It really begins in the sixth week (Dix), when the child, lying on its belly, supporting itself by its legs, occasionally jerks forward, and soon afterwards begins to slide backwards, supporting itself with its arms. In the second half of the first year this action is often performed when the child, in a good humour, finds itself on its belly, and it is accompanied by expressions of lively pleasure. It then frequently rolls by itself from a back and side position to a belly position from which it then gaily slides backwards. Sliding becomes real crawling with the use of the knees in about the eighth month. Crawling forward is begun at about this time. But it occurs completely, as an aim in itself, solely as a pleasure-activity, not in order to reach something or to escape from an unpleasant situation. The source of pleasure may lie in the kinæsthetic excitation of the belly muscles; the arm and leg muscles are certainly considerably supported by the tactual stimulations which are over the whole skin surface; the pleasure which is already connected with lying on the stomach is further increased. Only at a later time, in the ninth month according to Dix, is crawling, and indeed crawling forward, placed in the service of an aim: the child crawls toward an object that it wishes to grasp. The line of demarcation cannot be so sharply drawn as in the case of grasping, for crawling in itself apparently remains for a long time a remarkably pleasurable process, and pleasure-crawling cannot be distinguished from purposive-crawling, as the pleasure-movements of the arms can be from the precise, short grasping-movements for an object. The next weeks perfect crawling, especially with reference to distance and speed. Only in the eleventh month does crawling give way to the attempt to stand and walk. It is now used more as a means to an end, when it is necessary to flee from the disagreeable and to run away quickly. Crawling is completely given up toward the end of the first, or at the beginning of the second, year; it survives only in play in connection with its pleasure-function.

Perhaps more exact observations would also show us a discharge phase preliminary to crawling, for the movements which the infant in the stomach position makes in the first weeks have some similarity to its later attempts at crawling.

Watson has already found in a child " very shortly after birth a regression of as much as four inches." Yet no conclusion can be drawn from this, since the observations are too accidental and superficial. There are some who maintain that these early movements of the child are swimming movements, coming phylogenetically from the amphibian epoch. On the other hand, child psychologists, in their descriptions of the actual crawling processes, do not give enough fixed points to determine how far it is a question of real crawling, co-ordinated arm and leg movements. According to all indications, these occur rather late, generally only in the last phase of crawling, whereas that form of movement which we designate as crawling is more like pushing oneself or sliding. At least Watson, who uses the word crawling in its narrowest sense, finds it appearing rather late—toward the end of the first year of life—or not at all in its correct form. Finally, one may assume—anticipating later investigations—that the infants brought up under those forms of child-rearing which, contrary to modern European methods, prefer the positions of the child on its stomach, crawl earlier, more intensively, and " more correctly " than those infants about whom we have some data—namely, the European (American) infants.

A third way of extending the range of action of the hand is climbing. Although climbing cannot be directly connected either with sitting or crawling morphologically, it will be briefly presented here. For sitting, crawling, and climbing are extensions of the range of grasping which result from the typical child-rearing situation: the back position, the stomach position, and the braced position. The infants of those peoples among whom the infant spends the greater part of its waking life on the hips or on the back of the mother are in this last position. For these infants the climbing movements are made possible by the given conditions. How the development is formed in these cases has not been investigated. " Negro children spend their first year of life in a carrying bag, and leave it when they can walk." This statement from Franke is, of course, not to be taken literally, for even these negro children are given ample opportunity to crawl, to sit up from the back position. But extensive contact of the chest and stomach with the mother's body is part of their most important situations—and certainly of the pleasure-situations. They lie to a certain extent in a vertical position on the stomach, and every crawling movement which they make becomes a kind of climbing movement.

It is noteworthy that the children of our civilized circles have a very strong wish to produce a situation which is similar to the natural one of the negro child. I shall speak more in detail of this when treating of the wish to be taken into the arms, to be picked up, and the infant's manifestations of tenderness. Something of this seems to be contained in the child's efforts to climb. These efforts—often succeeding quite early—to push itself up on a chair or divan, or the knee of the seated parent and, in general, on all suitable objects, to pull itself with the arms and drag the legs after, usually become clearly noticeable in the fourth quarter. It seems that those objects are suitable for this which are, at least, as broad as the child, and to which the child can cling closely and raise itself; an activity which is decidedly pleasant, and which, when it is mastered, serves grasping too. But in the narrower sense this fact becomes secondary toward the end of the first year, at the beginning of the climbing period. Climbing occurs in the service of another tendency which will be spoken of later. Like crawling, climbing ceases to be a significant activity in the second year, but remains in play and in impetuous expressions of love.

STANDING AND WALKING

The developmental scheme which we found in other motor functions can also be established in essentials—indeed, very obviously—in the development of the function of the legs. The stages of discharge, pleasure, and purpose can be easily differentiated. The first begins very early; discharge phenomena of the legs can be established in the first hours of life, as well as those of the arms; and the legs remain for life the place for certain discharge manifestations, such as shivering and paralysis from fright. The time at which the pleasure stage begins in the legs is even less exactly defined than in the arms; for the legs are seldom seen by the observer, because of the modern method of child-rearing; more exact descriptions of early leg movements are lacking. Yet some authors note " comfortable " bending and stretching movements in the bath, which seem to be no more than discharge processes; Scupin notes it in the fifth week, Ischikawa and Queck-Wilker in the first month. "Kicking" or "exercising" (Queck-Wilker) the legs as a pleasant activity, containing its purpose in itself, is used during the whole infant period whenever the child's situation permits, even long after it has learned to use its legs purposively. This happens at first in crawling, then in sitting; finally, in standing up, standing and walking, or running.

Dix's memoranda are typical for the stages of standing up and standing: Fourth month: "During his bath he props himself up with his feet against the tub," which is not a purposive activity; an evaluation which Dix also implies when he speaks of "preliminary practice." Fifth month: "He makes energetic stretching movements to stand up in mother's lap." Sixth month: "Standing alone delights him, and is preferred to sitting. And he bursts into exclamations of joy." In the beginning of the ninth month he stands up, firmly holding on to a stool. "His continual wish to exercise by raising the knees high is crowned with success; for he raises himself to a standing position, alone. From now on he wants to stand all the time; when he is laid down, he stiffens, which expresses his desire to stand up. 8¾ months: "He dexterously lifts himself up alone in the following way: he supports himself by the soles of his feet, and draws himself up to a standing position; now he does it without kneeling. The joy over this was very great; he squealed." · 10½ months: "Standing alone was attempted, but he quickly clutched at something to hold to." 10¾ months: "Stood so securely that by holding on with one hand he turned on his axis. In spite of his security, in spite of the fact that as yet he had not fallen, he did not stand alone, he sought something to hold to." Eleventh month: "Stands alone, without holding on. This makes him very happy; he is delighted, shouts, and wants to be admired; he calls me and expels the sound *Ei*; the little fellow exudes pride." 11¾ months: "He stood alone for thirty seconds, and then angled for something to hold to."

The individual differences with reference to time in this development are considerable; thus Preyer's child stood alone only in the fourteenth month; the stages, however, are generally valid. This whole development is completely in the service of "pleasure": standing up, drawing the knees up, propping and standing are in themselves pleasurable, and are not exercised in the service of a purpose. On the contrary, the child kneels when it wants to grasp something, for it only recently learned to stand alone, and has known only for a short time how to use its hands. Standing up and standing become a purposive activity only in the second year. It is also worthy of note that the child must first overcome anxiety in order to stand alone. It is afraid of falling, one must assume—although, as Preyer also emphasizes, he has not had that unhappy experience. Whether the pleasure in standing and standing up is kinæsthetic, I should not like to decide at present; of course, it plays a part. Moving the knees up and standing do not, however, develop from the bending movements, and from kicking of which we spoke above, but from stretching the legs, which is less frequent at the beginning (Preyer), and from touching the soles of the feet upon a firm support. It is in decided contrast with the embryonic situation and with the mode of behaviour during the first quarter; whereas walking, if one may express oneself thus, in the newly-acquired position of uprightness, is a return to an earlier form of leg movement, alternate bending and stretching.

Kicking the legs in the lying position begins at 6½ months, even when the child is held under the arms, so that the soles of its feet touch the floor lightly (Dix). Again disregarding the variation in time similar observations are made of all infants. Before this time, this reaction does not take place; on the contrary, in the immediately preceding months, there is only a forceful propping up against a support. But it cannot be clearly learned from the preceding material how far these "unregulated walking movements" are only apparent, arising from the thenar reflex. But it is certain, that the child, when it has finally made progress in standing up—that is, when it has exchanged the thenar reflex for the opposite behaviour, alternating with pleasure—tries to lift his legs even before these movements are regulated, as is seen when one supports it under the arm in standing (Dix, 7½ months). The capacity (in the eighth month, Dix) is "accompanied by strong pleasure-feelings; he lifted his little legs directly forward, pushed forcefully with his heels; he was delighted by this, especially by the sound which the descending heels made; often he lifted both legs at the same time, and sometimes they crossed in front. The lack of co-ordination of the muscle movements, when he raises his legs too high and too vigorously as he often does, is very amusing to us." Soon both legs are regularly, and alternately raised, they do not trouble him any more, and held by one hand, he correctly places one foot before the other (ninth month). " He straightened up quickly in his play-yard and walked quickly along the rail. Then he held fast with his hands and walked sideways, placing his feet correctly, and drawing one after the other just as the adult uses the side step. Only a week later he used one hand to hold on, and turned his body so that he walked directly forward; then he brought it to a rather quick walk." This walking is almost exclusively a pleasure-activity at the beginning, and it remains so for quite a long time, but is soon used also as a purposive activity to reach a definite goal which is sharply fixed with the eye. It is noteworthy that the child is more anxious, or in general only anxious, when it does not hold on itself, but is supported. When the stage of standing alone is reached, the attempts to walk alone also begin, but for a few weeks longer they end in sitting down after two or three steps. In the meantime, walking while holding the hand of a guide becomes very sure, and is combined with great pleasure in walking. Besides the pleasure, the purposiveness of walking is obvious at this stage. Dix could " always notice the following four points: (1) He sets his eye fixedly at the goal; (2) joy and longing radiate from the eyes; (3) then he stretches out his little arms longingly; (4) seeks a place to hold on and goes forth, gracefully and quickly." Between 11½ months (Miss Shinn) and one year, the child overcame its anxiety, and walked quite freely, or, more correctly, ran (Scupin). " At one year," says Dix, " he suddenly ran alone to his birthday table, extending both arms forward for balance; made for his goal, a little uncertain, in a wavering line, but nevertheless alone." In walking alone, as in standing alone, considerable anxiety is seemingly overcome. This anxiety is the more remarkable because the child experiences it before it has fallen. Generally children fall, so it seems, only when they are able to run with comparatively less attention than they expend in the first weeks; Dix's son fell for the first time only on the three hundred and ninety-eighth day, almost a month after he first walked alone. This applies only to falling forward, for falling backwards is not real falling, but much more sitting down, during which the child scarcely expresses any unusual fright or pain.

Preyer finds the development of walking completely puzzling, and, as far as I know, no one else has solved this mystery either. Indeed, no one has suggested any solution, at least in so far as I am able to judge and review the situation, in so far as it is a problem of child-psychology. What I have to say with regard to this question is likewise not even the beginning of a solution; it is suggested in the foregoing pages and will be more thoroughly elaborated when we come to a general summary of the development of the mastery[1] (possessive) apparatus. This will not exhaust what perhaps can be gained from our principles for the knowledge of locomotor development, which really first begins after the infant period, but a detailed discussion of it would extend beyond the compass of this book.

MATURATION AND LEARNING

The mastery apparatus develops by stages and degrees during the first year of life. One organ complex after the other becomes part of the development: hand, upper part of the body, legs (by stages); within every stage various phases are reached successively which are divided from each other by plateau periods. Both of these principles of progression partially overlap. The successive stages are fundamentally as follows: discharge, pleasure, purpose.

We are now confronted with the problem of explaining the general tendencies of the motor development, too. In doing this we will, *a priori*, endeavour to avoid the rocks on which many explanations foundered. We will concentrate our interest on the question as to whether the functions under consideration are innate or individually acquired. In the history

---

[1] The relation of " mastery " to " possession," and the reason for selecting the term mastery for *Bemächtigung*, is perhaps explained by a few sentences from Köhler's *The Mentality of Apes.* " There is yet another form of greeting which appears to have special emotional value. An arm is extended with the hand flexed inwards and towards the ape itself, so that the back of the hand is toward the person greeted, and the fact that a *human* friend is especially often greeted in this way seems to give this greeting a special character. When a chimpanzee approaches another of the same species with whom he is on " difficult " footing—for instance, if they have recently been fighting—and is dubious about the possible reception of his advances, he will probably extend his hand with the palm turned *inwards* as described. I am not absolutely certain about the significance of this gesture, as it may also often be observed in circumstances of complete tranquillity. But one might, perhaps, guess that the flexion of the palm and the extension of the back of the hand are meant to reassure, by contrast to the grasping or hacking motion characteristic of attack."—*Translator.*

of psychology and its individual problems, nativistic theories alternate with empirical theories. The period of sovereignty of each one brings with it a profusion of facts, but no lasting satisfactory solution. This is not wholly valid for child-psychology, which is only now beginning to be a science, in the sense that it is seriously making use of theories. Its history up to the present consists essentially in an increase in the number and range of observations, and these observations are also becoming more precise. With all matters which go beyond the observations hitherto made, works on child-psychology have dealt only incidentally and, as a rule, very naïvely. This should not be considered a reproach; it brings with it the advantage of a great deal of material from observation, and may be explained by the tendency toward the popularization of almost the whole of child-psychology. But it relieves us from the task of considering opinions so incidentally stated. Among the German investigators only Stern, Bühler, and Koffka have adopted a carefully thought-out attitude toward this question, in so far as it concerns the period of infancy, an attitude to which we shall refer.

Stern rightly emphasizes that the problem is not whether a manifestation is acquired or inborn, but what part of it is inborn and what part of it acquired. And no one doubts that in the development of the apparatus of mastery the innate portion is fairly large and important. Certainly the experiment of allowing a child to grow up completely without stimulation and without an environment to imitate has not yet been made, and the very wise can object that we have no proof as to whether or not such a child would learn to walk and stand. I believe it would learn neither this nor anything else, nor would it develop at all. It would simply be destroyed, for the conditions of the experiment would be to allow the child to grow up completely isolated, and that is impossible. But to decide from this in favour of the more predominant factor of " acquisition " would be as wrong as to argue thus: If I allowed the embryo to " grow up " outside the womb, it would develop no leg movements, which are, therefore, not innate but acquired. The mother's care, which offers a thousand stimulations toward motor functioning, belongs absolutely to the infant; the care and the conditions which it offers are, so to speak, innate in the infant, just as is its capacity for sucking. No one denies the innate part of the motor functions; we ought, therefore, to refrain from this sophistry. But if we wish to give a more graphic description of the relation between these two parts we must first study the innate portion. And we can say that the child is born with the tendency to perform certain movements and actions as far as they are physiologically and socially possible, but it is also born with physical and social conditions which guarantee *a priori* the appearance of this possibility—of course in the normal case which interests us here.

But it seems as if this tendency were not only innate, but possessed also temporal regulation. For the successive appearance of the activities: raising the head, grasping, sitting, crawling, standing, running, is a constitutional one. Some of these successive activities are conditioned by the motor development; walking must follow standing, lifting the head must precede sitting. But this by no means applies to all; grasping and sitting could follow crawling, sitting could follow walking; one could think of forms of locomotion which are in general not indicated or only weakly indicated, and explain them phylogenetically. It is, therefore, as if that tendency—with which the child comes into the world and which forces it to adopt at definite times certain gradual advances, new ways of behaviour —were as effective as a post-hypnotic suggestion. Of course one is accustomed to consider the time when a new movement occurs among the acquisitions. It varies with the individual. It is, so it seems, dependent rather upon the external conditions, which converge with the innate (Stern). This is by no means obligatory. However variable the times may be, however obviously they are individually conditioned, nothing permits us to mistake the individual for the acquired; there may be enough of the individual innate tendencies. To this may be added that the variation in the time of appearance, as I shall show, is essentially smaller—and more comprehensible—than is generally assumed. We would have to assume tendencies which bring about definite movements at their due time. This would be a conception which is not without considerable difficulty, but there are only two ways open to circumvent it: either the motor functions prove to be learned ones and the sequence of learning can be understood immediately from what has been learned, or the development of the motor apparatus is intelligible from another mental manifestation which develops at the same time or earlier.

Bühler selects the first way. If anywhere within the realm of the innate there is room for the factor of experimental acquisition, it is certainly within "practice." If the appearance of every new movement, according to form and time, were innate, it would appear completely developed, it would not need completion through practice. The necessity for practice, however, is no proof that it must be learned. It may seem so, but there is a possibility in this case that, instead of maturation, learning of a movement exists. Here Bühler remarks: the law of selection of what is fitted for the purpose, by trial and error, explains the perfection of bodily movements in the main through practice. At first the purposeful movements which lead to success are copiously mixed with inappropriate ones which do not. And progress takes place in this way: movements unsuited to their ends are more and more weeded out, and the suitable ones are retained. By thought the adult is frequently able to come to this choice or to aid it. In the small child and in the animal, on the contrary, another factor serves as a substitute for thought—namely, pleasure and ' pain.' Success brings pleasure, and this pleasure effects the frequent repetition, impresses it firmly and permanently. On the other hand, lack of success brings ' pain,' which does not incline toward repetition; so that the movements unsuited to their purpose are not impressed and are thus eliminated. This principle is "rooted in the natural adaptation to training" (Dressur), " or, what is the same thing, associative memory." " One soon learns that for training ' an overproduction of movements,' ' aimless trials,' are necessary, so that there is room for the occurrence of accident which leads to success, and so that this latitude is then again limited, and finally abolished by the building up of a unified association." Under training Bühler considers in this chapter all the functions which interest us from grasping to walking. " All this is training, self-training in play, and gradually becomes practice."

This point of view would be well suited, if it could be established, to liberate heredity from the responsibility for determining the time of such complicated movements, as, for example, the appearance of walking toward the end of the first year. The new-born commands a number of simple movements which it uses either as reflexes or as discharge-movements, and from these by means of memory and association under the regulation of the pleasure-pain principle, grow movement-complexes which are suited to gratify the child's needs. At this point it can be added that the child can take its time for a year, since all its imperative needs are assured by well-developed inherited activities (instincts) and rearing measures of the mother. Their termination and sequence remain, of course, in any case not understood.

But, waiving all this, the number of objections (Koffka raises some of the following) to Bühler's views are very great, the more so because he does not test the usefulness, indeed not even the practicability, of his conception in any concrete instance.

1. First of all, it is not true that the infant makes numerous unsuccessful trials. The child's behaviour in learning to open the door—Bühler's example—may be an argument for Bühler; many similar examples may be found, but certainly only among older children, or only in that stage of perfection which Bühler himself considers among the intellectual accomplishments. The grasping child of three months generally makes no false trials, scarcely any which could with any degree of certainty be interpreted as false trials. · The six-months-old child who is learning to sit certainly makes vain attempts to sit up, but its position is not wrong, its means are still too weak; the same is valid for the child who wants to stand up from a sitting position; this is even more evident in learning to crawl. In learning to walk there are also very slight difficulties which have to be overcome, although they are really present, for example, when the legs get in each other's way; but these difficulties especially are overcome in a few days. But if one does not wish to accept these extreme formulations, which can be justified only later, one must certainly admit that the deviations between unsuccessful acts and successful ones are only minimal. Indeed, the over-production of movements, presupposed by Bühler's conception, is lacking in the infant period.

2. What is the motive of aimless movements ? Grasping is at this point very instructive. The motive is to stick an object seen into the mouth; this movement is performed with such assurance from the very first time, and the difficulty of finding the mouth exactly is so quickly overcome, that one must say: the principle of movement is grasped without trial or choice. Of course the hand has found the path into the mouth numerous

times before. What was the motive of these earlier movements of the hand to the mouth ? But this functions from the very first days; we have no reason for assuming that the backward and forward gesticulations of the hands are attempts to put the hand into the mouth. But if the motive of these earlier movements is to grasp " some object with the hand," then all back and forward movements are just the right way for grasping something accidentally. In the attempt to stand up from a sitting position, what is the motive ? Does the child know beforehand that it will be a pleasure to stand ? The law of choice requires an aim; for the most part, the infant cannot have this aim.

3. For this aim the pleasure-pain principle could be substituted to a certain degree. But since every movement is pleasant, since it must be pleasant in itself (for otherwise the child would not make any movements), the pleasure derived from function and the pleasure derived from success must come in conflict with each other, the consideration of which would create very great difficulties for Bühler's conception.

4. Finally, Koffka analyzes this, from the point of view of Gestalt psychology, very fully and, I think, very aptly: a movement is not at all a composite of single parts, just as the perception is not a mosaic of sensations, but the decisive factor of every complex movement—and all those movements here under consideration are complex—is the " melody of movement," which can hardly be made at all comprehensible by combining kinæsthetic and optic data, or by a mere concurrence of elements.

The gradual development of the apparatus of mastery is therefore essentially a process of maturation, which of course in its more delicate improvements is completed by individual learning and, it must be said, by " intelligent learning." There remains the possibility of assuming that the process of maturation is not autonomous, that, at least to a great extent, it is in comprehensible, necessary dependence upon other processes of development, if one wishes to avoid burdening the hereditary factor with too many concrete tendencies. Bearing in mind the object of this book, this second way is obviously ours.

As a prerequisite for this attempt some tendencies are assumed as innate modes of response of our psychological apparatus. The following are conceived as such: (1) The arms and legs are places of vigorous discharge-phenomena; (2) moving the arms and legs is capable of offering pleasure; the same is true of the broad belly-surface of the body under certain conditions; (3) certain primitive needs from birth correspond to certain complex movements which are suited to satisfy these needs.

The movements at the pleasure stage are subsequently fully comprehensible as a sexual instinct activity, as pleasure-gain, when the possibility of pleasure has finally been learned by experience. This first experience is an individual acquisition; it is the release for numberless repeated (and slightly varying) movements. This experience may be assured for kicking of the arms and legs, by the fact that from the beginning they are the place at which discharge-phenomena are seen; so this experience must necessarily be gained during the first days. (The question, how can the discharge-phenomena offer pleasure experiences, will occupy our attention later.) Let us first continue further with the arm movements. There is not a large variety of these; but two groups can be differentiated from the beginning. One group aims in the direction of the mouth, the other strives to swing back and forth rhythmically within moderate amplitude from every given position. Both groups are comprehensible, the first as a return to the fœtal state of rest, the other as pleasure-gain. Because the oral zone develops, the state of rest necessarily becomes a pleasure-situation and will be sought continuously. Here the strivings of the mouth zone seeking stimulation are co-ordinated with the strivings of the hand seeking a state of rest. For the present we can only deal superficially with the theory of coincidence in this differential co-ordination, but not without stressing the point that some conditions provide that a result follows soon and always. Of course grasping with the hand is in no way inhibited; it is a completed movement already during birth. The phase " putting the grasped object into the mouth " is from a motor viewpoint the same as " hand in the mouth." " Grasping the observed object and putting it into the mouth " is new in principle. Here two movements, both of which were performed earlier, are executed in combination and placed at the service of a wish. But even here nothing essentially new is to be noted with regard to motility, but only that the movements are now controlled; by what cannot yet of course be said. But the pleasure movements have found their master, who uses or inhibits them according to his purpose. We will describe the details of this process later; but one cannot free oneself from the impression that grasping from now on is an " intelligent " process. From now on it has an aim by which the result can be measured; from now on actual blunders occur which are corrected, and the child strives to make the correction. From now on the mode of acting occurs which one must designate as learning, and which, with Bühler, one can also call *Dressur.*

If we wish for the present to attribute to the instinct of mastery the indefatigable efforts of the infant to seize things and put them into the mouth in the second and third quarters of the first year (Sigismund's " Grasper " state), we would say that the pleasure phase of grasping ends (in principle) when the innate " movement melodies " of grasping fall into the service of the instinct of mastery. From now on the infant learns a number of corrections and improvements of the original movement melody, which go so far that they also can be designated, if one wishes, as new structures (melodies). The time at which this progress occurs is not autonomously given with the other innate grasping movements, but it is dependent upon the rapidity with which the instinct of mastery develops and also upon the resistance which the pleasure phase may set up against overcoming it.

Sitting up and crawling fit in well with this method of consideration, without any forced interpretation. Sitting up is a pure purposive act in the service of the instinct of mastery, which needs expansion. It therefore begins as a purposive phase after grasping. Its termination in contrast to its beginnings varies considerably with the individual, dependent upon the degree of development of the instinct and upon individual experiences. Sitting is learned, but not as typewriting, for example, is learned. It is a natural, a fundamental innate melody. It is perceived as pleasant by the infant in its mother's arms at a time when nothing in the infant tends toward the mother. One might say that to perform this remembered (and perhaps innate) configuration actively is a discovery of its instinct of mastery. And the result is generally successful without unsuccessful trials—provided only that the musculature already permits it. Crawling in its discharge and pleasure phases offers us no new problems for observation. As a purposive act it can be considered, like purposive grasping, an "intelligent" activity of the instinct of mastery. Its termination after grasping and before standing can easily be understood. Nevertheless, the material of child-psychology need not be widely varied for a definite understanding; only exact observations of children brought up in an environment friendly to crawling will teach us the natural termination of this function. In this respect, because of the forms of child-rearing in European circles, certain disguises prevent us from seeing clearly. In our children, crawling approaches more nearly to the functions of standing, climbing, and walking, which occur late, than is presumably the case in other cultural groups. Those factors which determine the later motor functions play a part in the development of crawling in obscure ways. Until we have considered the changes which comprise the whole psychic situation in the fourth quarter—to be referred to at present as teething and weaning—we cannot expect to understand more exactly the motor functions which terminate in the fourth quarter of the first year. It is, therefore, sufficient to refer at this point to one important factor. Our statements regarding the three stages are also valid for standing and walking, as this chapter shows, but they are a little obscured, because, in the last quarter, the instinct of mastery has already taken possession of all the motor functions; because standing, crawling, and walking are also permeated by purposive tendencies from the beginning—namely, from the moment when the various pleasure movements have united with the structural movement structure, standing or walking; and because some intelligent processes—but only a few—play a part. But it is the more remarkable that these functions in the first part of their development (from about the seventh to twelfth month) seem to have a common tendency which is lacking in grasping and sitting, and which has nothing to do with locomotion, the means of which later become the function itself.

It is as if an impulsion to touch its belly-surface on a foreign object arises in the child, as if it strived after a vertical actualization of the crawling position. Perhaps this sounds a little forced, and yet this impression results from observation and is not invented to conform with a theory; on the contrary, it represents an enigma, harmful to any theory. Clinging to an object which reaches to its armpits, and standing before it touching its breasts and belly, climbing on the chair from this position in order to enjoy again the same situation, wandering along the table and the edge of the bed—these are very obviously pleasure-situations of the child at this age, they are the aim of numerous efforts. This tendency is already clear in the second and third quarter of the first year, when the child vigorously demands to be taken up, when it calms itself quickly in the position, and when it puts itself to sleep in this position even when in pain. The new tendency is, in the fourth quarter, to seek this situation actively, and if it is not provided by the mother, to realize it with its own body against the side of the crib, chair, or table. It realizes exactly, even if symbolically, we might say, a primitive child-rearing situation in which the child, until the end of the first year, was carried on the breast, hip, or back of the mother, in the same climbing attitude and chest-stomach contact which it endeavours to attain when it wants to be taken up, and which it strives for independently in the first stages of standing, climbing, walking. ' Pain ' and anxiety are connected with the relinquishment of this situation. The final crisis consists now in overcoming this anxiety; clinging is given up, the child stands alone, it abandons the chest contact, it even rejects it; it goes away from it, in the actual sense of the word. It walks alone. It strives away from the mother's arm. What until now it had frequently to ex-perience with ' pain ' and anxiety, when the mother went away from it, it now does (symbolically) itself, and gains pleasure thereby: of course only a few steps at the beginning, and mostly from one support to another; but in a few days it walks with entire certainty and for a much longer time. The forms of child-rearing which are considered the more primitive show this connection clearly; for the scholars say that until the child can walk, it does not leave the sack or other cradle it occupies on its mother's body.

Let us turn again to those questions which we can clarify in this connection. Classifying the observed relationships, according to the ideas of the libido theory, permits us to make some more exact formulations. The psychic energy by which the movements in the pleasure stage are executed is libido. They serve the acquisition of stimulus-pleasure, stand in the service of the sexual instinct, are sexual instinct activities. This new terminology for already well-established mechanisms is simple enough, but it obliges us to ask the following questions: What relation has this libido to the psychic energy which is behind discharge phenomena and which urges the movements to a purposive stage ? In order to avoid a possible misunderstanding I wish to repeat that the relation between nervous energy and psychic energy will not be discussed in this book, and that therefore they are not treated as equivalent. We do not, therefore, ask about the energy process in the nerves during movement, regardless of whether this process is identical with the conversion of psychic energy or not; we are only concerned with psychic energy and its relation to movement, without concerning ourselves with determining whether these processes take place in the nerve fibres or elsewhere. In the pleasure stage of the development of movement, the organ—i.e., the arm—behaves like an erotogenic zone. Certain forms of stimulation of the organ under certain conditions call forth a certain amount of stimulus-pleasure. This form of stimulation is thereafter continuously and intensively sought. The organ is richly invested with libido, and in a very definite way. It keeps libido bound, which is denser than the cathectic energy (libido), as we said, but it never hinders the releasing processes. We will ascribe · the pleasurable processes of these erotogenic zones, since they are of a tactual nature, to the sexual process in its defined sense. If we see the organ in the purposive stage decreased in its value and in its imperative force as an erotogenic zone, we say that it has been desexualized; the quantity of libido with which it was invested has been decreased. It cannot, however, be merely a case of a simple decrease of libido; one surmises that at the same time changes in the ways of binding libido take place; but we have as yet no adequate idea of these processes.[1] We are, therefore, satisfied with what is comprehensible at present, and venture to say generally: maturation of motor functions occurs in such a way that the organs become erotogenic through suitable libidinal cathexis, and that definite pleasure-giving movements whose structure is essentially innate are performed numerous times for the sake of this pleasure and thus attain the effect of motor drill for these movement-melodies (*Strukturen*). Learning new nuances of these movement-melodies or completely new melodies presupposes a desexualization of the organ, and occurs by adaptation of the libidinally practised movements to the new aim, which in any case is no longer the acquisition of kinæsthetic pleasure. The

[1] Ferenczi (2) is also concerned with the idea of de-eroticizing organs, but scarcely goes beyond the formulation and biological consideration of this obtrusive assumption.

adaptation has the form of intelligent processes which are yet to be shown.

That it is a question of desexualization, at least a question of · a diminution of the quantity of energy in the desexualized organ, is manifest by the fact that after the consummation of this process the libidinal cathexis of other psychic factors is essentially increased. This displacement of the quantity of energy can be well studied in the example of the transition of the arm from the pleasure-movement stage to the purposive-movement stage " to put the seen object in the mouth "! We said that this transition follows when the instinct of mastery has become strong enough to co-ordinate the pleasure-movements of the arm. This strengthening becomes clearly intelligible when we—at present inexactly—retrace it to the so-called desexualization; that quantity of libido which was withdrawn from the erotogenic zone, the arm, flows into the instinct of mastery; it now disposes of this surplus of energy. The unprecise formulation will have to be corrected when the idea of the instinct of mastery becomes clearer. Linking up with Schilder's (1) terminology already shows us at this point the direction of this correction. The libido withdrawn from the arm increases the operative value of optical experiences.

The transition from the discharge stage to the pleasure stage is fundamentally obscure. The process can well be described dynamically. It offers us nothing new, but the wished-for confirmation that the principle which has been confirmed several times should already be proved in this case too. The movements of the pleasure stage (e.g., those which can be studied clearly in the arm movements) are slightly modified rhythms of the movements already existing at the discharge stage. They occur spontaneously—that is, independently of a shock-like stimulus—and in rhythmic sequence. On the contrary, the discharge-movements on the extremities are originally exclusively part of a shock-reaction—therefore, in principle, unpleasant—in so far as they are accompanied by *consciousness* at all; more exactly they are anxiety reactions. In the pleasure stage the ' pain ' (anxiety) seems to be overcome; it is changed into pleasure; exactly as in the case of the acoustic stimuli. The path of this transformation is spontaneous and rhythmical. And when we say above that the object of pleasure movements is stimulus-pleasure, that to seek these independently of excitations from the outer world would be the determination of spontaneity, then we may assume an earlier stage in which the spontaneous repetition of anxiety movements in rhythmic sequence, therefore its transference into pleasure, becomes the task. If we wished to reconcile ourselves to this possibility, it would be classified under the repetition-compulsion which Freud established in the psyche, and which, according to our terminology, belongs to the R.-instincts. We would then come to the following—but always dynamic—interpretation: phylogenetic factors determine the discharge of psychic energy freed during the act of birth in the movement of arms and legs. The repetition-compulsion causes the similar discharge-phenomena, as often as the stimulus situation of the outer-world reproduces the act of birth: frightening the new-born (with the development of anxiety, as far as there is any consciousness). These fright attacks are discharged in considerable quantities of energy. In the course of the first weeks the overcoming of this anxiety begins: the repetition-compulsion reproduces the fright movements—in short, rhythmic succession—independent of the stimulus state, and only with a limited quantum of energy. Here, to a certain extent, by the rhythm itself, not only birth proper but its completion, stimulus—stimulus pause, movement—rest, is represented, conditions which lead to stimulus-pleasure. If this is once experienced, it drives toward pleasure-movements instead of toward continuous reinstatement of the pleasurable conditions.

In the above I have made an attempt to build up a conception of the various grades of density of energy (libido), and we assumed that the frequent repetitions of the releasing processes which cause fright attacks in the new-born lead to a refinement of the density of the forms of libido in cathectic energy. This conception is valid also for the processes under consideration. In them the reverse process occurs. Cathectic energy is converted into denser forms, in the libidinal cathexis of arms and legs, which thereby become erotogenic zones.

Having engaged so deeply in theoretical discussions—many, I expect, will disdainfully style them " speculations "—we must venture yet a step further. It is not simple to reconcile our conceptions with the usual views on the nature of the discharge processes. One thinks of these as consuming psychic energy. Thus it is as if one imagined that the energy which the motor process requires is taken away from psychic energy;

this is consumed by the transformation into movement energy. Whether one attributes this movement to physical energy or not, it would be directly or indirectly a transformation of psychic energy into physical energy. I do not wish to pronounce judgment on the admissibility or fruitfulness of this conception, and nothing forces us to establish it here. We avoid discussing the relation of psychic energy to other forms of energy in relation to child-psychology. The stated view of the consumption through motor discharge binds us to the transformation of psychic energy to physical energy, which is implicit in that view. I would, therefore, prefer to speak of the release of motor processes by psychic-energy processes, without giving a prejudged decision about the mechanisms. What then happens to the discharge-phenomena? We do not need to modify what has been said. We will not, however, presuppose that discharge diminishes the level of energy by the consumption of a definite quantity, but we leave open the possibility that discharge-phenomena may also be the indication, means, or result of changes in density of psychic energy.

A few remarks ought still to be added about what happens to the libido, which—as we assumed above—is withdrawn from the erotogenic zone, the "limbs." In observing the child one certainly receives the impression that the moment at which it reaches the stage of putting "seen objects into the mouth" is very important for the child's development. It is as if this introduces a decisive step toward the psychic structure of the adult. Bühler makes this moment parallel to the earlier one, in which the child turns its eyes toward the source of the auditory stimulus, and, in fact, this is really a preliminary step in that advance. They are the earliest indications that the single groups of perceptions and feelings which the sense organs and erotogenic zones brought into reciprocal co-ordination are conceived as centrally unified. "Centrally" here does not refer to the neurological basis which is disregarded throughout this book, but only to a psychic centre. In the first hand-grasping, psychic processes of some kind are experienced in the oral zone, the optical sphere, and in the erotogenic zone the arm, in a reciprocal relation, and they are moulded into a unified process; thus the single zones attain a certain gradation, the optical zone attains a demonstrative function, the motor zone, an auxiliary function, and the oral zone functions as a goal. One cannot fail to see in this association the nucleus

of an ego. For, figuratively speaking, it is not as if the hand
and eye, impersonally without any compensation, exert themselves for an alien third factor, the mouth, in order to give it
sucking-pleasure, but it is as if all three act as partners of a
common firm " Ego " and are entitled to the profits because
the pleasure gained belongs to the ego. I do not wish to
assert that no beginnings of an ego exist before the grasping
activity, but rather am inclined to the opinion that from the
beginning the psychic zones and spheres stand in a certain
relationship to each other, just as, even from birth—and
naturally even earlier—all physiological functions are regulated
homogeneously as a whole, standing in close relation to each
other. But this primal-ego is more than a mere theoretical
postulation, particularly in the grasping activity. At any rate,
we can make this ego intelligible to ourselves in some respects
through this activity.

In this grasping activity the ego as a prerequisite is
necessary for the first clearly centralized regulation of motor
functions. This regulation occurs when the effect of the optical
experiences (perception) and the expectation of oral pleasure
have become sufficiently large to release or inhibit specific
motor effects. In certain perceptions and ideas a concentration
of psychic energy has occurred, placing the motor apparatus
in the service of this apparatus which has become unified by
common energy cathexis (Schilder, 1). Translated into the
conscious language of the adult, this moment means " I want."
The automatic consequence of this " wanting " is—for so this
process must appear to the child—that the wish is fulfilled; no
further psychic processes intervene between the energy
cathexis—formation of a wish—and the consequence, if the
cathexis was strong enough, if the effective value of the optical
images, e.g., was large enough to carry out the intended
movements.

One can obviously assume that the libido withdrawn from
erotogenic zones is used for the increase of the effective value
of a number of wishes. They serve to strengthen the ego,
the preliminary stages which only become the ego by this
influx of energy—and then only that of the three-months-old
child, which is a long way from the further development of
the adult ego. But when we speak of the strengthening of the
instinct of mastery, it is not a contradiction; for the wishes
and experiences the effective value of which at this stage is

increased, and which begin to develop into a central regulating group, belong to the instinct of mastery. We have, therefore, indicated the way of the increase in power of the instinct of mastery, and therewith broach questions which belong to later chapters.

THE FORMS OF MASTERY

The second and third quarter of the infant's first year may be characterized as a unified period. In spite of all disputes concerning the various groupings of the periods of childhood, this impression is nevertheless rightly accepted. Even child-psychology of the old school has a good part of this half-year under the name of grasping age (Sigismund). For us this period is marked off by two important events; grasping in the narrow sense, the grasping activity, occurs at the beginning; teething and weaning occur at its end. The first stage in the development of the apparatus of mastery falls within this time; it belongs, as will be yet more exactly demonstrated, to the instinct of mastery. And very many psychic phenomena occurring for the first time in the first months, or capable of being described for the first time, stand in a definite structural relation to the development of grasping—that is, to the pheno-mena which we ascribe to the instinct of mastery.

In order to make this instinct intelligible, let us observe more extensively and conscientiously than has hitherto been possible what use is made of the developed mastery apparatus and its continuing advance.

Two responses which belong here lead us back again to the first quarter. The lips open in response to suitable stimuli, embrace the stimulus-object, if it fulfils certain conditions, as if with a proboscis and perform the sucking act. The movement of the hand into the mouth very soon becomes a preferred act which persists even in spite of hindrances. From the first it is not a matter of a completely passive response, even if this by far predominates. Indications of turning the head, efforts at snapping the mother's hand, are not infrequent occurrences in the new-born. Both are more than mere passive functions, since they need the effort of the head, neck, and the cervical muscles, and the releasing of these movements takes place because of a perception which does not pertain to the organ of mastery itself; regardless of whether an optical, olfactory, or perhaps a tactual perception has served as a releasing stimulus (the perception of the cheek, for example, but by no means a perception of a part of the mouth zone in its narrowest sense) (Popper). We have thus already given in the new-born the prototype of the purposive activity with its factors: the organ aimed at (mouth), the apperceptive (demonstrative) auxiliary organ (olfaction), the motor auxiliary organs (muscles of the neck); all three in perfect congruence with relation to the object and final purpose of complete mastery: breast nipples— drinking (sucking).

It is perhaps worth while revising the development already presented in the first quarter in the light of these relationships. Thus facts which can be formulated without being forced into certain schematizations obtrude themselves, it seems to me. The co-ordinations of the various psychic spheres of oral possession given *in nuce* in the new-born are destroyed to a great extent in the following period. The sense organs lose their apperceptive auxiliary function, or more precisely stated they assume a rich development which is independent of this function, so that the function itself disappears almost unrecognizably into the background. So little is known about the olfactory organ and its mental development that its apperceptive auxiliary function cannot be studied during the process of mastery. All indications point to its existence at the beginning, and certainly it normally recedes very soon into the background or is obliterated completely. In its place, the eye, which played no rôle in the instinct of mastery in the first days, begins to function. Later it can have a secondary function, but for many weeks it develops without any relation to mastery, according to its own lines and only during the purposive grasping act, but after this it remains forever the leading apperceptive auxiliary organ of mastery. The function of the eye which is always visible in the first quarter of the year is: (1) its co-operation in nursing; recognition of mother's breast, bottle, face, of the preparatory actions in infant care; (2) the early seeking with the eyes for the source of sound; (3) every sensory act of attention, the optical not the least, may be accompanied by pouting of the mouth, grimaces, as if every sensory experience were first taken by the oral zone to relate to itself, and as if it were answered by getting ready to snap. Yet this is true of the tactual sphere, curiously enough, only in slight indications. Acoustic stimuli originally release only fright reactions; they do not exist, so to speak. Their transition into stimuli of pleasurable qualities, their further development, is independent of any direct relation to mastery. Disregarding the pursing of the mouth even during auditory attention, tones, as such, if their source is not seen, do not release actions of mastery, neither at this period nor later. The same applies from the beginning for the tactual stimuli, and for oral mastery for all of life. Only this restriction must be made, that the tactual excitation of certain parts around the oral zone (*e.g.*, cheeks) at first calls forth direct mastery actions (snapping, sometimes with appropriate head movements), a response which is obviously soon given up. Accordingly, for the infant the apperceptive auxiliary organ of mastery is the eye particularly. But it takes up this function decisively only relatively late, after it has enjoyed several weeks of autonomous development; whereas the nose, which has the rôle of the eyes in the first weeks of life, completes this rôle in this period, though it is as yet unobserved. This is not strictly valid, however, for the nose remains—at least for certain types —a truly secondary apperceptive auxiliary organ for sexual mastery, and the nose has an auxiliary function for oral mastery also—somewhat as in the psychological processes which we call appetite almost entirely.

We can see that similar autonomy takes place in the motor auxiliary functions in the first three months. Here it can be seen even more than in the apperceptive function, although it does not solve the relationship completely. The muscles of the neck and throat do not lose their significance for the oral act of mastery for a long time. For a time the infant continues to snap at objects which it has first grasped with its hand then placed in its mouth (Shinn). But already in the first weeks of life the head movement occurs very clearly and increasingly often in the field of optical apperception; whereas the hand, by far the most important motor auxiliary organ from the beginning of the second quarter, and the only one from the beginning of the second half of the first year, is active for months, independent of oral mastery. It is in the beginning rather the object of oral possession than the means. Of course, an object which by itself, so to speak, makes oral mastery possible and considerably easier—by its preferred directions of its spontaneous movement—frequently makes even the intervention of the head-movers unnecessary.

In the inborn grasping reflex, and in the aimless closing of the hand (during the first quarter), we have a response which we need not necessarily subordinate to oral mastery. It would not be difficult to do this, but it is not convincing in every instance; we can regard this response as a form of mastery which is to a certain extent independent, and we can designate it as grasping mastery (*haptische*) alongside of oral mastery. Inasmuch as grasping-mastery is independent of oral mastery, it should be described as a tendency: the infant clings to the mother. In human infants this tendency gives the impression of being very " piecemeal," while in monkey infants it is recognized as a conclusive response (Brehm, Mitchell). Thus grasping-mastery plays a subordinate rôle in the behaviour which is independent to some degree: grasping reflex; grasping during falling; holding to objects when they cross the path of the arms moved for pleasure, provided that the object is not immediately put into the mouth, but is held fast in the hands, and the arm follows out its pleasure-movements. We see grasping-mastery in relation to oral mastery when the embraced objects are brought to the mouth, and in the grasping and striking movements of the hands on the mother's breast during nursing, which are noticed very early and which, not infrequently in the first weeks, develop into holding the breast correctly.

The neurological facts, the established relationships and continuity of behaviour appear, according to this, to be arranged without any definite order in the first quarter, and seem to develop largely without centralization. If one understands the manifestations of the second quarter as a centralized mode of behaviour which tends toward mastery (chiefly oral), one sees also in the preceding weeks the diversely scattered beginnings of this instinctual response. And we can consider the stage arrived at in the fourth month (at the latest, normally) as the result of development. But one may also have the impression that the beginnings are fragments, and that their scattered quality and decentralization are the destruction of a phylogenetically given relationship. This view thrusts itself upon us when human infants are compared with monkey infants. Accordingly, the development of mastery (possession) seems specific for human infants. The firmly established relation which we can see in the new-born—nose, head muscles, mouth—is disturbed, a displacement in the formation of the instinct of mastery occurs; during the latent interval, which occupies the first quarter of the first year, the apparatus necessary for mastery becomes independent, more extensive, and more inclusive—in the way already summarized. In the fourth month it unites again with a newly-established behaviour in the service of mastery: seen object, grasping, grasped object into the mouth.

Oral mastery has no further important development; it is in principle terminated at the stage when the grasping activity is complete. We have already described the perfections which are consummated in the functions of the motor auxiliary organ —the hand. In this connection the head movements disappear almost completely. The eye as an apperceptive auxiliary organ obtains the undisputed leadership. And indeed in both directions: mastery occurs, almost without exception, only after optical release; and almost every optical perception releases efforts of mastery.

For many weeks, a predominantly greater part of the infant's waking life (till the fourth or fifth month) consists of nothing more than oral mastery activities, optically released, until gradually oral mastery recedes into the second rank, and until in later years of childhood it recedes more and more into the background, though of course it is not completely abandoned; for even in the mental life of the adult oral mastery plays a rôle, although a weakened one. That it remains latent, that it remains in the unconscious as an impulse of considerable strength, psycho-analysis assumes with good grounds, for it so often reveals just this repressed oral mastery as a decisive agent behind depressive states of all kinds, to say nothing of the effects of this impulse in the normal mental life as well. Only recently Abraham emphatically proved the significance of the oral impulses.

The preceding observations permit of no positive assertions on one point: what happens to the objects in the end-organ itself. Very often they are used for pleasure-sucking, often— appearing as unpalatable and uninteresting—they are scarcely brought to the mouth and are released again; often at a later time they are nibbled and sniffed at. A rule, an understanding, cannot be formulated. The only thing that is certain is that none of the numerous objects put into the mouth are swallowed. Not even an attempt to do so can be observed. If it does sometimes happen, the impression that it happened because the infant saw wrongly predominates; at least I know of no case in which a mistake in swallowing occurred before weaning. Thus oral mastery is not a direct preparation for devouring. On the contrary, it occurs at a time when, without exception, the incorporating movements, sucking and swallowing, appear only as a response to liquids of definite quality. At the time which ends the infant period, when solid food is chewed and swallowed, the result of oral mastery is not devouring, but pleasure-sucking, nibbling, holding the object for a short time in or near the mouth. Most authors speak of it as the infant's apperceptive interest; the mouth is a taste organ, oral possession is a perception, the child tastes every object that it can reach, with its primal taste organ (Stern, Bühler). Although I do not wish to deny that the mouth is a taste organ, this conception does not seem to me satisfactory. It gives the perceptive interest a rôle which cannot be attributed to it. The earlier developmental phases are concerned with instincts and affects. The interest in perception, which derives from the perceptive impulse, certainly does not occur at the beginning of development, but originates from the instincts and affects, in a long and complicated way which does not concern us here. There has been no conscientious research concerning the criteria in the infant (and one-year-old child), according to which it differentiates palatable objects from others, whether it has any such criteria at all even for strong spices, and how it acquires and perfects them is not known. Nothing certain, therefore, concerning the relation of oral mastery and "eating" (*fressen*) can be established. My opinion is that the child during or shortly after the weaning period is guided by such criteria, and that it is the result of a later development, which by the way does not seem to occur in all children, when it reaches the point of devouring everything, swallowing pennies, celluloid balls, and ink.

Mastery enters into a decidedly new phase with the relaxation of the close relation between oral and grasping mastery and its complete dissolution in the end. Scupin cites the following moment (from the fifth month) of the infant's life: "Today it held in its hand its favourite toy, a banjo with a wooden handle, then leaned forward and let it fall. The ring caused by the fall aroused its attention; it looked about until its eyes remained fixed on the coloured thing lying on the floor. The banjo was picked up and placed into its hands. It looked at it again, touched it again, then—plunk! The toy was on the floor again. Then the child leaned forward energetically and looked for the fallen object. This happened several times." Grasping-mastery is not a partial activity of oral mastery, but it serves acoustic pleasure. Similar instances may occur only sporadically, so that this one may seem to be accidental. Very soon, however, the infant's behaviour indicates beyond a doubt that the grasping of objects has as its purpose the creation of noise. In the instance cited above, the " intellectual " interest plays an important part; but in conformity with the programme of this book, the problem of intellectual development will not be discussed in detail.

In general, objects which are not suitable for use in the mouth, or can be put into the mouth only with great awkwardness, are used for making noise. Attempts are, nevertheless, made to use even these objects orally. Perhaps the oral use remains preferable throughout the whole of infancy. But yet there are instances in plenty in which grasping serves primarily the acoustic pleasure-gain. In such instances we have no reason to ascribe this action to the possessive impulse; we may list it under the purposive actions which are performed in the service of sexual pleasure, and note an important advance, viz., the possibility of using the hand in the service of zones other than the oral zone. Here the eye also undergoes an alteration in its function. It now has not only to look at objects which are suited for oral mastery, regardless of what their purpose may be, but also at those which promise possibilities of acoustic pleasure. Until this point, the infant knew two ways of gratifying the acoustic zone: by waiting until a suitable auditory stimulus is accidentally offered by the outer-world, or by deliberate formation of noise through the vocal apparatus (mouth). It has made frequent use of the last possibility, and now finds an increase of it by using mastery for the production of many varied sounds.

Other experimentations with grasped objects—for example,. attempts to possess hitherto unsuitable objects—have this in common: they do not lead to oral mastery, which is apparently in no way their purpose. Besides this, these activities seem to have little in common with each other. They are the favourite forms of behaviour: tearing paper or at least crushing it; snatching, tearing, crushing, kneading, scratching, plucking all possible suitable objects—covers, materials, wool thread, etc.; snatching at the nose, eyes, cheeks of the mother and other persons; scratching, tearing the hair, and other endless varieties of similar activities. It cannot be positively decided to what extent these activities bear no relation to the oral zone. There does not seem to be any necessity for thinking of them as independent of it. One can easily construct the relation if one considers that all these are actions of breaking things up into small bits, or may have that as their intention. If the child snatches at the eye—with special preference—the act may very well mean that it wishes to pluck the eye out of the socket, or to tear off the nose as an object for mastery; a piece is to be pulled off the cover, the teddy bear is to be broken in two, etc.—to put into the mouth all of these objects thus detached and thus formed: a purpose which cannot be realized, or at least not frequently. Thus the infant behaves in all these acts just like a young monkey, only more awkwardly and sporadically. The monkey also grasps everything in sight —with relatively less choice—leads it to its mouth and tests its palatable qualities; it breaks unsuitable objects into pieces, it peels, breaks off a piece, turns it around and around, in order to see whether it contains something palatable: an action which for the frugivora, who have to peel, separate the seed, break off and hull the fruit, is complete in itself and rationally purposive, and which has a direct relation to oral mastery. This is nothing other than the introduction to the nutritional act. In infants this same behaviour seems much broken up and changed, partly through the direct and indefatigable effort necessary and the positive influence of the environment.

That an acoustic pleasure plays a part in some of these activities, as in the tearing of paper, is only mentioned above, without detailed observation as to whether it is primary or secondary. In the same may it is only indicated here that in the attempts to take possession of the mother's body, a new motive may very soon be associated: the perception of the mother's serious and playful expressions of pain, which the child soon follows with great interest, and for the sake of which such actions in " play " are very soon and frequently repeated, enjoyed, and increased.

Active mastery, which has occupied us until now, is freely joined to a form of behaviour which one must designate as the passive form of the same impulsion, but one must not forget that a very close connection with the heterogeneous instincts will prove to be demonstrable. The infant is not always—even at a later age—in a position to satisfy its need for clinging, for it calls for mother and wants to be taken into her arms, in order to nestle up to her and to hold and cling to her. The interpretation of a component of this behaviour as a grasping-mastery impulse which cannot be actively fulfilled, but needs the help of the environment, is not a forced one. Stretching out the arms is the gesture of this wish, an expression which conveys quite generally the wish for grasping-mastery. It is nothing else than the effort to increase the range of the arms and to reach the distant object, to hold it close in order to subject it to oral mastery or one of the other uses described. In one instance this effort can experience an apposite fulfilment. When the child longs for the mother, it cannot draw her to it, but it is embraced by her, and thus the mastery impulse experiences its gratification passively, without muscular exertion. Certainly this is for the infant a remarkable experience whose significant mental consequences we have yet to consider.

THE INSTINCTUAL COMPONENTS OF MASTERY

For purely descriptive purposes, the term impulse of mastery, or instinct of mastery, which we have used so frequently in the previous chapter, is sufficiently precise. It describes a number of actual facts correctly and significantly. But if these facts are to be organized with relation to the other instinctual tendencies, mastery must be split up into components. The term instinct will thus not apply to them, and can at best apply only to these components; and the expression impulse needs closer definition. In accordance with the beginnings of a psychological theory of instincts, carried out in this book in the closest dependence upon Freud, the question to be asked is whether the impulse of mastery is an expression of the sexual instinct or of the R.-instincts. If it proves to be the results of a fusion of both, their parts should be indicated and, as far as possible, differentiated from one another.

Each complex can easily be separated from the impulse of mastery, as a whole, and sometimes can be classified under one of the two instinct groups. Parts of the nutritional instinct, which we attempted above to incorporate under the R.-instincts, are clearly recognized in it; and the stimulus-pleasure phenomena which we assigned *per definitionem* to the sexual instincts lose none of their force. But it would appear that some phenomena remain which cannot so easily be separated. And the relation of both of these complexes to each other and to the other miscellaneous ones brings up more questions than one need attempt to answer at present.

The description of the nutritional instinct attempted above, applies very well to many manifestations of the oral impulse of mastery. Putting the seen object into the mouth, making it fit the mouth (tearing, pulling off a part), and lastly looking for palatable parts in the thing which is seen and grasped (and found unpalatable as a whole) are three complexes of oral mastery which coincide with the nutritional instinct, which are doubtless manifestations of this instinct. These complexes are modes of response which are permanent, innate, to a certain degree accommodating to the oral conditions, capable of being released by a perception, and in themselves significant. There is no objection against designating them as instinct. If they run their course with consciousness—and it would be quite senseless not to assume this—the mental representation of an instinct would be expressed by the wish, which could be interpreted as follows: I would like to put the seen object into the mouth (and eat it). If the wish cannot be fulfilled dis- pleasure results; if it is gratified pleasure results, and indeed obvious gratification-pleasure, rest-pleasure. The absence of perceptions which release wishes will after a time produce motor unrest; this, experienced as discomfort ('pain'), will lead to attempts to change the situation, which indeed will continue until releasing perceptions finally appear. If after a time this does not happen, they are then hallucinated, and thus a concrete wish is built up within the general motor unrest.

This procedure represents in two directions all that we can expect from the R.-instincts. Their aim is, as everyone knows, the reinstatement of the disturbed state of equilibrium. The disturbance is here first an inner one: hunger. Hunger sets in when the organism has for some time had no opportunity to see *and to grasp* the palatable thing. (We disregard the infant for the present.) One must place special stress upon " and to grasp "; for if the impulse to possess objects seen were not dominant in the individual, then even if it were surrounded by the most appetizing food it would wait for acute hunger. In agreement with Claparède's (1) conception one can say: The possessive impulse, when free from acute hunger, under normal conditions prevents its appearance, which is very unpleasant and dangerous, since it may easily be too late. Nevertheless, in spite of this protective function of the impulse of mastery, the inner disturbance can set in. What the individual then does instinctually, such as changing its place, will in the end, by means of instinct energy, lead directly to oral mastery, to satiation, to the removal of the disturbance, and thus to the reinstatement of the disturbed state of rest. Only then will pleasure and indeed rest-pleasure set in, in the system Cs.-P. (Consciousness-Perception); the acts which lead to the reinstatement, the instinctual activities, will be—theoretically —'pain,' regardless of how it may express itself, for example, as greed, irritation, tension, etc.: *per definitionem*, as *R*.-instinct behaviour.

But the state of rest can also, secondly, be disturbed from without. Seen objects release the oral wish for mastery (appetite, in the broader sense of the word) before the nutritional state of the organism has made itself psychically noticeable by inner stimulation. That this is possible can be seen in the paradoxical result of the impulse of mastery, with its function of defence against hunger. In this case the disturbance is removed, the state of rest is re-established by annihilating the disturbing object. Thus it radically and definitely loses its disturbing power, its ability to stimulate "appetite." Annihilation occurs orally or—theoretically—in complicated instances by destruction, throwing away, etc. Oral annihilation is the definite removal from the range of vision; it is the most radical and enduring, the most assured way of holding off the disturbers of rest that is possible without the use of instruments. When oral annihilation does not occur, then a temporary removal from sight—hence not a durable and not an assured one, although sufficient for the immediate future—a rejection sets in, or that degree of destruction which reduces the effectiveness (disturbing quality) of the object, and, wherever possible, removes it altogether. Fruit on the tree, an object of highly disturbing quality, is converted, demolished into a small heap of peel on the floor—even when the fruit is not palatable. (A procedure which is true of visual animals; olfactory animals do not seem to need this procedure because of their precise capacity for choice.) A pure *R*.-instinct procedure occurs in each single concrete set: the disturbed rest-situation is again reinstated by radical annihilation of the disturbance, and a certain assurance against the most acute disturbance, hunger, is attained by the whole procedure.

This classification of an extensive part of the impulse of mastery under the R.-instincts is endangered at the outset—even for the manifestations in infants—by two conspicuous tendencies. Firstly, the expressions of pleasure occurring during mastery do not apply much here. Secondly, real oral annihilation takes place during oral mastery only in infrequent instances.

This second fact will be treated first. Applicable as it is, it nevertheless means no more than that the phenomenon under consideration is complicated in human infants; that complication has taken place in the infant which our discussion, since it had to be general, disregarded. There is hardly one case in the concrete, mental life in which R.-instincts are expressed pure and unmixed; they are almost always interspersed with components which are found to be classifiable under the sexual instincts, according to the theoretic separation which must be undertaken. Why this must be so, why this assumption is more applicable than the reverse, why the R.-instinct components are mixed with sexual instinct components, will later become more intelligible to us. But for the present, we must be content with remembering that all statements concerning instincts assert, not actual facts of concrete mental occurrence, but theoretical, limited concepts which serve the interpretation of concrete facts. But one need not assume the fusion of instincts in order to dispose of the second objection advantageously. Perhaps it is sufficient to generalize from the facts with which this objection is concerned. One can also interpret them as showing us a broken relationship. Oral annihilation, in its development, is not closely dependent upon oral mastery. Primally, and in accordance with the idea that component parts of one tendency belong together, both are separated from each other in ontogenetic development. The development of oral destruction is delayed, or that of oral mastery is premature. This is not the first time that we must assume such a severance of the primal and conceptual connection. What Freud (2) calls the duality of the development of the sexual instincts is clearly noticeable in other fields too. Unified modes of behaviour very often develop ontogenetically in such a way that they are split up into two components which appear successively, occasionally separated by a considerable period of time. The whole of oral mastery, which includes annihilation and mastery, begins its development with mastery alone; it does not at first reach the terminal phase, annihilation, which is brought on only after a few months by a new start in the development. We understand the earlier stage, which in itself has no meaning except with reference to the later phase. The mixture of the impulse of mastery of the R.-instincts with libidinal components gives activities an individual function even in the first stage: pleasure. Thus the R.-instinct activity, oral mastery (without annihilation), may appear as a pleasure-activity. We learn that this is only appearance, upon more exact consideration of the pleasure itself.

With this statement, we have touched the first objection again. Mastery is bound up with pleasure. The expressions of strongest pleasure are linked with it, indeed the very same expressions which we know from stimulus-pleasure coming from the most varied causes. Observers repeatedly describe it with pride and joy. Where this audible, excited pleasure is expressed, one might easily be tempted to assume the fulfilment of the sexual instincts. After all is said and done, at least one may prefer the impressions that rest-pleasure,which we found in sleep and satiation, must be the typical form of pleasure of the R.-instincts. But we know too little of pleasure in general to dare to set up the two extreme forms of pleasure (which are distinct from each other, and which in their most extreme expression are classifiable under one of the two instincts) as the only and typical forms. That the forms of pleasure cannot be separated simply according to their modes of expression can be seen in pleasure during pleasure-sucking, which certainly belongs to stimulus-pleasure, and certainly to the sexual instincts, and is nevertheless as quiet and intensive as the rest-pleasure in falling asleep. On account of the complexity of the question, still so vague, it would not be advisable to take the ways of expressing pleasure as the decisive criteria of the instinct under discussion. The similarity between the expressions of pleasure in mastery, and the expression of pleasure in hearing rhythmic sounds, is no reason for arguing that both are the result and not the aim of the same instinct.

If we wish to try by reflection to see into this vague question, the following facts offer themselves. Oral mastery and anni-hilation does not exhibit any expression of joy or genuine pleasure. The impression is that the pleasure accent in it was placed upon the completed action, the removal of the disturbance, just as we expect *a priori* from rest-pleasure. Here, of course, a complication intrudes: the oral zone begins to function, as it necessarily must, and secondary sexual pleasure thus mingles with R.-instinct activity—or at least can mingle with it when a prolonged functioning of the oral zone is necessary to the completion of the oral mastery, annihilation. The important expressions of joy are dependent on grasping mastery regardless of whether it was the means to oral mastery or to other mastery, or whether it exists for itself. But this is certainly not stimulus-pleasure; in all these expressions of pleasure it is not a question of rhythmic control of anxiety or ' pain ' of any kind. In specific cases where such conditions appear to prevail—for example when a child, in a lively manifestation of pleasure, bangs the grasped object on the table—we come to the simple conclusion that pleasure is to be ascribed to the sense perceptions, to the kinæsthetic perceptions, and to similar sources of pleasure, which have nothing to do with mastery itself.

If pleasure after a successful effort appears as joy, triumph, it can be easily understood, regardless of whether the intended success was striven for in the service of the R.-instincts or of the sexual instincts. In any case, the purposes of the result in a single case would be criteria for making the decision. If pleasure occurs without this preceding effort—and that is how it most often happens in the case of joy at having grasped something—nothing remains but to maintain that the realiza-tion of an instinct—that is, the success of every instinct activity—must bring pleasure. But it is surprising that this pleasure also appears when only one part of the instinctual activity has run its course. We understand grasping mastery as a stage of oral destruction. If we recall the assumption which resulted above, we would then understand this pleasure as the consequence of the withdrawal of libido from the organ to the ego. This means that the pleasure of grasping mastery is a feeling of self-regard (*Selbstgefühl*), the kernel of the feeling of self-regard as it can be attributed to the kernel of ego. But it is bound up with the same conditions with which the feeling of self-regard will always be bound up: uncomplaining submission to the world, subjugation of the organs of its own body to the wishes of the ego. We experience this as pleasure, and the infant no less than we.

The ego can now—at least to some degree—be precisely described in its attitude to R.- and sexual instincts in this situation, mastery. It serves the R.-instincts as opposed to the sexual instincts, it serves grasping mastery as a means to oral mastery, as the forerunner of oral and grasping annihilation, and really as their beginning as opposed to kinæsthetic stimulus-pleasure. But in the service of this function, the ego draws libido to itself; the sexualization (erotizing) of the ego which will become noticeable in the second year of life, begins perhaps already at this age.

Thus we see the impulse of mastery as an instinct fusion of R.- and sexual instincts. The R.-instinct portion can be recognized more clearly the younger the child is, as a complex complete in itself. It is, however, obscured in three ways. Firstly, by adapting and developing itself ontogenetically in two (or perhaps more) periods; secondly, by varied fusion with libidinal and, in a narrower sense, sexual (pleasure giving) components; thirdly, by an anticipatory factor. We shall understand the second factor more exactly when we have studied the libidinal structure of the second and third quarters (in the next chapter). We indicate the third here only in passing. The social situation of the infant determines that the ego and grasping-mastery develop earlier than is at all possible for oral annihilation. It is not through the infant that hunger is gratified or prevented, but through its mother. A conspicuously important part of its R.-instincts is satisfied by the existence of definite instincts in the mother and definite psycho-social conditions. This also applies to the animal infant. As soon as it is weaned, however, it needs a whole number of possessive activities, in order to satisfy its hunger independently. It practises these actions in anticipation, even while it is being gratified at the mother's breast. Even for the portion which appears prematurely, the severance of the original nexus of the instinct is thus an anticipatory manifestation. This is valid for the human infant to a greater degree, because it is far from independent with regard to the procuring of food by the time of weaning. The complexity of the conditions of life expresses itself already in the complication which the simple and primal unwinding of the instinctual activities experiences in the infant period. Here we agree with Groos (1) with respect to preliminary practice and later practice; thus we may call the mastery activities, collectively and separately, play. Only one must bear in mind that preliminary practice and play are not explanatory terms; on the contrary, they create a problem and, moreover, a teleological one.

THE LIBIDO DEVELOPMENT OF THE INFANT AT THE GRASPING AGE

In the preceding section frequent mention has been made of the libidinal strivings of the grasping age, so that so far as the presentation of facts goes, we need only summarize and supplement them. A part of the libido adheres to definite regions of the body: the erotogenic zones. The number and significance of these regions undergo, during the first nine months of the infant's life, certain changes which can be easily designated. During the first three months, the oral, the auditory, and kinæsthetic zones are the most important. Of these three zones only the oral zone has retained its primary significance, perhaps even intensified at the end of nine months. The kinæsthetic zone has given up a good portion of its erotogenicity. The arm musculature responds completely to the wishes of the ego, but undue rationalization has been applied to its movements. They are no longer directed exclusively toward the aim of winning pleasure from the arm itself, but they are used for the sake of pleasure-gain (instinctual gratification) from other organs or from the whole ego. The same process is already well advanced in the leg muscular system. The ear as an erotogenic zone has so far retreated into the background that it is almost unrecognizable as such; it is no longer a question of its excitation—pleasure as well as 'pain.' Certainly it is no longer a question of tactual pleasure, but the libidinal cathexis at least in essentials has been transferred to the auditory perceptions (and ideas). The ear behaves for several weeks with relation to the libidinal processes, like the eye which from the beginning is related through its perceptions and ideas to the libidinal phenomena. This is an indubitable fact, which our detailed discussion cannot stop to establish at this moment.

The complete absence of material in the previous chapters

on the anal zone (see above) was intentional. We know nothing about the libidinal processes of the mucous membrane of this zone during the infant period. Nevertheless, it should not pass unnoticed that often, even in the third month, a certain regularity of defæcation is successful, which reveals that a definite relation between the local irritation processes and the ego is established.

No detailed solutions can be derived from the available records of observations concerning the erotogenicity of the whole bodily surface, the skin (Sadger). We know that immediately after birth, under definite conditions (perhaps in a warm bath), pleasure of a considerable intensity is derived from it, and that this fact remains true during the whole infant period; while the infant scarcely gained pleasure from a local defined rhythmic excitation (tickling) unless the stimulation was applied to one of the erotogenic zones.

So we see brought about a diminution of the erotogenic zones and their significance in the course of the first nine months. On the other hand, during this period one zone develops erotogenicity, which in the first weeks of life played no noteworthy rôle. I refer to the genital zone. Exact proofs —as we have already shown—are lacking or almost completely lacking; nevertheless, it cannot be easily doubted that the sensitivity of the genital zone is of importance even in the first weeks. Watson records erection of the penis in the first weeks of life. There is no evidence to contradict this possibility. But this zone cannot play a rôle in the first three months because the specific stimulation cannot yet be applied by the child itself, and is prevented by the mother as much as possible, or remains unobserved. Only when the hand has attained the ability to make definite manipulations is the psychic possibility of using the genital part as an erotogenic zone present. One cannot therefore *a priori* expect masturbation as a general phenomenon before the fourth month. As far as our information in the scanty and reticent literature goes, masturbation has been observed as early as that, but not yet incontestably.

Authors are at opposite poles over the interpretation of the act of masturbation; they describe and date it inexactly, but no one denies its occurrence; for when personal experience is lacking, we rely then on the indubitable observations of others which occasionally have been made. Moll, for instance, who utilized not only his own experiences, but correlates the scattered moralistic literature, emphasizes that erection during the infant age, manual manipulation of the genitals and masturbatory acts occur through pressing the thighs together, etc. It seems to him far-fetched to interpret all these actions as sexual, but he does not strictly repudiate this for all cases. He says, moreover, that the sensual feeling " happens even to the small child, perhaps even to the infant. When a child lies with moist eyes wide open and presents every external indication of sexual excitement, as they have been observed in the adult, we are justified in assuming sensual pleasure. But in these instances, at least in young children, the orgasm which occurs at the moment of discharge in the adult is naturally missing. Several cases have, however, been reported to me in which it has occurred even in infants " (Moll).

The number of cases as yet published is not sufficient. Friedjung (2), however, was able to assemble a whole series of his own observations, and his literature survey (3) shows that the number of case reports can no longer be overlooked. The earliest dated case of masturbation in this literature is in the sixth month. Friedjung (2) describes a case in which masturbation began in the fourth month. But this case is reported by the parents; the physician's observation was made in the sixth month. In general, the end of the first half of the first year would be, according to this, the earliest period for the beginning of masturbation. There exists, relatively speaking, so great a number of observations for the third quarter of the first year, that one may cite that as the usual time for the beginning of infant masturbation without thereby committing oneself to any opinion concerning its frequency.

We do not hesitate for a moment as to whether we should ascribe infant masturbation to the sexual life or not; for it cannot belong to the R.-instincts. Before we can decide on principle not to add the genital zone during infancy to the erotogenic zones, before we are able to see the motive for masturbation in something other than pleasure which acts as an intermediary, we must have proven arguments. Such have, however, not been presented. It is characteristic of literature on child-psychology and pediatrics, that it seldom considers a scientific problem earnestly and impartially. Arguments are lacking; one must construct them by reading between the lines of the authors.

Let us see, for example, how Moll resolves this problem. I do not agree with him, but he has written the only detailed book on the subject of the sexual life of the child. Naturally, it cannot be expected that he should confine his attention solely to the infant, which would be a form of *petitio principii* from his standpoint. He does not deny the facts which we advanced, in part from his statements. But erection and masturbation, Moll thinks, could "not be conditioned by sexual processes." Erection can be caused, for example, "through a tightening of the foreskin or through infections of the genital organ. Now and then a full bladder leads to erection." In interpreting the meaning of the act in the case of the infant and child, Moll thinks, "we must be careful." It happens that children stimulate various parts of the body. . . . There are those who press their ears with their hands . . . those who have the hateful habit of picking their noses, and obviously these and many other similar habits of children stand with other instances on one plane in which the child irritates the genital zone manually. . . . The child does not wish to release a specific genital sensation, but it is a matter of one of the mentioned analogies, perhaps pathological, though not a sexual activity. In many instances it need not be pathological at all, and it merely signifies that when the child begins to become conscious of its organs it touches them. It touches its nose and ear as well as its feet, and it is quite self-evident that in the processes the sexual organ will be touched. . . . It is naturally correct that out of this non-sexual touching, genital onanism can follow. Only one should not immediately classify every manipulation of the genital organ as a sexual action. Certainly, Moll reduces the possibility of such non-sexual manipulations if he shows that these non-sexual irritations draw the attention of the child to the sex organ and its excitation.

Moll's arguments are not very decisive, clear, or final. We have already repudiated the over-estimation of " touching." In this case they are equally unenlightening. The one thing that remains is the acceptance of manual excitation on the same plane as the picking of the nose, tugging at the ear lobe, and similar habits. All these actions are unfortunately thoroughly unintelligible if they are not perceived as derivatives of sexual activities. To wish to treat masturbation on this plane would make it completely unintelligible. It is not a commendable procedure to classify intelligible actions along with unintelligible, and then not to attempt to explain the unintelligible in the light of the intelligible, but to abandon the understanding of all—*e.g.*, not to perceive tugging at the ear as a compensation for onanism. Such a procedure could be justified by some very special exclusive reason, but no such evidence is adduced by Moll or other writers. Moreover, this explanation would still be faced by the difficulty that " picking the nose," etc., seldom occurs in the infant, while masturbation does. But all these half-confirmations and half-denials are only necessary when one has an affective motive, the possibility of clinging to non-sexual masturbation. If this motive is absent—and it should be absent in scientific thought—one need not say: masturbation in infants exists, but one should not suspect every infant of this (*sc.* improper) action; it is perhaps in this case not sexual. But one will be concerned with the origin, the form, and the meaning of these activities; the idea that they are not sexual could not even occur.

In one respect the limitations Moll makes are justified. Because masturbation is not present from the very beginning, touching the genital organ which leads to actual masturbation must first occur. All these irritations named by Moll, accidental grasping of the genital by the hand, the excitations from defæcation—*e.g.*, the fæces in which the child lies for a long time, the urinating, *e.g.*, touching the urine, and finally all these manifold excitations which arise out of the manipulations occurring during child-rearing, come under consideration (Freud, 2). It seems that all these manifestations of erotogenicity of the genital zone only awake in the course of time, but this is really not certain; in any case they effect in part the formation of the genital zone as an erotogenic area. Before ' this is attained and the pleasure function attached, manipulation of the genitals may be wanting. As soon as this phase is reached, masturbation in its proper sense begins. This does not consist in occasional accidental placing of the hand on the genital for an instant, but in prolonged and repeated manipulations which have their specific rhythmic form and their habitual placing of the finger, thigh, etc. Interrupting this activity is disliked by the child, and after it has been prevented or stopped masturbation is again resumed. Masturbation is accompanied by all the expressions of indubitable pleasure. The child is completely absorbed, just as in intensive " pleasure-sucking." Sometimes phenomena similar to the orgasm have been observed. Townsend reports thus " of an eight-months-old child who flung his right thigh over the left, closed the eyes, and clenched the fists convulsively. After one or two minutes of perspiration and blushing of the face, complete sleep followed. This was repeated once or several times during the week " (Moll). It is naturally impossible to interpret such instances as anything but sexual, even if the word had not the further Freudian significance which we attribute to it.

The fact that the genital zone as an erotogenic area first makes its appearance during the third quarter of the first year in no way excludes the possibility that it has dispensed pleasure earlier. But the erotogenicity of the genital zone which appears first at this age causes a clear, visible, well-understood, established manner of behaviour.

A complete final decision as to the ubiquity of this development cannot at present be ventured. What is certain is that it is not a question of an infrequent or of a pathological phenomenon. One should not conclude that because of the infrequent published instances, masturbation is an infrequent occurrence. On the other hand, mothers, midwives, and nurses know that erection in infants, as well as masturbatory measures, are very often common. They also know that stimulation of the genital zone calms the infants, puts them to sleep, and that they react with pleasure; but investigation of the question, which could be easily decided statistically, has not been undertaken. An argument to refute the ubiquity of this phenomenon can scarcely be found. The genital zone, which very soon, certainly in the second year, will begin to play a very significant rôle for the whole life, can hardly attain its libidinal cathexis in one day. It is much more probable the above-mentioned forms of behaviour are not isolated instances but the usual ones, and the development of the mental significance of the genital zone had begun during the infant period. There is no sign that the infants who were observed in masturbation developed in any way differently from or more pathologically than others in which this form of behaviour was not explicitly proven. The assumption of the general insensitivity of the genital zone, to which the published and implicit instances are exceptions, would be a complete fabrication contradicted by the impressions of the observant layman. But without this assumption, the possibility that masturbation is not a wholly common phenomenon is not to be defended. But, on the other hand, the stimulation is so frequent and so unavoidable—and the conditions for the production of spontaneous pleasure through masturbation are provided in some way for the infant in the second half of the first year—and it is so easy to be attained by the baby; it is represented in numerous actions, which serve the attainment of other purposes by gaining other pleasures.

We shall have to assume here with Freud that the genital zone behaves erotogenetically during the infant period and shall have to assume further that it begins generally from the sixth to the tenth month and that the attainment of this pleasure is achieved by means of the masturbating acts. One can perhaps concede a large part to individual factors; not, however, with regard to whether and when the erotogenic zone causes pleasure-activities on the genitals, but perhaps only with regard to what the nature of these activities is, how frequent and how intense and with what relation of intensity to the oral and anal zones.

The following examples from Friedjung (2) may illuminate the discussion for those readers who have not made their own observations. Here are several instances between the ages of seven and fourteen months: " At each undressing the child grasps toward the genital with apparently purposeless movements of the finger. . . . In a baby girl six and a half months of age I saw apparently already co-ordinated purposive movements: she led the right hand to the genital, pushed the forefinger into the vulva, placed the thumb and middle finger on each labial and directed rather quick rhythmic movements with the finger. . . . A girl fourteen months old: since her sixth month one observed about three times daily that as often as one puts her to sleep, she crossed her legs, rocked her body until she became red, then with glazed eyes she lay on her belly and did not respond to calling, and finally fell asleep."

These observations are simply the occasion for mentioning a point, by way of supplement, which until now has scarcely been observed. One may rightly be surprised that the masturbating act is even at such an early age completely developed or is indicated in all essentials, and that masturbation up to that of the adult has remained constant from this early act during the infant age. And one must ask whether one is not here dealing with an inherent fixed form of behaviour.

This raises the question whether or not an unobserved component of the sexual instincts does exist which one could call outright masturbatory.

I believe a short consideration will be enough to repudiate this possibility, and will call attention to a few interesting details. One part of the masturbatory activity consists in pulling, tearing at, pressing the genitalia. First of all, the child behaves towards its own body as it behaves toward the external world: it attempts to take possession of the prehensile parts of the body evidently to bring them to oral annihilation. For this end hands, fingers, toes, feet and penis are suitable. They are actually seized and an attempt which we have met with before is made to pull apart those which cannot be brought to the mouth and to break them up. This applies primarily to the penis. In this play the discovery of pleasure in the penis is made which finally becomes the motive for the action. On the other hand, rather large tactual surfaces because they cannot be seized are from the very begininng dedicated to tugging and breaking up activities, etc. This is valid for the feminine genital, on which on these occasions the same experience of pleasure is established as in the penis. Stroking and rubbing is a repetition of those activities which were conducive of pleasure and which the child experiences as mastery; imitative actions, which first of all have nothing to do with the erotogenic zones themselves and whose repeated performance on the erotogenic zones leads to sexual " pleasure."

It is, therefore, not a specific instinctual masturbatory behaviour habit, but in a notable manner even here it is the application of R.-instinct activities to the erotogenic zones exactly as in "pleasure-sucking," which also develops in dependence on hunger-sucking and becomes independent of it. At this point it ought to be mentioned that perhaps a residue of masturbatory activity remains unexplained: inserting the finger into a hollow in the case of the girl and building a cavity around the penis with the hand in the case of the boy. We cannot conclude from the previous observations whether this behaviour refers to the infant period. In any case it comes soon after. In the last analysis the essentials of the sexual impulse are on the whole contained in this behaviour; it would not astonish us if it were established as an absolutely certain fact that it is inborn and is already expressed as an impulse-activity in the first months of life

In addition to this it is further fortified by its dependence on the aims of the R.-instincts, for hollowing the hand belongs to grasping. But because the penis is rhythmically moved to and fro within the hollow hand, it represents the " pleasure-situation " of the " finger in the mouth," the hollow hand appearing as a symbol of the mouth, the penis as a symbol for the finger. Masturbation is a form of " pleasure-sucking "; here too the mouth (the hollow hand) is generally active, the finger (penis) " passive." In the case of girls the finger remains unsymbolized, but the vagina symbolizes the mouth— in truth, an inactive mouth. One need not stress the difference of sex too much here, because the girl at this age hardly masturbates in the vagina, but on the clitoris and labials; but this symbolism, which later becomes very important, can be traced back to the primal period of the infant age. Whether these symbols have any meaning for it will be considered in another connection. We here note facts of symbolism which for us are very apt: masturbation is oral mastery on a symbolic level with a similar pleasure on the real level of the bodily zones.

All erotogenic zones attain complete independence of the external world during the grasping age. This applies to the oral and kinæsthetic and anal zones from the very beginning; the genital zone is added to this group as soon as the masturbatory activities can be performed; the auditory, which is to be partially disposed of here, fits in well when the child has become capable of producing, actively, oral sounds and noises with the hands. Despite the fact that the child remains completely dependent upon the mother in the most important item in the gratification of the R.-instincts, the satisfaction of hunger, exactly as it was in the first days, nevertheless it attains the desired pleasure of excitation from all the erotogenic zones: thus its sexual instinct in its most important phase remains autonomous, independent of the mother and the external world. Freud (2) designates this phase of the development of the sexual instinct as auto-erotic. The sexual instincts participate on the erotogenic zones of their own body without any help from the outer-world. According to Freud, this phase is the primary, original one. We have seen that this is not generally valid, in that some of the erotogenic zones must have been externally stimulated for a long time before the auto-erotic participation becomes marked.

Freud also calls attention to the following fact. He speaks, as we have already indicated, of the dependence of erotic gratification on the vegetative functioning and child care. The libido, which is concerned with these auto-erotic acts, Freud calls narcissistic. And he has incorporated this formulation into psycho-analytic literature: the primary form of organization of the libido is narcissistic, a given condition in the infant. The meticulous study which for the first time is devoted to the infant period in this book closely confirms the grounds for this formulation. But one need not succumb to the idea that the entire libido is narcissistic even in the grasping period.

On the contrary, some of the infant's behaviour which can be ascribed to object libido (as the antithetical idea to narcissistic libido) has already been clearly noted; the transition from narcissistic libido to object libido cannot be exactly specified. In the first days of life we already see the phenomena of cathexis which are exacted with libido and which are not enacted on the erotogenic zones; in fact, not on the body at all, but upon perceptions and ideas—that is, upon the outer-world, upon objects. Besides this we must theoretically separate object libido from narcissistic libido. There is at present no other theoretical possibility. But one must not even then forget that the first beginnings of this transition are noticed very early—so early, in fact, that we can assert with almost complete accuracy, that from birth (from a few days after birth certainly) definite small quantities of libido are used for object cathexis.

These early libidinal object processes are to be studied in connection with perceptions and the ego and we must be patient until we reach a description of them. Among these objects of earliest childhood love (for how else can the relation of the child to its rattle, its blanket, its many lights, be named ?), one object, the mother, takes a very special place. She is not only the possessor of the breast but also the amplification, one might say, of the very earliest recognized and loved object, that object toward which the new-born first turns. Balzac expresses this beautifully in the following words: " The small creature knows nothing besides the mother's breasts; it loves them with all its might, it thinks only of this fountain of life; it comes to them from and deserts them for sleep; it awakes only to return to them " (Compairé).

They are quite evidently a very special object, a part of the external world of particular incomparable importance even for the "little grasper." First of all, the mother is the bestower of gratification and excitation-pleasure in a high degree. She probably plays a very important rôle in the mind of the child, as a condition of innumerable situations of gratification. I do not believe that an analysis of the love relations of the infant can find a final explanation in this factor. This view is just as near at hand as the hope of the final analysis is distant.

Compairé briefly summarizes the position of knowledge, accentuating his standpoint of course. "Love of others, except in its childish form," is by no means " simply one of a number of pleasant impressions grouped through association of ideas around one and the same person. . . . But these pleasant expressions are the occasions, the circumstances, which rouse the need for affection and which guide it in one or another direction. The analysis, which purposes to give an explanation of the perceptible tenderness which the child shows toward its mother, can enumerate the visible and external elements, so to speak, of childish feelings: gratefulness for services rendered, the memory of caresses received, the whole series of impressions which has flattered its useful impulses or bewitched its senses; but there is another element here which analysis has not reached: an heirloom of nature, the tendency to love which emanates from the depths of the soul. In other words, we can well give an account of the reasons for which the child's heart is drawn toward one or the other person, just as in the case of the growth of a creeping plant, we can say, it twines more on one shrub than on another because it is nearer to the first; we have the possibility of explaining the child's love for its mother or its maid , but we cannot say why the child loves."

Admission of ignorance on the part of the scientist has a sympathetic effect. Unfortunately in this case all efforts to seek necessary insight are lacking. Authors satisfy themselves throughout with two statements: First, " When one sees how the infant of six or eight months, at the sight of its mother, jubilantly opens its arms to her, and when taken into her lap, how it clings to her, it is impossible to view this as mere egoistic joy, which is in no way different from the joy taken in a many-coloured, sparkling toy. On the contrary, it

is the first stirring of a personal emotional relationship which ;
spins itself out from the child to other people." And, second,
" Further deduction does not appear possible. '' One should
deplore this gap, even if one has no hope of offering an ultimate
contribution for the solution of the problem. Perhaps a
point of view is already discernible in the criticism. This
viewpoint must, I believe, be linked with the desire of the
author. For Compairé, Stern, Buchner, for example, it is a
question of defending the infant against the reproach that
he is a complete egoist and incapable of any altruistic yearning. A reproof which hardly hurts the infant and a vindica-
tion which is of just as little use to it. But our knowledge
thwarts this tendency. For in such discussion it often
happens that the approval of an action for the mother
is confused with its meaning for the infant. Because having
one's hair pulled is unpleasant and being stroked on the
cheek is pleasant, it is not to be supposed that therefore one
action is egoistic and the other altruistic. This false conclusion is only possible if one overlooks the fact that egoistic
and altruistic are solely ideas of moral worth, but neither is
descriptive nor illuminating for real psychological facts.

It would be well to emancipate ourselves from these unprecise words and to delimit the question. The impression
which we as well as other observers have received from the
behaviour of children is that the mother holds a privileged
position among the child's objects. In what this privileged
rôle consists we shall now attempt to establish.

The child comes to know when the mother is present and
desires a close physical contact with her. That is the way
we should like to interpret our impression, for with this interpretation really essential elements of all love are actually
established in the "grasper." It remains to be proved
whether this exhausts all the activities in question and whether
these demands pertain exclusively to the mother, in a greater
degree and different manner than to other objects. One must
confirm the first statement. Whatever the specific wishes of
the infant are, for the gratification of which its own psycho-
physical mechanism is insufficient, they will run in one way
towards the mother as the aim or means or will begin from
her. All these wishes, of whatever sort they may be, demand
the presence of the mother. When it is not a question of
imperative necessities, such as nursing or relieving pain, the

presence of the mother is satisfying and an occasion for joy. The infant's idea of the mother's presence means, of course, seeing her face and hearing her voice. It is apparent that her presence very frequently culminates in physical contact. The " grasper " wants to master whatever it sees. It wants to grasp the mother; it wants to be grasped by her. We have already said that tearing, pulling the hair, clutching with the hand, being taken into the arms, are in this sense identical activities; which means the activities of tenderness are activities of mastery. A catalogue of these affectionate activities cannot be established for the grasping age. But to those already named scarcely more need be added than the following: twisting the arms around the neck, thrusting the head and body on the mother, and seeking some form of contact. Kissing and caressing are certainly wanting at this age, but caressing could probably be taught to some. Clinging, flinging itself and caressing are to be regarded as the specific acts of tenderness. Perhaps a diverting of these specific actions of tenderness might, in an emergency, succeed from the actions of mastery. Caressing in particular can be easily understood as a weakened form of striking and according to its origin is also chronologically verifiable. I do not believe, however, that this interpretation would be useful.

Three considerations differentiate this group from the other as real activities of tenderness. (1) They are obviously not a means, but an aim. They are, it seems apparent, more an aim than let us say pulling is, which leads to a goal but not as a means. Pulling, for example, is practised on the rattle, but the child cannot by this means break up a celluloid pacifier; but it is easy to understand that the pulling is for this purpose and is given up when finally the futility of this conduct is recognized. It should not be denied that even in the embrace of the infant something similar to the tendency to smother, to overpower, can be included as a primitive phylogenetic property, but the activity is severed from this and independent of it. It gives pleasure and nothing more is sought for. (2) The activities of tenderness bring pleasure in the erotogenic and tactual sense; differently from and in a greater degree than the overpowering activities. Pleasurable contact with the bodily surface is its outcome. (3) The noticeable rest which results from the tenderness activity in the case of the infant is conspicuous and is more or less a contradiction of them. For some children, in some situations these activities are exquisite producers of rest and sleep; they are conditions for rest and sleep for all children.

The problem of the infant's love must now be confined to the understanding of the infant's wishes for the mother's presence through physical contact and of the specific activities of tenderness. But before we attempt to clarify this problem, we shall examine the second question, as to how far this relationship is specifically concerned with the mother.

As far as these activities of mastery are concerned, all objects are used with approximate equality. One qualification must be borne in mind—namely, that normally there was only one object in the child's realm, which opposed every overpowering, every attempt at destruction: the mother. She has a choice in these actions directed against her, in that she defends herself or hinders those which are painful to her by regular, consistent methods. If the child tries to master its well-tucked-in red blanket, he is not successful. But since these objects only interest the child in so far as it can master them, it will after a while give up its vain efforts. The object recedes into the uninteresting " gray " background of the perceptual world. The mother arouses a variety of interest; if the child cannot overpower or possess her, she does not step into the background, but remains an object. One cannot say, however, that the mother alone can be used for no other purposes than for oral annihilation. She shares this versatile utility not with many but still with some objects. She is, however, the most utilized and most varyingly utilized object of the grasping infant's world.

Until now we have considered too schematically the pragmatic value of the visible things in relation to mastery. In this connection it is necessary to refer to one condition of mastery. The wish for mastery occurs only when the thing seen arouses no anxiety. If it produces anxiety, flight instead of mastery results. The mother belongs to those well-known objects which produce no anxiety. For the " mother with the new black hat " (Bühler) is not the mother, but a strange object. Even this quality of not producing anxiety is not exclusively hers; she shares it with a few other objects.

The specific activities of tenderness become attached to objects of very definite qualities. They must arouse tactual pleasure; for instance, they must have softness, resistance, temperateness, etc., and certain qualifications of size and form; and above all, they must be capable of being mastered by the child. In other words, the tenderness-activities can only be directed towards grown people. Later the child will learn how to substitute playthings, cushions and whatever similar examples there may be from the inexhaustible variety of objects as compensations. To my knowledge such substitutes have not been observed in the grasping age. But even if this were the case, we are still faced by a secondary process, a substitutive one; for in the primitive forms of infant-rearing a basis for such substitutes is not to be found. It cannot be doubted that these activities of tenderness are not directed toward the mother only, but toward adults of the child's environment in general. Preferences, however, appear very early in life, but from the previously discussed observations it cannot be learnt exactly when these are made. And what was said of the objects of mastery is still valid.

The first condition is that the person concerned should arouse no anxiety. But very soon one of these persons who arouse no anxiety is decidedly preferred, certainly as early as the grasping age. We know nothing specific of the motives and criteria of these preferences; it is easily possible that odour plays a part in the decision; but certain it is that the preferred one is the child's nurse, really a psychological mother. With our present knowledge the possibility is not to be excluded that the woman in childbed, if she occupies herself with the infant and becomes known to it, and even if she is not its nurse, offers conditions not yet known to us, which necessarily lead to being preferred. We are also unable to decide whether all infants can build one, two, three, or more groups of preferences or whether these are infrequent single instances. It is certain, however, that the nurse and the personal attendant belong unconditionally to the preferred ones. In this sense it can be said, in fact, that the mother is the primary object of the activities of tenderness. But one must not out of love for schematic simplicity overlook the fact that apparently the ability to carry over evidences of love is considerably frequent and relatively easy the younger the child is. Perhaps the end of the first half-year is one of the turning points. The older the child is the more limited this ability, but the range of the sphere of objects becomes larger. But even for this from the sixth to the seventh month seems to be the observable limit.

A definite understanding of these tendencies of the infant will be reached in a later connection. Here only a few apposite remarks which will lead us quickly into the " theory of the libido " and the ".theory of energy," can be presented. I have briefly shown that the object which can be mastered stimulates the child's interest. This fact, theoretically very important, should not be inserted merely in passing, but must be duly discussed. For the time being we must content ourselves with the interesting and inevitable inference that consequently the objects of annihilation are at the same time objects possessing libidinal cathexis—that is to say, in popular speech, the child loves what it wants to eat.

In the simple case of the working out of the R.-instincts we have a complicated situation in that the R.-instincts action and the R.-instinct object have libidinal components. One can here use the unprecise formulation of instinct fusion. If one wished to describe the state more exactly, one would have to find a really complicated expression, whose essential content would reveal that libido is used in the service of the R.-instincts and attains pleasure-in-rest. It becomes obvious to imagine that, since there is so compact a fusion of instincts in a simple case, the higher combined phenomena are not more simply constructed. And actually a certain portion of this fusion is sustained for the whole of life. Love will be closely tied up with tendencies toward possession and mastery; and the tendencies directed at oral annihilation which are retained in the repressed portion can be shown: those in the manifest portion of love are reduced to the activities of tenderness—as kissing, for example. The reduction and changing of the course of an R.-instinct tendency into a sexual instinct activity has not yet begun in the "grasper." It has not learned to kiss instead of putting things into its mouth, it can scarcely caress instead of striking and scratching. The original use of object libido is in the service of mastery, of oral annihilation.

The libidinal cathexis of the external world, a very radical change of the prenatal situation—the mental analogy to the radical change in the method of feeding—finds its original use as the motor for the unwinding of the instinctual activities, which wish to annihilate the environment by eating it up, by incorporating it into the organism. The libidinal cathexis of the external world exaggerates the value of these as disturbances and increases the individual's activity, which is directed toward removing the disturbance. Projecting the adult affects back, one would say that the grasper's " love " expresses itself in the forms of " hate." The primary ambivalence consists in this, that the force of the sexual instinct is subjected to the R.-instinct mechanisms. One might venture to formulate from this the characteristic of the mental behaviour of the mature undomesticated animal, whereas the human adult must succeed and normally does succeed in overcoming this primary ambivalence.

The groups of tenderness-activity are the connecting link of this development. We say they are passive activities of mastery. The older the child becomes, the more " activity " becomes differentiated as an essential attribute; passive mastery is transformed into the opposite of mastery. Equivocally expressed: it tends to become in the last analysis " being annihilated." The result of this is the dispelling of the potency of disturbance of the whole environment; of cancelling birth, but not by the overthrow of the integrity of the external world, but by a form of dispelling all libidinal processes: they are detached from all katergic behaviour habits. Sleep occurs as an indication and result of composure which is experienced in the mother's arms. But acts of tenderness by themselves are not sleep, but a libidinal process. One object, the mother, retains libidinal cathexis, and indeed the cathexis is in the physical contact zones of both individuals. The external world which separates the two bodies is destroyed; the contrast between the autoerotic libido and object libido is to a certain degree removed. The embryonic situation is again recreated, though of course it is transferred from the katergic to the libidinal.

D. TRAUMA AND FRUSTRATION

In our presentation of the infant's development in the first three-quarters of its first year of life, we have pursued some manifestations very conscientiously from their first occurrence; some of these we have followed even into the fourth and fifth quarters. But other large groups of phenomena have been studied only up to the beginning of the grasping age, and we were not concerned with their further development, their further vicissitudes. Others have been mentioned many times, but have not been discussed connectedly, so that they break through the more thoroughly observed phenomena rather as an obstruction to understanding than as a deepening of it. The reason and excuse for such digression is perhaps that not every mental manifestation can be understood at its beginning. Sometimes the understanding of its origin comes only in the course of a retrospective consideration of a more developed phase. Other phenomena lead to a more inclusive survey only when they and their consequences, side by side, are compared after a long period of time, or perhaps when a definite answer concerning this or that general psychological point of contention is assured. This applies to the idea of the trauma of birth, which at first is continually used hypothetically, but more positively in the course of the presentation but which was nevertheless only mentioned in passing, without discussing and affirming the ideas, its implications and its application. We shall soon see that a certain relation exists between trauma and frustration, therefore those manifestations which are connected with frustration and even the frustration itself had to remain unconsidered, for they can only be built up on the definite idea of trauma. The infant period ends with a frustration, weaning, so must the presentation of the psychology of the infant end with the psychology of frustration. And now it becomes necessary to describe, in this connection, the development of frustrations, which ought to begin with the trauma of birth. There will be much repetition which, because of the difficulty of the material and novelty of the point of view, may not be as disagreeable to the reader as it is to the author, who feels this repetition awkward from the point of view of presentation.

Freud (11) has suggested the concept of birth as a psychic trauma; since then this idea has been repeatedly taken up in the writings of psycho-analysts, although no one has seemed inclined to attribute more significance to it than one does to an interesting idea whose value lies in the possibility of its throwing some light on the puzzling nature of anxiety—a light as yet unfortunately small and weak. Recently two papers, by Rank and Ferenczi (2), appeared simultaneously. These papers contradict each other only slightly, and supplement each other to a great extent; they take these Freudian ideas as the starting-point of their views and develop and establish them in two different directions. This book of mine does the same. It is in contradiction to Rank and Ferenczi only on a few points; in essentials it supplements them and is supplemented by them.[1] Objections to the application of Freudian ideas and to the ideas themselves have not yet been raised, because it has not yet been possible to object to them; but objection to the ideas themselves represents the attitude of official child-psychology, which has not even once considered Freud's principal ideas, still less an idea that seemed to have been proposed casually.

But certain objections are sure to be raised. It may, therefore, not be useless to answer them in advance, even if they be only objections which the author himself creates. Such objections present themselves even before recognizing the material and before checking the possible conclusions, because the whole method of consideration is a little unusual. One finds that it overestimates the importance of birth. Psychologically birth is an arbitrarily given moment as every other is, regardless of what significance this particular moment may have for social phenomena. But even this assertion

---

[1] Of course, I do not wish to establish a priority. Anyone who has cause for delaying publication of his views must be content that these causes should also have their consequences. But in order to excuse the inequality of the consideration of Rank's and Ferenczi's books in this work, it should be mentioned that it was being written at the same time as these and was complete in concept, but for the most part, written and finished when these books had been published, so that consideration of them could be indicated without essential changes only in some chapters.

may not be correct. It is true that birth may be quite irrelevant psychologically. We would gladly agree to this conception if there were no manifestations of life after birth which remained unintelligible, unless one had decided to understand them as the effects of birth. And the psychic importance of birth will be estimated by the number and significance of its consequences. I believe that I have shown in the foregoing, and I hope to show in the following, that there are such phenomena and that they are important. But an opponent might be right in saying that birth is of manifold importance for psychology, and these various directions must be differentiated. We know so little about the mental life of the embryo that we cannot make even a vague statement about it. The hope of considerably increasing this knowledge is very small. A developmental psychology which traces psychic manifestations back to their first origin will in the end extend back to birth as a boundary exceedingly important to methodology. Although the meaning of the following assertion may be very problematic: the first phenomena of the life of the new-born are psychic; although it may be conceivable to exclude from a psychology *sensu strictu* the first days of life, the first hours of life; although it may perhaps be excusable to cover the first weeks of life with this exclusion—nevertheless, all the manifestations shown by the child which are established after birth remain characteristic for the psyche for the whole of life. If these are the preliminary stages of the mental life, they are such that one cannot say when they merge into the actual mental life because they are so similar to it. There are preliminary stages which very soon—in weeks certainly, in days, in hours perhaps—will pass through the whole puzzling change which makes it permissible to diagnose them as undoubtedly mental. Now if one completely abandons, as we are doing in this book, the equating of conscious and mental, then there is no other way than to trace the mental phenomena back to birth. Perhaps sometime later we may, with our knowledge of the mental, penetrate beyond birth into the fœtal being. Then birth will no longer necessarily be the beginning of developmental psychological thought. But *a priori* it is probable that the fœtal mental life will prove to be so different from the post-fœtal life that birth even then and truly then will retain its methodological and systematic significance. Presumably the rhythm of sleep and waking, the predominating part of the stimulus world after birth, is lacking in the fœtal life. Above all, the organization of the need for gratification is still different from that immediately after birth, different even from that given fundamentally by birth. Perhaps one can here gain a precise idea of the mental preliminary stages. Thus birth is the initial point of all developmental psychological consideration. Historically, all phenomena of adult mental life must be traceable to birth.

But this historical description does not offer any lasting satisfaction. The point in the line of development from which a phenomenon becomes intelligible is more important. For example, the end of the first quarter of the first year is such a moment in the development of the ego. In spite of its systematic (historical) importance, birth need have no reasonable significance; one will justly attempt to show its historical importance as a relative factor, both significant and reasonable. We must ask whether the conditions which make intelligible the mental manifestations of the first months of life—even if they are still germ-like—are present in the birth situation; and must further see whether·"memories " of this event are found later (in the next days, or years), and what the phenomena of later life were which first become comprehensible with reference to the birth situation. Such an attempt is certainly legitimate from the standpoint of method. Whether it will reveal any evidence cannot be decided beforehand.

Of course, one must guard against giving a causal significance to an historical significance. In order to make no error here memory helps, for birth has next to the undoubtedly historical (methodical-systematic) and the questioned causal significance, undoubtedly a third, a conditional significance, which should not be confused with the causal significance. It is a conditional factor of the first order because, primarily through it, the individual attains to that psychic milieu in which the psychic, in the strict sense of the word, may be said to exist at all. In this sense, birth is, of course, the " cause " of all mental phenomena; the word " cause," however, is not used precisely. The completed birth is the condition for the post-natal mental life—a self-evident statement which must nevertheless be kept in mind. If one wishes to understand the significance of birth, then those manifestations, besides the historical and the conditional ones which have a special relation to it, must be described especially accurately. For example, when Rank concludes that the course of certain of life's subsequent vicissitudes is determined by the fact that the individual had either a difficult or an easy birth, he was referring to this. The individual consequences of birth, however, will not occupy us particularly, but the criteria for the relationship remain, nevertheless, approximately the same.

If one has become acquainted with the theoretic possibilities of such individual and general consequences of birth, a simple deliberation will show what kind of consequences are to be expected first of all. The fœtal mental manifestations may be preliminary stages, but even these undergo some development. The mental preliminary stage of the first day embryo will be further removed from post-natal mental manifestations than that of the last day embryo; but the development from the first embryo day to the adult mental life is not equally constant. On the contrary, the fœtal mental life is separated from the post-fœtal mental life by a sudden, radical alteration in the environment, birth. If birth has consequences (more than the historical and conditional) we may *a priori* expect that they will be connected with the characteristics of suddenness and radicalness which is inherent in birth. We would not be surprised to discover that there is a specific consequence of these characteristics of birth—namely, that the individual reacts to birth as it later will react to such sudden disturbance of the existing psychic balance, which we call trauma. Of all the possible consequences of birth the traumatic will surprise us the least. We understand this consequence immediately because we, as adults, respond with traumatic manifestations at least with violent fright, to fundamentally less radical and sudden occurrences. The absence of this reaction is the astounding and improbable occurrence.

BIRTH AS A TRAUMA

If birth runs its course under psychic processes similar to our consciousness, or if one could recall it as one recalls other early experiences, it would then certainly be described as a sudden tumble into the depths, as pressure and compression on the head and whole body as in passing through a narrow channel, as a choking fit, crying out, relief, a renewed fit of choking, exhausted relief and falling asleep; to which may be added cold shivers, noises, and floods of light, vigorous heart beat and asthmatic breathing (Garley). It would be a complicated, more difficult state of anxiety and, indeed, the first anxiety the individual experiences. Of course, we do not know which of the experiences have conscious representatives, but this is quite irrelevant to the problem which here interests us. Birth is characterized by a series of given factors, which are intelligible biologically, and which result from the birth situation itself; no problem exists here. But the most interesting result of our previous presentation is to be formulated thus: occasionally after birth this whole complex of physiological states recurs, and some essential parts of these recur even more frequently. As was shown, and is still to be emphasized, in these instances, the consequences (the complete or partial reproduction of the birth situation) are completely unintelligible from this releasing situation. We understand the dyspnœa during birth; but we do not understand why, for example, an adult registers this dyspnœa on the sphygmographs when he is frightened by the experimenter. Not only does unmotivated, unintelligible, physiological reproduction occur, but this physiological syndrome is accompanied in the post-fœtal life by a definite affect: anxiety. One without the other is impossible; the affect and its appropriate physical expression belong so inseparably together that one might say that the complex of physiological tendencies is the affect itself. According to this idea, birth would be an anxiety state; but I do not think this is a very happy formulation. It forces us to question only whether birth and its first "reproduction" are represented in consciousness and not how they are represented. With the confirmation of whether they are represented in consciousness, the answer to how they are represented is given. It is certain that this soon occurs; exactly when cannot be said with certainty. In this sense every anxiety state is mentally and physically a repetition of birth. To be sure, the anxiety states of the later life are not only reproductions, or reminiscent scenes of birth, but they have also enriched, changed and displaced, their motives, their significance, their value; like every mental process they have various levels, but the lowest level of all historically remains, the reproduction of birth. That the anxiety state, as such, first becomes intelligible from this lowest level is decisive for psychology. It must not be forgotten that I mean the lowest individual level, which, of course, rests on a much deeper one, the phylogenetic level, but this one need not concern us further in this book.

If we wished to raise this view to the rank of a universally valid and positive psychological fact, we should have to devote a basic study to the so-called bodily gestures of affects (emotions). The theme has been treated very often; it is not my task to summarize the extensive literature devoted to it. Such an interpolation would extend beyond the province of a psychology of the infant. And the conviction that the literature treats the decisive questions inadequately excuses us from all further consideration of whether this extension be justified. In order to investigate this question from the point of view of child-psychology a long series of new experimental investigations is necessary. But one can sustain the position that an understanding of the hitherto completely vague field of expressive bodily manifestations of affects results from the observation of the traumatic effects of birth. There are above all two organic systems on which the effects play, the organs of respiration and of circulation. Particularly these experience in birth a sudden, radical alteration in their functioning. The alteration in the normal function, such as its weakening or strengthening, is also the essential content of the expressive gestures. The bodily manifestations accompanying the polar affects and emotional states are themselves not completely opposite, for there are very remarkable disguises and differentiations. The assumption that these antithetical states are differentiated from each other or from a primal state, and that the manifestations in the respiratory and circulatory apparatus preserve the history of the affects, is obvious if we could only understand them. The assumed primal state would be the unwinding of bodily manifestations which accompany birth; it seems that the expression of anxiety reproduces birth with the closest exactness, whereas pleasure and 'pain,' as well as the manifold affects, would designate various ways of overcoming and repeating the primal anxiety.

How fruitful this hypothesis will prove to be for the understanding of the general problems of psychology may be left to future research. We have only to establish how far it proves true for infancy. Unfortunately not even this restricted inquiry can be answered satisfactorily; and this is the more apparent because experimental research is lacking. Nevertheless the few attempts which have been made can be evaluated from the following standpoint.

The physiological birth situation contains the following elements most important to us. (1) The sudden transition from the state of apnœa to the choking fit, its alleviation followed by deep inspiration; a new fit of choking followed by vigorous expiration. This complete rhythm continually diminishing in strength is repeated till stabilized and automatic breathing is attained. (2) The specific change of expiration and inspiration which crying represents. (3) The modifications of the functions of the circulatory system, consisting of a paralysis, followed by increased activity. (More precise details are not positively enough established to be taken into consideration here.) (4) Convulsive movements, twitching of the arms and legs; jerking, shivering of various parts of the muscles. (5) Cold shiver of the skin. To these can be added as less important: the downward movements of the whole body, falling; and the varied pressures which the body experiences. The nucleus of bodily expressions of affects is throughout life the reproduction of this physiological birth situation; briefly stated, it is the reproduction of birth as a whole or of an essential part of it, manifoldly varied, and indeed varied according to the cause of the reproduction—that is, according to the affect. The expression of anxiety is a pure reproduction of the birth situation. One might imagine that the pleasure and ' pain ' affects are differentiations of the anxiety affect, for the pleasure affects would show in the foreground those portions of the birth situation which correspond to the overcoming of birth anxiety; the progressive symptoms, accelerated life activities; the ' pain ' affects, on the contrary, can be interpreted as regressive, in that the degrading life activities emphasize components of the situation before birth. The facts are perhaps even more complicated, for pleasure and ' pain ' have their own specific bodily modes of expression which fuse with the undifferentiated anxiety reaction.

The unintelligible nature of bodily expressions of emotions in general and of certain affects such as anxiety and fright become intelligible as such to a certain degree if they are thought of as the reproduction of a situation once really experienced. This understanding of them is increased because the reproduced situation is universally valid and highly significant biologically. But the facts of this reproduction itself need explanation.

As far as I see there are scarcely more than two possibilities. One could first refer to those numerous manifestations in the biological field which can be formulated as the repetition-compulsion (Freud, 9). We do not understand the compulsion further; but we see it continually in operation: it is immaterial whether we wish to speak of a general memory function which has, so to speak, made itself independent and expresses itself in a given instance as a meaningless reproduction, or whether we want to assume that an unwinding of energy having taken place once determines all others, by striving to accomplish it again when a release is given, or however else we may formulate and classify this fact in a larger relation. Of course, such an incompletely satisfying explanation must suffice in numerous instances; but only when a more powerful, less general one cannot be constructed. But I think that the second way, —namely, the case of the reproduction of birth—is open to us. We must, however, interpret birth as a trauma which *a priori* is not a paradoxical conjecture. Thus the reproductions—meaningless in themselves—are of the same kind as all repetitions of the traumatic situation in traumatic (accident) neuroses, which appear so frequently and apparently so senselessly, like the well-known repetition of agonizing experiences in phantasy and dream (examination dreams), etc., in direct contradiction to the pleasure-principle. With the understanding of these repetitions of the traumatic situations we have at the same time gained an understanding of the reproduction of birth without having recourse to the general psychic-biological tendency toward repetition. Freud (9) has presented an assumption which brings us very close to the understanding for which we strive. In the present state of our knowledge we can apply only this attempt at an explanation to our problem. And we find ourselves in full agreement with the trends of infant psychology, staying within the limits of those theoretical views which we have had to construct in order to arrive at the first, inadequate organization of the mental manifestations of infancy.

The Freudian attempt at explanation is of course economic; it builds everything upon the assumptions of energy. It cannot be otherwise, although even today the change in the point of view as the explanation develops is still easily found repellent. The dynamic consideration necessarily leads finally to biology. One must, therefore, abandon it at this turning-point if one is to remain in the field of psychology in the strict sense, and proceed from the economic consideration. This of course leads directly into the hypothetical, but nevertheless into the hypotheses of psychology—into theoretical psychology—from which a consistent investigation of problems in developmental psychology cannot possibly escape. Freud's economic point of view mentioned above is simple enough. From the point of view of energy the trauma consists merely in this: the sudden supply of a quantity of free energy so considerable that the protection against stimuli is broken through and the mental apparatus is thoroughly flooded with it. In this situation there is only one saving task: the quickest binding (discharge) of these disturbing quantities. Whether an outer stimulus operates traumatically is determined by the absolute strength of this stimulus as well as by the height of the level of energy attained by cathexis in the receiving apparatus. The apprehensive preparation should be considered as such a heightening of the level of energy; the conditions for a traumatic effect of an outer stimulus would be the absence of anxiety-cathexis, or low anxiety-cathexis. The repetition of the traumatic situation in dreams has this as their function: " These dreams are attempts at restoring control of the stimuli by developing apprehension, the pretermission of which caused the traumatic neurosis " (Freud, 9).

In the birth trauma it is not a question of the absence of apprehension: on the contrary, we understand birth quite especially as the anxiety state. In spite of that the apprehension, so to speak, is not great enough and not sufficiently extensive. The control of the new mass of stimuli therefore occurs in numerous small attacks. In order to make this more concretely intelligible let us refer to ideas discussed before. As we said, the control of a mass of stimuli occurs by their binding or their discharge.

What this binding consists of cannot at present be conjectured, but we must imagine that it is probably the mental phenomena, introspectively so well known to us in its resultant form as perception, imagination, impulse, pleasure, ' pain,' etc. The binding of quantities of energy which flow to the mental apparatus from the outer-world is presumably linked in the inner part of the apparatus as a condition to certain energy situations. The optimal situation is the investment of the stimulus-receiving organ with cathectic energy. The embryonic state may have stabilized a definite system of such cathexis suited to control the stimulus not entirely lacking even in the embryonic state. This organization, however, is not adequate to perform the controlling function in the post-natal life; it must undertake an extensive reorganization. We are not surprised to see that this transposition is not con-summated at the moment of birth. A part of the stimulus-receiving apparatus is not capable of binding the new quantities of energy. They are therefore vigorously discharged. But simultaneously with these discharges a part of the new cathectic organization is established. This state therefore is a highly *labile* one; it is a certain temporary balancing of energy between two discharges, anxiety attacks. The first days of life are spent, so to say, in the repetition of birth. For from the point of view of energy the mental situation resulting from every new stimulus is similar to the birth situation. In this repetition the excess energy mass which the outer-world trans-mits respectively to the structure of the receiving apparatus and to the fœtus-situation, is gradually controlled by the completion of the reorganization of the cathexes. These new cathexes prevent the repetition of the unexpected breaking through of energy, as it occurred in the actual act of birth. And every anxiety has such a preventive tendency; this is its rationally intelligible portion. .

A difference between the anxiety of the first weeks of life and the anxiety of later life should be established, and it is advisable to differentiate the former as primal anxiety. The experience which takes place during birth should be designated as primal anxiety. It is distinct from the anxiety which prevents the child from letting go of the table edge and from walking around the room alone, or from the anxiety which someone feels during a storm, or from which a neurotic suffers. I do not speak of the difference of the conscious experience, for we do not know whether the primal anxiety is represented in the *consciousness* of the new-born or how it is represented. But anxiety is more complicated than primal anxiety. In primal anxiety the supply of a large quantity of uncontrollable energy from without plays the decisive rôle; in anxiety the accent is placed on energy relationships and displacements in the inner psychic apparatus. It aims at the prevention of the release and the repetition of primal anxiety. It is simultane-ously a repetition of these, in the physiological expressions—at least perhaps weakened, certainly varied, but because of this it is able to prevent the intolerable primal anxiety consisting in the unexpected overflow of stimuli from all sides. If we consider primal anxiety as the forced reaction of the mental apparatus to quantities of energy from the outer-world, anxiety is then an action of the mental apparatus with its own energies—an action which makes impossible the repetition of the former passivity during the birth trauma.

We have seen that the energic cathexis which serves the control of outer-world stimuli is to be understood dynamically as libidinal; we have also—though not sufficiently clearly— tried to imagine certain gradations of accumulations of libido (their binding relationships) and have thereby assumed that the libido of the fœtus is all bound to the organic, and that these bindings, figuratively speaking, are loosened by the shock of birth. Now we can make this great process of delivery more intelligible: a considerable quantity of libido is suddenly freed to oppose the assault of the outer-world stimuli, to serve the cathexis. But it is as if this occurs unwittingly without an ordered plan, so that only the chaos of the primal anxiety appears. But nevertheless organ-libido is transformed into libido which of course does not immediately find its adequate use. This libido, freed from the previous binding, and not yet newly bound (and indeed insufficiently accumulated), is the medium of the component anxiety (in the real sense of the word) in the primal anxiety situation. Anxiety is the primary form of libido, and is convertible into libido at any time: the ego experiences unbound, undischargable, free libido, as anxiety. Anxiety is the state of libido at birth; the state in which it was found at birth. Perhaps it is also the state in which, and out of which, it was born, if one wishes to consider the difference between organ-libido and libido as a principal difference. And this also throws light on the assumed function of anxiety—namely, that it aims to prevent primal anxiety. Whereas the anxiety which threatens during release from bindings is a conserving factor, anxiety once developed with its impulsion to new bindings is a stabilizing factor, and it can well protect the mental apparatus partially or completely from the chaos of an absolute freeing of libido such as occurs during birth.

If we wished to follow this range of ideas to its conclusion, it would lead us deep into the psychology of anxiety, which had better be left for another connection in which concrete material will check and establish speculations which I think are necessary to fill out in detail the bounds of the psychology of anxiety definitely delineated by Freud. The next chapter will supplement this.

Freud (11) occasionally[1] calls this root of anxiety the "separation from the mother" by birth. Rank uses this designation very frequently and fundamentally. The expression is convenient and plastic; I do not wish to avoid using it; but it must be clearly understood that this expression does not mean that the new-born experiences the separation from the mother, and that the child at a later age repeats this experience in anxiety states. It means that it is a question of the recathexis of energy (libido) which is completed at birth or shortly after it, and which really objectively signifies the separation from the mother. Subjectively it implies the separation from the fœtal situation. But since we know nothing about the conscious experience of the new-born, the expression "separation from the mother" is doubly metaphorical. The possibilities (consummated by Rank) of the misuse of such metaphorical phrases justifies a minutely accurate analysis of a concrete application. The frequently mentioned year-old child who will not move unaided from the table is repeating, one might say, the birth experience of the "separation from the mother." This expression is relatively rich and fraught with meaning if in its concise form it means something in the nature of the following. The child's behaviour seems well motivated, it apparently is afraid of falling; its anxiety may not be without objective cause, perhaps it has not yet attained sufficient skill in walking; and yet this reasonable explanation, immediately self-evident to us, is insufficient. How should the child know that walking by itself offers greater dangers than supported walking? An inherited fear instinct of this kind would perhaps be very useful, but unprejudiced research shows beyond a doubt that the child is not afraid of actual dangers. This anxiety does not deal with the fear of the outer dangers —real or imaginary—nor with *Realangst* in Freud's sense. One cannot say that falling is evaluated as a danger or an

---

[1] The essentials of the psychology of anxiety which I have developed above are also given here. The details of my presentation, which were not discussed explicitly by Freud, for which I therefore bear the responsibility, result from a comparison with Freud's *Introductory Lecture*, chapter xxv.

injury by the child when it does happen; but in most instances
the child behaves as if this were scarcely agreeable but an
obviously unavoidable obstruction to the efforts of walking.
Actual harm in learning to walk, in comparison with the
anxiety existing universally, is so infrequent among children
that it is insufficient motivation for fear. From a merely
phenomenological psychology there remains no other explanation than to approach anxiety from the new and unfamiliar.
How and to what should it be referred ? Here developmental
psychological consideration goes one step further; and it will
discover that numerous states of anxiety preceded the one
discussed, and will find the first expressions of fear " of the
unfamiliar " in birth. Dynamically applied it will mean that
in the anxiety situation given above, the anxiety of birth is
repeated. Introducing the idea of energy gives further clarification. It tells us that the new situation, the new energy
cathexis, requires the child to walk alone; just as at birth, so
now it relinquishes the stomach support and the assurance
from grasping—both are usual responses representing definite
energy cathexis, that is one relinquishes a mode of behaviour
(therefore a portion of energy) which has suffered no great
alteration since birth.[1] Accordingly the energy situation is
given at birth and with it the most general condition for
anxiety whose dynamic function is abreaction by repetition, and
whose economic function is the prevention of primal anxiety.
The point of view of energy is a limited one; it tells us nothing
about the specific conditions which are added to the most
universal conditions, and which in a given case cause the
anxiety. Here the libido concept helps; for if the libido
which exists in this energy situation is involved, anxiety is
experienced. The libidinal cathexis of the stomach support
wants to be given up, the libidinal cathexis of " free space "
is not yet perfected in its stead: anxiety results. This is the
birth situation too. It can be quite concretely shown on the
plane of the libido theory. The mother's body is invested
with libido after birth, after the fœtal cathexis is disturbed
by birth. The cathexis of the mother's body is easily
transferred, displaced to objects that are similar to it in important qualities (in any case to the body). Now this binding

---

[1] This was discussed earlier; and is especially obvious among those
people whose children are kept in a carrying sack on mother's back from
birth until they walk alone.

of libido must be released; a real separation from the mother
is to be attempted, independent movements away from all
" mother bodies " are attempted. It is a real repetition of the
libido process at birth, and runs its course with anxiety (which
ensures it against a complete repetition of primal anxiety).
We should like to prognosticate that this time it runs its
course spontaneously. At birth the *endoparasite* became an
ectoparasite (Ferenczi, 2); it should now become independent.
Thus occurs a repetition of the " separation from the mother "
which happens at birth; however in this case the actual
separation in contrast to birth can only metaphorically be
called " separation from the mother."

I have shown that in the expression trauma of birth we
unite a series of complicated facts and supplementary assumptions. These are separated into three fields. First, psycho-
physically, birth is the moment of radical alterations in the
circulatory and respiratory systems; the traces of this sudden
transformation can be recognized throughout life in the bodily
expression of affects; secondly, the primal anxiety affect
(showing itself in physiological expressions) which relates to
an ingress of large energy masses from the outer-world to the
mental apparatus; the outer psychic trauma, if one wishes to
name it separately; thirdly, the recathexis and new energy
cathexis which become imperative for the new stimulus and
need-situations, and last, but not least, from the necessity of
controlling the external trauma. They are in closest relation
to anxiety in so far as they are of a libidinal nature.

Two restrictions should not be overlooked which, although
they scarcely decrease the significance of the trauma of birth,
can protect it against exaggerations. (1) There are a series of
factors which lessen the suddenness and strength of the alterations and stimuli. We have already mentioned a few at the
beginning of this book as psycho-physical retardations.
They must be recalled once again. And the note should also
be added that birth does not occur suddenly, but always
extends over a period of several hours. It is, of course, not
impossible that the stimuli of these birth processes which the
child encounters *in utero* and *vagina* are at the same time also
releases for energy displacements and freeing of libido, which
decrease some of the traumatic effects at the moment of birth.
In any case the process, presumably decisive, of breathing
after apnœa is always a matter of a few seconds.

2. The following question has been raised: to what extent are the individual vicissitudes of birth decisive and important for the further course of the individual life ? Freud (11) is inclined to consider the trauma of birth in principle as the inherited attribute of such stability, that in comparison with it the individual vicissitudes are not of great weight. Macduff, for example, would not remain free of anxiety throughout life. Rank maintains that the most specific situations of birth greatly determine in the unconscious the character and fate of the individual. Better established facts for deciding this question are not as yet available. Freud is undoubtedly correct about Macduff (Shakespeare notwithstanding). For whether the child is cut from the mother's body or enters into the world in the usual way, it must exchange the fœtal situation for the real one suddenly, in an instant. This is not in contradiction to Rank, who at most can expect that such a Macduff ought not to exhibit a hysterical headache. The birth trauma must be experienced by every one at the beginning of his post-natal mental existence; nothing else is conceivable. The hereditary basis, therefore, need not be taken too broadly; that it is present càn scarcely be refuted. Fundamentally, nothing can be said against Rank's conception; but the empirical basis for proving it is lacking. The psychology of the infant in general lacks this basis for any study of individual differences, their genesis and conditions. Only after weaning can child-psychology even today venture any positive theories about them. The psychology of the infant must resign itself to the more general problems. But there is no reason why it should be more than merely cautiously expectant if a scientist suspects the roots of individual differences to be in a process which varies individually but which is in general generic as birth particularly is.

All that has hitherto been said about the actual traumatic effects or consequences of birth summarizes those mental manifestations which are explained by a definite relation to the birth situation. If one wants to delimit the whole mental significance of birth as a trauma, one must also give one's attention to those phenomena which are only indirectly related to the birth trauma, and in which is to be found a causal, not merely an historical, a special and not merely a general condition. I mean all those manifestations which serve to overcome the birth trauma without being a part of it—as, for example, anxiety. In the course of the presentation we have encountered such manifestations continually and have discussed them more or less in detail. A summary of them will be more appropriate in the concluding supplementary chapter. One part, however, will be repeated here in a short paragraph.

Anxiety as the most significant component of the birth trauma is contrasted with stimulus-pleasure as the most significant factor in the overcoming processes. And the path which we recognize as leading to pleasure, rhythmatization, remains for life, and is of the greatest importance. And where processes run their course according to this scheme we can speak, in the same abbreviated way we permitted ourselves in the expressions " repetition of the birth trauma," and " separation from the mother," of the " repetition of the overcoming," of the trauma of birth. Rhythmatization is the primary characteristic of this " overcoming." We see the nature of this rhythmatization in the quick and frequent repetition of the whole " course of birth." This repetition is, so to speak, symbolic, if we apply the economic consideration; for it runs its course on a minimal quantum of libido (energy), of cathectic energy. And the transition from passivity to activity, from accident of external relationships to the restrictiveness from inner spontaneity is contained potentially in this repetition, gaining greater and more decisive significance after the first few weeks.

THE WEANING PERIOD

Strictly speaking, weaning concludes the period of infancy; for as regards the child and its mental development weaning is not an external and indifferent date as is the time when one dons leather shoes over one's stockings. But it is a very incisive change of all the infant's life habits. Weaning is generally not easy; its technique and the child's behaviour create many difficulties. It is a critical time and as such is considered as an important period of life both by doctors and popular opinion. How and with what success the weaning is carried through is by no means unimportant for the infant's health and for its further physical development. A number of special difficulties are bound up with this period (Hochsinger). Psycho-analysis finds good reasons for assuming that besides these difficulties a series of psychic disturbances in the adult can, in the last analysis, be referred to the process of

weaning (Starke, Abraham). How correct nursery superstitions, popular opinion, medical science and psycho-analysis
are, must first be established. In any case the weeks of
weaning are a period which deserves some attention in child-
psychology; even if it were only because in weaning lasting
and very far-reaching alterations of the mode of life, of the
habits and needs of the child take place. The child's development shows only a few such clearly described periods of
transformation. Those interested in developmental psychology will find, to their surprise, that psychology—true child-
psychology by no means excluded—has hitherto completely
neglected to describe the facts systematically; to say nothing
of organizing, interpreting or explaining them. I cannot
undertake the task of atoning for this neglect in this book; it
is not my intention to publish my own new observations here.
My present task is only to collect from psychological literature
which is not specifically devoted to children, as much factual
material as it possesses, without special study, outside its own
field, and to see whether within the limits of all the views presented up to this moment this literature will give unbiassed
material which might further our understanding.

A review of the last quarter of the infant's first year shows
us that the transformation, which we call weaning because of
the active intervention of the adult, contains three varied
processes. (1) Teething as the prerequisite for the alteration
in the mode of life. (2) The consumption of more solid food;
biting and chewing. (3) The deprivation of the mother's
breast or the substitute for it, the milk bottle, and with it the
relinquishing of sucking in so far as it relates to nourishment.
These three phases are to be distinguished from each other
not merely phenomenally: they are also separated from each
other by time, and have separate psychological significances
and should, therefore, also be considered separately in the
following discussion. It is not merely an accident that walking alone, which is so rightly taken as the symbol of attained
independence, starts the period under consideration here, and
is the symbol for the second separation from the mother,
consummated in the weaning period. Walking, chewing, and
speaking are the three main conspicuous approximations to
the adult state, which are acquired in a relatively short time
during the end of the first year. Learning to speak will not
be treated in this chapter and only slightly in this book; it

belongs more appropriately to the psychology of early child-hood than to infant psychology. On the other hand, we shall have to give some attention to the paradoxical fact that this termination of the infant period is forced by the intervention of the outer-world, that it is parallel to the event from the out-side which initiated infancy, birth.

1. *Dentition*

Teething, the prerequisite of the weaning process, naturally begins much earlier than weaning itself—namely, from the seventh to the ninth month (Vierordt). The average sequence can be briefly expressed thus: " The eruption of the milk teeth begins at the centre and proceeds toward the back; that is, the central incisors come first, the two molars appear last, so that only the canine teeth, which erupt after the first molars, are skipped " (Vierordt). This eruption is consummated in differ-ent periods, three of which usually fall within the first year; the two lower central incisors from the seventh to ninth month; the four upper incisors from the eighth to the tenth month, and the two lower lateral incisors and the first four molars from the twelfth to the fifteenth month (Biedert). Yet all these terminal points are subject to extreme individual and family deviations; retardation as well as premature teething, even during the fœtus life, has been observed, so that some children are born with teeth.

Early medical opinion agreed with popular superstition that " teething " was a dangerous affair; numerous clinical pictures, some with the worst prognosis, were brought into a causal rela-tion with dentition. Hufeland, a relatively enlightened mind, shows that teething is not an illness but a " natural function." But he, too, speaks of dangerous risks which are associated with dentition: " Diarrhœa, fever, nervous fits, choking, coughing, breast obstructions, rashes, convulsions." Modern medicine, even in the popular books on advice to mothers (*e.g.*, Georges), repudiates any relation between these usual infant sicknesses and teething; they do not appear during the dentition period more frequently than at other times nor less frequently. Teething itself runs its course without any symptoms of sick-ness, with scarcely any discomfort; at most, a short high fever immediately before the eruption of the tooth is perhaps the rule. Conditions somewhat more difficult can be expected from rachitic children.

As a rule a certain restlessness, irritability, or apathetic behaviour indicates the psychic reactions to this event. Hufeland gives a good description of the child's condition: " Very often the child suddenly begins to cry vigorously, at the same time pulling at its mouth, and just as suddenly stops crying; it keeps its finger in its mouth all the time, biting everything that it is given; it spits continuously; in places the gums are swollen and red, and either it does not allow one to touch the painful spot or it likes to have the gums massaged— as the itch itself proves."

The Scupins have made similar observations which apply to the normal case:

" In all probability the first little tooth is to be expected soon. Often the child huddles together suddenly as if from cold, presses its gums against each other and expels an ' m-m-m ' through his nose. He puts every object within reach, most preferably the finger, into his mouth and rubs his lower gum wildly, moving his head vigorously from side to side. This occurs several times a day; in the intervals the boy is calm and happy as ever."

" Three days later Bubi was somewhat cranky and un-friendly; he demanded a great deal of attention and change," or: " Frequent, vigorous spasms preceded the eruption of the tooth, and the child was also somewhat tearful. The boy sleeps less, and more restlessly, than usual. His impatient groans make us take him out of his bed earlier than usual in the morning. Catching sight of the different objects in the room, he emits a satisfied ' ach ' or ' aha.' It seems as if he is happy to find everything still in its usual place."

Let us visualize the teething child's situation: what must it feel now that one part of its own body, which until now was the ever dependable source of pleasure, suddenly becomes the source of painful sensations ? One is naturally disappointed at the insignificant records of the mental expressions. One will, therefore, a priori, be ready to assume that the attention of the observer was not actually directed to these physiological events; or one will suppose that the psychic course in well-raised, well-nurtured, lovingly cared-for children —and such are the subjects of the child-psychologists' observations—is more hidden, than in the case of children who do not have these compensations. For it is hard to believe that the loss of an erotogenic zone should be overcome with so little complaint. Those who assume the libidinal cathexis of the oral zone will be inclined to ascribe a certain importance and significance to teething—and suddenly find themselves in remarkable accord with the beliefs of all peoples and ages. Of course, these beliefs and superstitions are now more important as arguments than the concept of modern child-psychology. But the surprising coincidence that our conception leads us to consider as important a definite process which has always been so considered would call attention to these popular medical usages, and stimulate the desire to study them more closely, even if they were contrary to science. It would then be time enough to examine a *priori* the expectations and to reduce them reasonably.

"The conviction of the significance of difficult dentition as the cause of a number of more or less dangerous child sicknesses is very deeply rooted among the masses." (Hovorka). How much this is feared can be seen from the numerous conscientious and strict remedies which vary greatly among peoples, and which are found in some form among all, and which aim at making teething easy, painless, and safe. Among the Bavarians (Hovorka): "The yellow blossoms of the barberry-bush (*Berberis vulgaris*) are first sewed into a linen bag, then sewed with red silk thread into a large red silk bag. All the sewing materials, needle, thread as well as the blossoms, must be put together into a special box. The sewed-up bag is hung around the teething child's neck, and is changed every four weeks on the same day of the month and the same hour. The pendant must never be removed from the neck—not even during the bath—and must hang down the back. The old bag must be burned immediately while the *Pater Noster* is being repeated three times. Should one forget to take the bag off on the appointed day it must then be left hanging until four weeks have gone by and only then can it be renewed in the manner described."

Long before teething threatens the infant it is already prophylactically fought. Thus in Franconia during baptism the midwife secretly dips her finger into the baptismal water and rubs the infant's gums in order to make later teething easier; in Prussia, the father during childbirth places a pail of water near him, puts his finger into the child's mouth, and then dips this finger into the water, saying: "Pain into the ground!" (this is done three times); while in Hessia on the wedding day itself the mother must think of the future teething of the future child and must preserve three crumbs of bread from the first meal in the new dwelling with which she will silently stroke the gums of the teething child. Sympathetic magic contrivances and amulets are numerous. Among these the mouse is most frequently resorted to in various ways as a specific remedy against dentition dangers of children: thus in Styria (Hovorka): "When the papillae swell, the mother should bite off the head of a live mouse and hang it around the child's neck"; while in Mecklenburg (Hovorka): "If one draws a linen thread through both eyes of a living mouse, and then lets it go, and if one then binds the bloody thread around the neck of the new-born, it will teeth easily."

These proofs of remarkable and complicated customs give us little hope of easily unravelling them, and it remains questionable whether it would offer child-psychology anything of importance if they were elucidated. But since the programme of this book bestows some attention on the customs of civilizations, and since dentition customs are certainly within our field, I have considered them more closely, knowing full well that we can do no more than enumerate them, and then be compelled to return without help from folk-psychology to child-psychology.

The notes of explorers collected by Hovorka and Ploss (2) show us the extraordinary extension of closely similar customs among people geographically, linguistically, anthropologically and culturally, completely different. If we seek a principle for ordering the material, the degree of rationality adhering to the custom presents itself—that is, how far we find it simply rational upon adapting ourselves to the assumptions underlying it.

We understand most easily those groups of customs which are adapted to the conditions of the physiological-psychological nature of dentition, or those which in a rational way tend to minimize the pain of the teething. To these belong the pacifiers of various materials and designs, wolf, boar, or dog teeth; these are put into a setting and hung on the child's neck, so that the child may bite and rub its painful gums on them. To these also belong those soothing palliatives which, according to Dioscuri, the Romans used; they soothed the itch with honey and butter (Hovorka). All such remedies give support to the childish instinctual activities that set in as soon as the child has acquired an object suitable for biting and rubbing.

We are not surprised that the mother rejoices over the child's teething, for it is a new sign of a healthy progress in development. An indication of this attitude is the felicitation of the Maronite mother with the repeated formula: " Its tooth has appeared, may his mother be rejoiced " (Ploss 2). The bestowal of gifts upon the teething child which is customary among the old Germans is comprehensible in this connection. In the same way the symbolic content of this event, the beginning of puberty, becomes one of the important festive occasions for the tribe, as for instance among the Bataks in Sumatra (Hovorka). The joy may be diminished by the thought that soon the vigorous imbiber at nature's source will become an equally vigorous eater for whom the means of sustenance must be provided by labour. Thus the Fellah wife in Palestine greets the event somewhat ambivalently: " Its teeth are out, hide the bread in the house."

The importance ascribed to teething, which is proved by the mere existence of these customs, regardless of their content, certainly has its root in the significant rôle which teeth play in the unconscious mental life. We cannot follow up this significance here. Psycho-analysis of dreams and neuroses proves it of existing peoples, as well as of the puberty rites, of the mutilation of the teeth and the pride in pretty teeth among primitive peoples. Part of the cares which superstition and custom seek to banish relate to the wish that the child should grow strong, pretty, and sharp teeth, similar to those of the wolf, boar, and the mouse. Thus the Maori mother of New Zealand, wishing her child to have teeth like a rat's, sings during teething (Ploss 2):

> " Sprouting, kernel, sprout,
> Sprout, that you may
> See the world complete !
> Come, you sprouting kernel,
> May the teeth of men
> Be given to the rats,
> And the rats' teeth
> To men !"

The rituals on which we dwelt at some length at the beginning are a warning to us not to trust the rational content of even the most seemingly simple and transparent customs. Biting rings, wolf's teeth, and similar contrivances have, for example, not only their rational ritual content, but they are simultaneously charms, spells, sympathetic mediums. They are not now simultaneously all these things, but they were so originally and previously. This is seen in the fact that very often they are hung around the child's neck before they can have any rational purpose, and that among some peoples they are not intended for this use, but are placed under the child's pillow, or on the side of the cradle, etc.

And, in conclusion, objects which are completely unsuited to their rational purpose are used no less frequently as charms quite in the same way as wolves' teeth. In Bavaria and Austria, the seed of the peony, called the "pearl tooth" (Ploss, 7), is very much beloved and preferred, because its seed pad is conspicuously like a tooth with roots, although it cannot be used for biting. It is not surprising that a deeper stratum animated by thoughts of demons, charms, and magic art is hidden behind the rational façade of all these customs and rituals. For this is so in all fields of folk-lore, and it is therefore impossible to interpret and explain an isolated group of customs detached from its background and native soil. But since we do not wish to go into the history of civilization here, and since the teething rituals interest us not as proofs of the belief in demons, but as symptoms by means of which we wish to make comprehensible the unconscious or unexpressed attitudes of the adult world toward childhood—and that means studying closely the history of civilization of childhood—we will be satisfied with this general reference, this reminder. It calls our attention to the fact that the demons in this case too are projections of unconscious wishes (Freud, 14), that the worry concerning the fate of the teething child that possesses the adults is a protection against their aggressive tendencies towards this child, which is treated so solicitously and sympathetically. We have had to make similar assumptions in the methods of child-rearing. It would be well to illustrate aphoristically the unfamiliar ideas which recur here.

In some respects this material is fortunately very accommodating. The expressions of anxiety seem contradictory to the parents' wish that the child should have strong animal-like teeth, and to the joy over the first signs of approaching independence and maturity. The old Hindus valued the dentition period as an especially important one in the life of the child. The following hymn (from *Avesta*) shows us that this period derived its importance from the psyche of the parents, from the psyche of the adult members of society (Ploss, 2):

" They, having become large, wish to eat the tiger-like father and mother, make both these teeth, Brhaspati, beautiful. O Jata vedas.

" Eat rice, eat barley, eat beans and sesame: that is the food for you both, do not injure father or mother.

" We call to both teeth united to be mild and bring joy; teeth, turn your ferocity elsewhere: do not injure father or mother."

The German custom of giving teeth as gifts can be understood from this as a *captatio benevolentiæ* and not merely as an expression of excessive joy.   When the negroes of Jamaica request the gift from the child, " so that the teeth shall not rot," one thinks almost immediately that the gift is intended as a compensation for envy.   The latent fear of the future use of the infant's teeth which are just breaking through, the latent feeling of uneasiness which attaches itself to the child, becomes most easily when something contrary to the rule occurs in the course of teething.   Many tribes therefore fear evil from those children whose upper incisors erupt before the lower ones.   This evil is two-fold.   In Uganda when this happens they are afraid either that something will happen to the child, and the magician is immediately called and the child is protected by the performance of certain dances, or that something will happen to the relatives, in this case the evil striking the child itself afterwards: among many tribesmen, the child is instantly and relentlessly killed (*e.g.*, in Mkulwe, German East Africa).   " If my mother knew when my first teeth would cut through, then she would prepare a shroud in readiness for me," is the proverb among the Maronites in Lebanon, which refers to the physiological dangers, and seems simultaneously in this connection to indicate the aggressive tendencies of the parents.   A residue of this weird idea about irregularity still exists in sections of Germany, so that in Berne when the child's teeth grow with a broad space between them, it indicates that the child will travel far (Ploss, 2).

The uneasiness which is released in the primitive mental life (and in deeper levels of the so-called cultivated mental life) by the phenomenon, child, may be mixed with fear of retaliation and repressed aggression, both of which are based on the identification with the child; the ego defends itself against this identification as against a dangerous regressive tendency. The *Avesta* hymn expresses a good part of this tendency. Here utterance is given to the fear that the child will devour its parents—which is a projection of a wish (deeply repressed) on the part of the parents to devour the child, and also a " recollection," as it were, of their cannibalistic tendencies as children against their own parents, whose place they now occupy. The theme of this book makes it necessary to con-dense these references and present them merely in passing, with difficulty, obscurely and inconclusively.

Thus we would rather emphasize the impression of the existence of one factor, aggression, by showing that a large group of specific tooth customs become comprehensible from this factor; they are those in which the mouse plays a part. These customs have remained very puzzling, although they are very frequent, and are found among completely different peoples. The fact that the mouse is a holy animal does not explain its relation to teething, since there are many other holy animals. That its sharp and destructive teeth are desired for the child leads us a little further, but it is still in the sphere of the rational, of the rationalized. This wish, however, contains an easy and partial identification, child —mouse. But this comparison, still detectable in the rationalization, has its cause and probability in a far-reaching identification between child and mouse, which psycho-analysis can prove to be a very common one. " Little animal " is a pet name for a small child; the infant is often enough called " mousie." The formation of this symbol, whose *tertium comparationis* cannot be the element of smallness only, is certainly complicated enough, and by no means completely fathomed. But one line of thought connects mouse—penis— child, another one may refer to the ground (or its substitute), mother earth; invisible in the mother's body as the haunt of the mouse: with the corollaries which lead from earth, fæces, child—penis (Freud, 3). A third will, in conclusion, be con-nected with the mouse-hole, from which the mouse suddenly jumps, into which he disappears again, as symbols for birth and general regression (Rank). If the mouse can represent the child in the *unconscious*, then a ray of bright light is shed on the significance of the mouse during dentition. The main tendencies are acts of violence against the mouse; there are others besides those already mentioned—mother or father biting off the head of a mouse, of a live one, and knocking out its teeth. Hanging a mouse's head around the teething child's neck may indeed protect it little from pain and may not be a comfort in its teething sicknesses, but we can easily understand that it actually does protect the child from death; for the aggression of the parents has been transferred to the poor mouse, has been expressed and therefore loving care and sheltered rearing remains for the child.

Some other considerations should not remain completely unmentioned. We learn from the anticipation of the puberty rites during the teething rituals, that the castration wish of the adult is already directed against the teething child. The mouse head, the teeth of rabbits, wolves and dogs may have this unconscious significance. And at the some time the tooth, the child's as well as the animal's, may symbolically represent the child: for it grows buried in the dark hollow, and suddenly breaks into the light accompanied by pain. What part the various aggressive aims may play in the ritual cannot be determined in detail—certainly not without comprehensive conscientious investigation; but they become very conspicuous: castration, killing, and perhaps also killing by eating up (oral annihilation). As soon as the child's teeth, the tools for its future oral annihilation, castration, and cannibalism begin to grow, the aggressive aims become overpoweringly actualized for the child, so that the preventive measure, assurances, distortions, symbolization, and repression become necessary.

We have come to the same conclusions as in the attempt at analyzing the forms of child-rearing into their *unconscious* "content." It can easily be understood how the father—that is, the masculine element in society—would be made responsible for the aggressions against the teething child. But this is not possible; it is more likely that the mother plays a part in this aggression also (*e.g.*, when she gives the present, and when she has to bite off the head of the mouse); but this, too, is not definitely determinable from the material, since it came to me second-hand. The problem must, therefore, remain unsolved. We shall, moreover, recognize motives in weaning which also make intelligible this aggression of the mother.

Last but not least we have concerned ourselves in such detail with these customs because we suspect in them a kind of age-long introspection, which might be a source—if we could only deciper them—of the mental life of the child which lies beyond the threshold of repression. And we are not disappointed. It is as if all these customs said: with the first tooth the original sin arose in me; teething is the epoch between two periods, the harmless infant period in which, peacefully in harmony with nature and society, I had no wishes which could bring me into conflict, and the early childhood period following upon infancy, in which instincts of conquering and murdering wildly dominated me, so that I and the world became enemies that fought each other, and I was beast and cannibal. But simultaneously with this viewpoint the study of rituals warns us against assuming that great pains, revolutions, and dangers, etc., are connected with dentition; they are, so to say, phantasies, which have their psychic and social functions, but need not have any objective content.

Why, then, are the diaries of child-psychologists in complete contradiction with former introspection? Why do they not show any new infant reactions immediately after the eruption of the first tooth? This question is raised only in order to give a self-evident fact direct emphasis, because the first tooth has only the claim to symbolic value as the beginning of an essential change. The ability to bite, the incentive to give up sucking, or the inducement to limit it considerably, or modify it, is not due to the first tooth but to a number of them—of course, to an undetermined number. But if we accept the first tooth as the symbol of the fourth quarter of the first year, then indeed alterations which the diaries clearly show take place simultaneously with it. We have already spoken of them and will later elaborate them.

But if we examine more closely the phenomena coinciding with teething in the first period, the following results:

First of all the transformation from the hitherto existing forms of behaviour (sucking) to the new one (chewing), does not occur suddenly. A series of small thrusts, one might say, advance the development unnoticeably. The process which begins with the eruption of the first tooth is in principle ended only with the eruption of the second upper incisor, and only at this time does actual biting and chewing become possible. This addition of small thrusts is, as we have often found, not an increasing but a weakening of the psychic injury. The transition to the new form can therefore be consummated without symptoms evident to the observer; indeed, the symptoms which are observed are unrecognized as having any relation to teething and to the alterations accompanying it. A slight indisposition, for example, is confirmed, but whether it has another significance for the later development cannot be decided. This applies not only to the manifestations which can perhaps be ascribed to the resultant effects of teething, but also, even to a greater extent, to many phenomena, which will later claim our attention in connection with weaning.

Indisposition, pain, fever—all these generally in a very mild form and of short duration—are as a rule processes accompanying teething. It is not difficult to reconcile them with the views presented. We as yet know very little, and nothing positively, about the psychology of pain, and it is not necessary for me here to elaborate in passing the complicated problem; but one fact, and one which is very important for our inference, is not contradicted: pain imperatively draws all the available attention to itself: " The soul lives alone in the narrow cavity of the molar tooth," says the profound psychologist, Busch, concerning the prototype of pain—teething pains. The cathectic energy is concentrated in considerable quantities on the system causing pain, and the libidinal cathexis is correspondingly removed from the rest of the world (" even long-standing love grows rusty "—during a toothache). On the other hand, there is no better remedy for a toothache than the withdrawal of this cathexis from the painful system—but unfortunately this contradictory case seldom comes to pass. The teething child behaves throughout as anyone else suffering from pain: it is restless and above all irritable; its relations to the *outer-world* are disturbed, and small interference is sufficient to withdraw the cathexis from the object, whether it be mother, ball, or its own body, and to direct it to the pain. The restlessness becomes motor which is always the case when an established way of gratifying a need does not attain its aim. Of course there is no other aim than to remove the pain, thus it is an *R*.-instinct reaction. Moreover, hunger is the prototype of all pain. The motor unrest finally accumulates to the point of crying and weeping, the primitive, universal activity. All in all the behaviour during pain signifies a regression to ways of behaving previously abandoned. The adult, too, cries, weeps, and behaves inexpediently and irrationally; un-teachable in such a case, he regresses just as the infant does to the stage of the new-born. During teething this condition is aggravated. For other pains the infant has at its disposal the consolation of the oral zone, pleasure-sucking " diverts it "; the cathexis of the oral zone minimizes the cathexis and in-tensity of the pain. And now the pain adheres to this very zone. Here is given the actual condition which we must call disappointment. The objective facts of disappointment are, so to speak, given, regardless of how the child considers it. But we have no reason for not assuming that the child experiences this event as a kind of primal disappointment. And it experiences this primal disappointment in these months several times in close succession in the same place. In the average case this will result in the child's dislike of this dis-appointing object, to a certain extent in the withdrawal of libido from this zone. In any case this is the normal course: that is, the norm which is required as normal, independent of the empirical percentage it represents. For the maxilla are not permanently erotogenic zones; they will soon have no capacity for offering ' pleasure,' they will soon have to give up their function in the service of the sexual instinct completely to the R.-instincts, the satiation of hunger.

The alternative fate of the freed libido is formulated simply enough: it will be bound to the skin, the lips, or another zone, or to the nascent ego. Instances, which can be interpreted according to one or other of these alternatives, are known. Kissing learned during the later infancy period, and the new intensity of articulation during speaking, or its preliminary stages, indicate new quantities of libido bound to the skin portion of the oral zone. The strengthening of the ego, which we see at this time in " mastery," and which we shall later see in perception, shows that the second alternative is traversed. The sixth month has become known to us as the beginning of masturbation; as closely as modern methods of observation allow us to expect, decrease of eroticization of one zone coincides with the increase of the other. The disappointment in the oral zone helps towards its partial desexualization. Perhaps this is merely a convenient literary turn, but it may also contain some information; in any case there is no contradiction of the facts in the formulation that this zone, desexualized by disappointment, becomes the primary carrier of hate—of the annihilation of objects.

Fever which accompanies teething is rightly and prudently perceived at this time as a purely physiological process. Nevertheless, Deutsch's investigations encourage us to mention another possibility. The fever will perhaps later be attributed to mental manifestations. Should this prove to be valid, it would be intelligible. We are familiar with the very puzzling transitory fever of the new-born; it is not dissimilar to teething fever (sc. B. Reuss). In so far as the latter or the former fever is psychogenic, it should be designated as a regressive manifestation.

The spitting of the teething child due to the increased secretion of the salivary glands which starts during the dentition period and which soon becomes a favourite sport of the child along with the use of the biting ring, finger and all other objects suitable for alleviating pain, can be better discussed under biting and chewing.

2. *Biting and Chewing*

Children practise biting and chewing even with toothless gums. Preyer's son bit in the seventeenth week long before the first tooth; Dix's child also bit in the eighteenth week. Of course this biting is naturally nothing more than clamping the finger or other objects between the gums. That this occurs approximately at the time when the Magitot membrane recedes deserves some attention; if this is true—and it has so far not been confirmed by the literature—we should be confronted in the fourth month with a kind of preliminary teething-period, in which begins the first desexualization of the gums and a certain modification of intense sucking. But it is certain that these first biting exercises come at the time when the mouth begins to develop the function of mastery. In this sense biting is a more firm gripping, analogous to grasping with the hand. But it really becomes a frequent response only during teething; and only after teething does it become an equally productive and enthusiastic activity exercised on all objects which are adequate in any degree—just as sucking is exercised earlier and also simultaneously with biting. Kissing is usually learned toward the beginning of the second year of life. It evidently must be learned as a moderation of biting; for it is not an instinctual activity but apparently learned and used to please the beloved persons, who coax for it in place of the impulsive biting which they forbid. This is a typical instance of the reduction of an activity of the instinct of mastery (an aggression) to an expression of tenderness.

Chewing begins even earlier; Dix noticed it in the second month and the eleventh week; Preyer also saw it " before the first tooth." The real stimulus for chewing as well as for biting is given when teeth begin. The chewing mechanism is obviously innate. But since it has not been studied in detail, it cannot unfortunately be recognized exactly. Above all, nothing is known about the relation of the chewing movements to sucking, and, on the other hand, of their relation to the releasing stimulus in the gums during and after dentition. Not even a vague impression can be established. It is as if at the beginning chewing served to overcome a disagreeable stimulus in the mouth, which cannot be or should not be removed either by spitting or swallowing. Preyer, too, seems to have this impression.

Nor has biting been studied any more closely than chewing. We see the completed act, and we must be resigned to our inexact knowledge of the relation between the biting process and the releasing stimulus, which, as is continually emphasized, is chiefly given for biting during dentition. Very soon chewing and biting pass wholly into the service of mastery. In particular they serve nourishment and in general the oral mastery of the world by annihilation and incorporation—in so far as the world permits it. And biting serves to protect its own body, as, for example, when the child on the defensive tries to bite its mother. We do not know the processes of this transformation. Of course, only the minutest details thus escape us; but they are nevertheless the processes existing during the loss of an erotogenic zone; and, indeed, the first loss of this kind which the child experiences. It would perhaps be worth while to describe them more carefully and positively than is possible at present. Nevertheless, this is not the most grievous hiatus in our factual knowledge which we—very unwillingly—have had to overlook.

The analogy with our losses later in life is astounding, almost ludicrous: displeasure increased to the point of pain takes the place of the pleasure which existed before. The child behaves toward this disappointing, this previously erotogenic, beloved and caressed part of its own body, in the same way as it will later behave or will want to behave towards objects in the outside world. It removes and annihilates them. It rubs and pushes (chews) them with the tongue and gums; it spits as if the gums, and the teeth, were a troublesome foreign body; it presses, rubs, pulls with its fingers; and finally bites. Of course in vain, for the irritation cannot be removed and the disappointment remains. It will behave in the same way throughout life, in anger and especially in emotions of powerless anger.

What makes the analogy so apt are the words, disappointment, annihilation, rage, etc. These words do not have for the infant the fulness of recollections, feelings, complicated intellectual and emotional processes which they have in later life. They denote very simple responses which are the crystallization points around which the later experiences organize, and which continuously carry back to the primal stages of the race.

The mouth, originally the seat of innately fixed responses that serve the R.-instincts, became during the first days of life in the performance of its nutritional function an erotogenic zone. The sexual function of the mouth assures, promotes, one might say, its vegetative function (R.-instinctual forces). It soon becomes the chief, the dominating erotogenic, zone. As such it becomes the promoter of the new responses of mastery, of the R.-instinctual· forces. Now it steps wholly into the service of the R.-instincts by the desexualization of its inner parts; the sexual function (sucking, kissing) remains bound peripherally. The libido is partially withdrawn and utilized otherwise; it is changed in part into katergy. The gums, originally objects of libidinal strivings, shortly become objects of hostile strivings and then the carriers of them. It is as if a process of projection had taken place; a kind of repression of the death-instincts from its own body into the *outer-world*, as Freud postulates for sadism. And actually, of course, oral sadism (cannibalism in its psycho-analytic meaning) is the most primitive form of sadism.

In the light of the oft-mentioned fusion of both instinct groups, it is not surprising that, in spite of all, the erotogenicity of the inner part of the mouth is partially retained, or that it is again acquired secondarily. This is frequent in pathological cases, and is also not infrequent in the realm of the normal. The former occurs in speech. It is not accidental that the decisive progress in the development of speech in the child falls within the dentition period. Speech is very closely related to oral sadism. It is an expulsion process which will only later become wholly clear in many details. In conclusion, as far as its motor process is concerned, it is merely an organizing of all those movements which we considered analogous to a sadistic treatment of the formerly erotogenic zone. What we call speech is a kind of chewing, spitting, rubbing, and crunching of the teeth and gums, with the tongue, teeth, and gums; and indeed a complicated and indefinite kind. Just as laughing and some mimical expressions are organized discharges of diffuse shock reactions, or defence phenomena, so speech is organized chewing, biting, gum, tooth and tongue movements.

A brief reference to a detail which has not wholly escaped any observer deserves mention. Biting of the painful spot (*i.e.*, pressing on it) is one of the devices which the child uses to moderate the pain during teething (usually slight). This can hardly appease the pain; on the contrary, it must increase it. We meet here a paradoxical form of behaviour, which has been insufficiently observed and which is universal. The adult, too, very frequently behaves in this way, particularly when he has a toothache. It is a strange pleasure that lies in this increase of pain. It is my impression that this pain receives its pleasurable character through the activity which the ego thereby displays. There is no doubt that early childhood has many such tendencies, and that the scratching of an itching irritation which the child even in the infant period carries to a point of bleeding belongs here, and that the sadistic tendencies directed against itself are the basis of this activity. One might call this masochism (Hug-Hellmuth) if one were less careful of one's terminology. In all these instances the erotogenic zones, or the former erotogenic zones, supply the " pleasure in pain." I know no reason for not considering the universal situation of the teething child as its nucleus, for it fits in quite well with what has been said. We shall find support for this concept in a later connection, but the complete darkness in which pain and "pleasure in pain " are enveloped prevents us from taking a definite stand.

An easily anticipated resistance to our point of view will be overcome in the following chapter. The reader will have sensed that the analogy is more serious for the author than for didactic reasons he wished to show.

To require the reader to regard as projections those processes which lead to biting and chewing, is to place no small strain upon his psycho-analytical allegiance. In connection with mastery the desexualization of arm musculature paralleled with repression, and now projection is called in. Philosophical and methodological objections to such procedure are plentiful. I believe one can rob them of some of their weight by the following considerations. Of course, repression and projection are concepts which were built on the mental processes in the current sense of the word. The ideas of libido and energy, which undoubtedly belong to the domain of the ego, were built up on the instincts.

Of course the processes which here interest us are more closely bound to the body. They are purely physical. They are phenomena easily accessible to physiology. In conclusion it should be repeatedly acknowledged that the application of psycho-analytical terms to organic processes may have its difficulties. But (1): Here only the erotogenic zones interest us. They are indeed parts of the body, but such parts which doubtless stand in some connection—it is unnecessary to be more precise—with psychic energy (with libido). They are at the limit of our field of view. (2) It must not be forgotten that the statements about the libido processes in the erotogenic zones give us nothing definite about the localization of these processes. I should be of the opinion, if I were forced to admit it, that real libido is found in real parts of the body, the erotogenic zones, and there undertakes and experiences real alterations; but I will not insist upon this view; there are others worthy of discussion. Both of these considered, it is very interesting to see that the unwinding and transformation of libido, which we credit to the most densely bound libido of the erotogenic zones, and which seem to be very similar to organ-libido, follow the same mechanisms as the more lightly bound libido which coalesces with the ego itself and on which Freud based his original idea. It too has repression and projection which, by the way, must be told directly only to pseudo-psycho-analysts. To be very exact in terminology, one might distinguish this from repression and projection as primal repression and primal projection. (What, then, really forces us to identify the terms primal repression and desexualization or to differentiate them ?[1]) Closer study of the organic pro-

[1] See Schilder's books.

cesses will soon teach us not only that the so-called Freudian mechanisms can be detected in the denser libido of erotogenic zones, but also that the biological courses follow them. With reservations, of course; but this need not concern us in child-psychology.

3. Taking the Child from the Breast

Our interest in the factors of weaning is not in the change in nutrition which is a medical dietary problem, but in the withdrawal of the breast in weaning. It is always a difficult event in the child's life, which is forced upon it from without. The child would hardly give up the breast voluntarily, at least not in the first year. Proof of this can be seen in the fact that, among those peoples who wean their children rather late, the mother's breast is taken gladly and regularly, even after other food is enjoyed, and even when the child helps to obtain and prepare it. This is easily understood; the conservative tendency in the mental life does not reach out gladly for new modes of behaviour, certainly not when there is no urgent motive; surely not when the old modes of behaviour are bound up with such deep and varied pleasure as is sucking the mother's breast. Before beginning this special presentation one must clarify a point of view that in colloquial usage is prejudiced. Suckling is not just a simple infant habit, and therefore giving up this activity, the central one of the first year, connected with many gratifying experiences, with a great variety of pleasurable experiences of considerable intensity, must be a psychic transposition of a deeper nature than the word weaning perhaps leads us to assume. The adult's attitude shows this clearly. The adult will experiences a repugnance, repudiation, occasionally even physical nausea at the unreasonable demand or the mere thought of enjoying milk from a woman's breast. This does not exist where a habit is given up, but where an instinctual impulse with reaction formation has been repressed—radically and fundamentally repressed. We may therefore expect to learn something about the origin of early repression as a by-product of the study of weaning which is prescribed for us within the scope of infant-psychology. To be sure a glance at the literature of child-psychology unfortunately reduces our expectation considerably. Whether the manifestations have escaped the observers, or whether they belong in that category which is consummated without important symptoms or expressions, the authors of comprehensive works have taken no notice at all of weaning. Authors of child-psychological diaries mention it only very sparingly and inexactly. Relatively speaking, the most detailed communication—aphoristically and not sufficiently thorough—that of Scupin is also limited in its value, because Bubi became sick with measles not quite two weeks after the beginning of weaning. His bad humour was thus influenced by his latent sickness. Nevertheless, Scupin's observations agree with the experience of doctors, mothers, and nurses.

The observations indicate that the child at first refuses the new nourishment more or less vigorously and consistently; it refuses above all the new method of feeding (bottle, spoon, cup, etc.). Only after much crying, fighting, and hunger does he compromise with the new method. There are many and varied indications which show that the child hankers for the mother's breast; thus Bubi tugs at his mother's blouse as if he wanted to open it. Such actions are sometimes actually carried out, even when in other respects the new method of feeding is accepted. Thumb-sucking is carried on with renewed intensity. In general the child appears restless, irritable, ill-humoured; he falls easily into fits of crying, occasionally is in a state which cannot be described better than by the words depressed and sad.

It can be seen that child-psychology tells us very little about this important incision in the child's mode of life; science tells us nothing, nothing that extends beyond our general knowledge. Before we begin a closer discussion of these findings, and before we supplement them by questions; before we complete the gaps by assumptions, or stimulate new investigations—we wish to gather in this case, too, apperceptive impressions from the age-long introspection which is preserved in ethnic customs. We feel impelled into this new venture beyond the boundaries of child-psychology by a new reinforcing motive. Taking the child from the breast is an event, the nature and time of which is determined wholly by society. It is the first of an endless chain of conscious interventions in the child's development on the part of the environment, which will be treated in a separate volume. After this intervention we no longer deal in the further mental development of the child with manifestations which can be related to the individual and merely to the individual mental functioning; but each manifestation is in the future to be understood, firstly, absolutely as the product of two different, although not always antithetical, series: First, the individual mental reactions developing from inheritance and from general immanent mental laws; second, the environment operating actively through its aims, values, and attitudes. We must know this environment in order not to overlook most of its influences, which are often exercised surreptitiously, in order to be able to evaluate the consequences of the influences. Of course, the infant lives in an environment to which we have made occasional reference, and which we will summarize in the next chapter. But the environment is passive for the child adapting itself to the infant's needs. In fact, birth was a heteronomous intervention in the fœtal situation; but it meets the undeveloped autonomy of the infant and is a biological force. Weaning is the first social force which opposes it heteronomously without destroying, drowning or killing it.

It is very striking that in the beginning of our study of the customs with which we are about to interest ourselves for a while, we notice that the time of weaning among various peoples ranges over several years. We have, indeed, often seen great differences in the behaviour of isolated peoples, but they were related to the details of the customs, not to the time element. Weaning is, as we can see from this fact alone, largely a social convenience which is independent of biological and individual-psychological points of time, which in child-rearing otherwise settle the immovable boundaries within which the social and social-physical motive can be freely accomplished. There is in early childhood no moment in which—in the normal individual psychic course—an aversion, to say nothing of nausea, occurs from hitherto customary feeding on the mother's breast, so that the infant spontaneously gives it up. In this question we see that children follow exactly the habits of their progenitors and that these habits do not come from a knowledge of the biological, physiological, or psychological situation.

And indeed the variation between the earliest and latest weaning time as found in the observation of ethnographers is incredibly great. Bartels has given a survey which we will make use of here because of its comprehensive nature (Hovorka). "The children are breast-fed: Less than one year by the educated classes of Europe, the Samoans, Kuloschan,

Tlingit Indians, Mayas Indians (Ecuador), Hottentots. One year by the Bugis and Macassars (Celebes), Gilan, Massawa. One and a half years among the Dacotahs, Sioux, Loango Negroes, Tamenbar and Timor Laut Islanders, Parsis. One to two years among the Armenians, Tartars in Erivan, Esthonians, ancient Romans, mediæval Germans, Karakirgiz, Waheli. Two years among the Persians, Nayar, Tshud, Aeta (Philippines), Ruchuru Islanders, Russians in Astrakhan, Turks in Fezzan, in Morocco, in Egypt, in the Nile countries, Mandi, Uganda, Wakimbu, Wanyamwezi, in East Africa, among the ancient Peruvians (also ordered by the *Koran* and *Avicenna*). Two to three years among the Australians, in China, in Japan, in Laos, in Siam, among the Armenians, Kalmuks, Tartars, in Syria, Palestine, Abyssinia, or on the Canary Islands, among the Kamerun, Mandingo Negroes, Old Calabar, Basutos, Makalaka, Tlingit Indians, Apaches, Abipones (Paraguay), Sweden, Norway, Styria. Three years among the Luongo and Sermata Islanders, among the ancient Jews. Two to four years among the Pennsylvania Indians, in Lapland. Three to four years in Greenland, among the Warrau Indians, Kamtshatka, Mongolians, in Madras, Kabyles, Naples. Three to five years among the Kanikar, Japanese, many Brazilian Indians, Ostyaks, Samoa, Palestine. Four to five years among the Serbs, Indians in Oregon, in California, in Canada, Maravi, Australia, New Caledonia, Hawaii, among the Kalmuks and on the Gulf of Guinea. Five to six years among the Samoyeds, the Fellah in Palestine. Six years among the Australians, in New Zealand. Six to seven years among the Indians of North America, in Canada, among the Armenians (Kuban). Seven years among the Eskimos (Smith Sound). Ten years among the North American Indians. Fourteen to fifteen years among the Eskimos (King William Land)." A glance at this tabulation shows that the decisive determinant for the behaviour even in this case cannot be the height of cultural development and the degree of medical insight, because the educated classes in Europe behave like the Samoans and Hottentots; and the Chinese and Japanese like the Eskimos and Indians.

One must not draw a false conclusion from the fact itself. Of course, there is no question but that the same conditions are covered by this citation of the time of weaning. Extremely late weaning is covered only by occasional observations, and does not indicate that among these people the child is nourished exclusively on the mother's breast; on the contrary, we are only concerned with the fact that the five, eight, or even ten and twelve year old child is permitted to imbibe at the mother's breast. These people differ from others, from the Europeans of the educated classes, only because they do not consider it counter to their good morals to permit the older child to partake of a drink during the youngest child's feeding time. Thus, for example, it is observed among the Motu, '' that often an older and the youngest child fight for the breast, thus weighing it down. The children are not weaned. They wean themselves whenever they wish. Consequently it is not unusual if the children run to the breast '' Ploss (2). This freedom which the mother and child enjoy may become a wholly legitimate rule among some peoples as, for example, among the Japanese. One derives this impression from the remark of Ploss (2): '' The children wean themselves. Like a lamb in the herd, the little ' gamboller ' suddenly deserts its playmates and, standing or kneeling, takes a few vigorous drinks at its mother's breast, which is never refused him.'' And the impression is strengthened when one notices that the Japanese speak of the use of the woman's breast (milk) by the adult more frequently than is customary among us (Ploss, 1). These peoples have not imposed repression upon sucking, nursing, mother's breast. They have no repulsion, no nausea, for the idea or act. They do not force this repression in their children. In general, the child is not taken away from the breast. On the contrary, along with the food which is tendered to it at a certain time—sometimes very early (e.g., German East Africa, after the third day, (Ploss, 2)—it continues to suck the breast as long as it wants to; until it voluntarily gives it up. This obviously never happens at the end of the first year. of life, but in the course of childhood—at the latest, at the beginning of puberty. Till then it enjoys the breast according to its opportunity and inclination. Here, as Ploss (1) and Franke expressly remark, the individual factors in the mother and child are the deciding ones. We need not consider the motive and nature of the disinterest occurring spontaneously in the mother and child; they belong to a later age, and can be understood from this mental situation and the social attitude.[1]

[1] One should not over-estimate the difference between these races and us. I myself have observed in a public park in Vienna a nursing mother offer her other breast to a boy who was perhaps six or seven years old.

Even among those who do not as a rule undertake weaning it is sometimes necessary for personal reasons, as when the lactation is insufficient, and probably when a new child is born. Among some people this is usually the end of the nursing period for the older child; but among others one can imagine that while the younger child is still cared for, the older child does not experience complete privation of the breast, although it nevertheless gets it more infrequently and for a shorter time if the quantity of milk is not sufficient for both children. Cases are reported in which the third born during the suckling period is killed (Bushman, Kalahari) (Ploss, 1). Some non-weaning peoples have the custom of discontinuing the nursing of the child as soon as a new pregnancy occurs. Accordingly, one can say: many tribes permit the child to imbibe from the breast regularly until a new-born takes its place. Even then access to the breast is not completely denied the growing child. Occasionally the former is, of course, not permitted. This was forbidden among the ancient Jews, who used to nurse the child until the third year; the child once it was weaned was not given the breast again (Feldman); a similar custom prevailed among the Lithuanians (Ploss, 1).

Where this is the custom, the transition from regular to occasional nursing takes place from the second to the fourth year; but not in the first year, although there are exceptions. Giving up the breast is not a condition originating in the child's psychology in the first year, and must therefore be accomplished forcibly in a certain way. Where it is done there is no lack of superstitious methods to make it simple and safe for mother and child; rubbing the breast with bad-tasting substances, in order to spoil the child's appetite is an ancient and widespread custom. Explorers are in the habit of inquiring for the motives for the prolongation of the nursing period. Ploss (1), in agreement with other authors, cites the following motives: 1. The motherly tenderness and weakness toward the children. 2. And though, of course, this is incidental and only occasionally valid, "the mother's milk, even if bad and insufficient, nevertheless supplements nourishment and is therefore a pecuniary saving." This motive is certainly a consideration for many peoples and classes; but we may overlook it because it is certainly not a primary motive. 3. The mother's well-being, for "nursing decidedly calls forth pleasurable sensations in the mother." 4. "The extraordinary widespread assumption that as long as the mother nurses her child she can engage in coitus with impunity—namely, without becoming impregnated." Ploss (1) considers this the most important instinctual release. This is contradicted, however, firstly, by the fact that there are a number of races suckling their children for a long time, among whom sexual intercourse is forbidden during the suckling period; secondly, that this view is not valid, for it often enough happens among the peoples who suckle their children a long time that they simultaneously suckle several children varying in ages, or that customs exist which forbid this, and which are based on the correct knowledge that suckling in no way hinders impregnation. Such a notion, empirically false, cannot be the motive of a form of behaviour; it can, however, be maintained for a long time in a rationalization of this behaviour. I should interpret these beliefs thus: they cover the pleasure in suckling—hypocritically, one might say; they reduce the woman's need for coitus, impoverish her heterosexual strivings, and strengthen her auto-erotic, narcissistic gratification;[1] the rationalization veils this condition for the men and imputes to intercourse a nobler motive than really is the case.

But this means that long suckling needs no special motive. It offers so many delights for mother and child, pleasure in the narrowest sexual sense (passion), as well as sublimated bliss, that if the mother gives the child her breast as long as the physiological conditions permit, and if the child takes it as long as it is offered, this is to be understood as the natural state. That this relation ends before the mother grows old has its social (psycho-social) reasons for mother and child. Besides these there are perhaps psychic reasons, which we do not know, and which we need not inquire into in this book. Although the sexual motive—on the mother's part—would perhaps suffice as an explanation, it should not be forgotten, that the mother already has libidinal gratification in this most primitive of relations in the mother-sucking-child relation which is independent of the pleasure of the narrower breast zone. The mother loves her child with greater quantities of libido than is bound to the erotogenic zone. And this love, like all other love, aims at lavishing pleasure to make the beloved object happy. There is scarcely

[1] A psychologically profound proof perceived by Balzac in *Two Women*.

a situation in which the bestowed pleasure is so obvious, so completely accepted as by the suckling who peacefully falls asleep at the breast or greedily imbibes at it. The love for the child is here completely realized and is enjoyed doubly by the identification with the beloved object. It is the perfect return, the gratification of all regressive tendencies simultaneously with the gratification of pleasure strivings, both enjoyed in harmony with reality and with the demands and values which are in the *unconscious* and the *conscious* of the nursing mother, or can be if no opposing influence exists. This seems to be reason enough for holding to such a situation as long as possible. Man does not lack an intuitive understanding of this situation; he can, of course, only express it indirectly: in the adoration of the Madonna.

On the contrary, the problem lies in the ways in which suckling is cut short. Astonishingly enough the most primitive peoples, Samoans, Hottentots, as well as the most cultured, even specialist physicians, face this problem. One must *a priori* willingly assume that the motives for these groups are very different. And there are a series of facts which prove our measures to be objectively correct. At least this is asserted, and I do not gainsay it.

Let it, however, be conscientiously noted that whether or not we have recognized the facts conclusively, they are not beyond objection and doubt. The statements of physicians about the dietetic quality of the milk during a period of an extended lactation belong here. Surely the question of weaning is not one of the regulation of the quantity and quality of the milk but of the complete withdrawal of the breast; the quantity and quality can be regulated otherwise. Furthermore, it is cited as a fact that lactation ceases. But the instances of the peasant women of the proletariat of some neighbourhoods who used to suckle their children far beyond the time recommended by physicians, speaks to the contrary. Teething and the digestive capacity of the child's stomach point to the fourth quarter of the first year as the time for weaning. Both of these, along with appropriate nourishment, do not exclude regularly continued suckling. Of course, the economic conditions are not without their rational motivation. The under-nourished mother's milk will become increasingly worse than the wealthy mother's. But the duration of nursing does not run parallel to the economic situation. Poverty occasionally becomes a motive for long suckling; and the wealthy classes particularly abide by the requirements of the pediatrist dietician. But with all that I do not wish to be arrogant in deciding about the objective validity of rationalization. I only wish to show that we need not be so impressed that we neglect to investigate its psychogenesis.

The fact that the mothers of the educated middle classes develop a common and extensive aversion from suckling in general applies above all to the psychic motivation of the behaviour of civilized nations; their inability to suckle the child is very commonly given as a reason, and this perhaps in part arises from these psychic causes. This fact cannot be explained yet; for first of all a careful, comparative confirmation of the fact itself is still lacking. It is, of course, based on the complicated alterations which the feminine mind in the ruling classes of society undergoes, alterations which at present we sense rather than know, but indications of which—in the relations under consideration here—are based on the changed attitude toward husband and child. The homosexuality of women seems to unfold more dominantly in this civilization, shifting the important accent from Weininger's mother-type to the prostitute type.[1] The breasts as an erotogenic zone will undergo by this displacement a very changed rôle which is indicated by the woman's justified worry that, by suckling, her breasts become disfigured. And the attitude to the child undergoes a still greater change, for the child is brought up with greater ambivalence, if not with open repudiation. The specific feminine situation of the nursing mother is repudiated —this situation produces unconsciously the much-lamented cessation of lactation—because the dominating direction of the sexual life of the woman is displaced by an identification with the father and not with the mother. This type of woman will try to dispense with suckling; a wet nurse and artificial feeding are the most usual substitutes. But when they do feed the child, suckling becomes the source of conflicts which in any case, however else they run their course in other respects, will tend toward the quickest possible shortening of the task. As individual phenomenon there are such women

---

[1] It is perhaps not entirely superfluous for me to stress that the use of this word is not intended discourteously, but merely as a convenient term which abbreviates very complicated actualities completely independent of Weininger's psychology, and moreover, if possible, of his evaluation.

in all civilizations, among all nations, classes, and strata of society. But it seems to have become the dominating type which makes custom and rationalization, to have become the norm, only in certain relatively infrequent and complex civilized ruling classes.

The discussion must lose much of its plausibility when we remember that the Samoans and Hottentots behave in this respect like races " which are very far advanced." Shall one assume the same complicated psychic conditions among them ? I think it would lead to difficulties. We know little about their attitude towards children. But some details are reported of the Samoans which offer us a point of support for the speculation—I repeat, that this is not meant discourteously, but only provocatively. Thus we learn from Ploss (2): " Weaning usually takes place in the fourth month if the father has no special instruction from the family god that nursing must be continued. If the father receives instructions, then the child prospers excellently and receives the title ' banana of God.' " This is significant enough. It teaches us perhaps that the insufficient duration of suckling is effected despite their knowledge of its harmfulness; that this attitude emanates from the men; and that it needs a compensation. Woe be, if the children are allowed to develop robustly (into a banana of God). The possibility of listing this behaviour among the established and accepted facts above is the result of this meagre report. The men fear their progeny; they keep them weak—to a certain point; they venture robust children (unified in love with the mother) only when a special protective relation to the Divinity is established. (The women in extreme capitalistic societies obviously act as men in this respect.)

I cannot assert that the study of all these customs has helped us at all in our problem of child-psychology. On the contrary, we now find ourselves in a deluge of new problems. But that need not worry us. If, in the present state of psychology on the road to theoretical condensation we succeed merely in stating problems, it is perhaps more useful than all the speculations which always have another and a lesser significance in psychology than they have for example in physics perhaps, or indeed in modern psychology which, as yet has grasped so little of the multifariousness of the phenomena. We console ourselves, therefore, the more easily with the value of stimulating further investigations, because the customs

—also independent of the constituents of their psychological knowledge—belong within the field of our efforts, and hold firmly to the one fact which resulted with striking clarity: weaning, undertaken in earliest infancy, is a frustration imposed upon the child from the *outer-world*, and contradicts the autonomous conditions and the phylogenetic path of development (presumably) previously indicated. The time recommended by modern pediatry moderates this heteronomy. Teething, which the infant usually undergoes towards the end of the first year, disposed it perhaps to some kind of compromise with this frustration; the infant is very cross with its oral zone which has disappointed it; it withdraws its libidinal cathexis. Perhaps from another angle a sympathetically effective tendency can also be assumed. The end of the first year is also the time in which—apparently spontaneously, autonomously—a certain " turning away " from the mother occurs: the child overcomes its anxiety of walking without protection, of walking alone, and it voluntarily goes away from the mother. And finally one reflects upon the fact that in the same month speech too progresses significantly. In any case, speaking offers a potentiality· for using oral libido; how far this potentiality is realized, to what degree and on the basis of what mechanism, has not been more clearly investigated.

Among our children the temporal coincidence of this phenomena is generally certain. It would be necessary to present weighty arguments if one were to refuse to see a relationship in this coincidence. Unfortunately at the present time one cannot decide how to co-ordinate these phenomena causally. We do not know anything about the exact time when children who are not weaned begin to walk and speak; we also know very little about the delicate structure of this phenomena of our children, and nothing about their reciprocal correlation.

In spite of moderations, everyone who is of the opinions presented in this book will estimate the profound effort of the frustration very highly, either from conviction or from well-disposed scientific curiosity; for it is indeed a radical frustration of the gratification of the infant's most powerful libido striving. This expectation is still further increased wherever possible, when we repeatedly find to our astonishment from analyses—one's own, and Starke's, Abraham's, Rank's—the rôle of weaning in the Ucs. system which cannot be overestimated. This expectation, apparently well-founded, is fully contradicted, it seems, by the experience in the infant. Of course, weaning manifests itself, but for such a short time and, in comparison with our expectations, so weakly, that we feel inclined to revise fundamentally the suppositions which led us to entertain unjustified expectations.

The available facts are scattered, acquired accidentally with insufficient exactness, and offer room for criticism in every respect. Nevertheless, these facts will be examined next. If we do this in the light of Scupin's reports reproduced above, there is no difficulty in understanding them from the economic viewpoint. We see the expressions of 'pain' which we understand and interpret as the unfulfilled gratification of an instinctual aim: the coveted breast is not attained. Crying, attempts corresponding to grasping and mastery, are undertaken. They do not attain their end. Substitutive-gratification is sought, pleasure-sucking, etc., and it does not lead to gratification. We will explain anxiety, restlessness, irritability, as symptoms of a greater quantity of libido, which cannot be bound, discharged, or satisfied because the instinctual aim cannot be attained. When we find ourselves in a similar situation we feel a yearning and behave like the infant. On the one hand, we are gripped by restlessness, and incline towards irritability and substitutive-gratification; but, on the other hand, a certain apathy takes possession of us. The reason for this is that a good part of our mental energy, of our libido, is turned to phantasy, to phantasy-gratification of our yearning, which may give us partial gratification. We see the same in the infant too; it, too, becomes, to a certain degree, apathetic— " sad," one might say, resigned. We do not, of course, know what takes place in it, because we can only infer its inner processes from its actions, and these particularly are not evident in this situation. We can do nothing but assume in it a process equivalent to our own. We shall yet have to bring forward certain conjectures about the imaginative life and its relation to the gratification of the instinct. Here the following assumption suffices: the libido directed at the frustrated gratification, which is withheld for an interval, turns immediately to wish-hallucination; it is not at the disposal of activities, new cathexes. The activities, the interest in everything in the *outer-world*, ceases for this time, or seems decreased, inconstant.

There is no objective difference between sorrow and longing. This difference exists only in experience; and only in one element: longing is hopeful, it has not given up its instinctual aim, it expects gratification at some future time; sorrow is without hope, it occurs when we are convinced that the object seen is unattainable, that the momentary frustration has become definite, has become a loss. It is characterized entirely by the cessation of the drive to activity, using a still greater quantity of energy much more consistently toward phantasy activity and toward certain transformations still little understood, the results of which we recognize as the overcoming of the loss, out of which an important mechanism has through Freud (7) attained for us a high degree of precision. In overcoming the loss, identification with the lost object plays a certain rôle.

Sorrow and longing are surely not differentiated in the infant. Both are very similar. Perhaps it seems to the infant when he has cried in vain for a half-hour that the breast is lost to it; but if after a short nap he sees the mother again the hopeful longing springs up anew. Romantic as it may be, there is no sense in projecting oneself into the infant's feelings, for we should learn nothing about the phenomenology of its life in that way. But we see the infant behave as if it would like to attain its instinctual aim, then again as if it has given it up. And indeed it takes a long time for it to make efforts to gratify its longing when it is hungry, or when it sees the mother or her breast, or is taken up into her arms, or in some other way is objectively placed in a previously gratifying situation. As far as I can see, varied individual differences underlie the child's concrete behaviour. In many children longing and sorrow are scarcely noticeable; others show an obvious mood which can be interpreted in this way, but it continues only for a short time; while others maintain it for a relatively long time. Occasionally this apathy goes so far as to refuse nourishment completely (Hochsinger). (It is interesting to see that all through life sorrow shows a tendency to refuse food.) We need not speak of this form of behaviour, since it produces the correct clinical picture, the nutritional neurosis (Hochsinger). But refusing food as such is usually indicative of trouble during weaning, and is really astonishing. It indicates in any case that the R.-instincts, which we consider responsible for all measures which serve the stilling of hunger, become to a great extent invested with libido. What the child strives for is not to obtain suitable nourishment, but to enjoy it in definite ways. This enjoyment has become part of the gratification situation. Indeed, this definite way seems foremost in the instinctual aim. The instinct is directed upon this gratification situation, so that the odour of milk, for example, as familiar as it may be, does not act as an incentive towards drinking when offered in the bottle. But here the relationships are very obscure. For we still do not know whether the behaviour of children who have had additional nourishment before weaning, and those who received for the first time at weaning food other than the mother's breast, can be differentiated.

It is noteworthy that the weaning in certain instances is not consummated smoothly; that in these cases this is the beginning of a mental development, so different from the normal that we must call it pathological. Our knowledge of the possibilities of individual variations is so small, that any statement about it is particularly rash. Perhaps there are some stages of development already in the first year at which a number of individuals remain fixed. We do not know; psychopathology gives us no information. And even more worthy of note is the fact that weaning is the first obvious cause which can be established and from which pathological mental development branches off—those nutritional neuroses which in extreme cases continue up to puberty, and which, in all cases, are contributory factors to the predisposition to neurosis. Thus weaning can occasionally become a psychic trauma. That means that the psychic situation in which frustration takes place, and the latter itself make demands on the plasticity of the instincts which cannot always be fully met.

But in general—particularly in so-called normal cases—these demands are quickly and well controlled. We see the child after a relatively short time free from irritability, apathy, etc. We do not see it behave either at the sight of its mother's breast or during a meal as though it recalled any consequence of the alterations in the form of nourishment. Ultimately we see it exercising the new activity, apparently libidinal, and we hardly ever find that the mother's breast is an especially preferable instinctual aim.

We are accustomed—rightly—to estimate the intensity of

a mental impression according to the duration and extent of its after-effects. It seems to us that the facts force us to say: if weaning creates a state at all similar to sorrow, it is a short and mild form of sorrow. And this necessitates the statement that the mother's breast is not an important aim of the sexual instinct, and that the libidinal components are not present at all, or only to a small degree, in the oral activity. All this applies at least to the normal case; it is generally valid.

I do not believe that this in any way strains the facts, insufficient as they are. One can perhaps explain them thus if they are approached with a definite presupposition. One need not, however, interpret them so if one does not agree with these suppositions, nor with the angle from which they are approached. The facts are even more ambiguous, for we do not as yet know the determining factors. After a little reflection we come to the conclusion that the consequences of weaning, of frustration in general perhaps, when these are present, must lie in the field of the phantasy life. The mental processes which we call frustration, longing, sorrow, overcoming of sorrow, loss, resignation, cannot be objectively confirmed. They show themselves ambiguously and incompletely, or tardily and indirectly, after they have run their course. Moreover, the mechanisms, repression and identification, which are active according to psycho-analysis, work noiselessly during this overcoming, and as processes are imperceptible and only recognized when consummated. This means that a conclusion about the extent of the effects of weaning will have to be drawn from an intimate knowledge of the child's reaction to its world and its activities, which are the expressions of its phantasy life, or at least are the nucleus of it. The next division presents the material for such judgment; we must therefore delay the conclusion of this chapter till the end of the book.

We will indicate here only one factor, with the aid of which we may perhaps foresee the geometric point from which, as it were, the understanding of weaning is to be concluded. Out of the profusion of alterations which the child's reactions to the *outer-world* at the end of the first year reveal coincident with the consummated weaning, one is especially obtrusive. The child discovers a remarkable game, described by Dix as follows: " At five months he apparently accidentally throws his rattle out of the carriage. He was much surprised at its disappearance and the ensuing noise, for I saw that he looked, inquiringly, with open mouth in astonishment. But he was helpless in the situation. He did not know where to turn. And several days later I noted that he threw everything out and looked after the fallen objects. At six months he continued this exercise, which became his favourite game at this time. An advance . . . was also observed: he held the object far out over the carriage, bent after it, let it fall, and looked fixedly for it. At nine months he was indefatigable in ' throwing ' things out." If the child discovers this game earlier, either by accident or by looking for the source of the sound, the game acquires new intensity and significance during weaning. If we try to relate this game to weaning, if we recall Freud's (9) ingenious paragraphs citing a similar game, of a somewhat older child, and of all that is scattered throughout this chapter, we get this insight: a spontaneous, rhythmic repetition, changing the passive form into an active form, as a method of mastering the trauma. The child has ceased to be an infant, it begins to be grown up; it has learned to separate itself from objects instead of desiring to incorporate them all into its body (orally, or by pressure); it has gained a world, a something separated from itself. But perhaps this is only an idea which cannot be proven.

E. THE INFANT AND ITS WORLD

BODY-EGO AND THE OUTER-WORLD

THE undertaking, which we have imposed upon ourselves in this book, to relate the development of the child to its instincts centrally, leads by two routes directly to a border which we cannot pass but must mark clearly. On the one hand we must assume heredity, which cannot be analyzed further. Sometimes it appears in the form of general tendencies and characteristics, so that there are two instinctual groups, and the mental course is oriented according to the pleasure-principle. More exactly expressed, these are all, of course, mere formulations in which we group and unify (interpret) the given facts, but we cannot ask any further questions about the determinants of this procedure without exceeding the scope of child-psychology. We cover all possibilities by assuming some phylogenesis or other, and are inclined to expect that the more general the facts the deeper are their determinants in the phylogenetic sequence; we speak of characteristics of the psychic apparatus, of general tendencies of the mental life. Furthermore, we must realize that a considerable part of the special reaction of the instinct is innate—innate with reference to the time of its appearance, of its instinctual aims, and of its instinctual objects. In general we will assume here that the determinants operate from the early parts of the phylo-genetic sequence, that perhaps they belong to humans only and do not extend further back. But in any case an investi-gation of the infant from the viewpoint of developmental-instinctual-psychology will be rather close to the phylogenetic border; and therefore it is well to bear in mind that it has perhaps often, certainly occasionally, unwittingly, overstepped the boundary, and has sought causal or other relations in the individual instance, and has found them with a display of genius and acumen which, in truth, are phylogenetically conditioned. Moreover, this crossing of the boundary still remains within the field of the living; it may have found mental determinants instead of physical or biological ones, but there still remain some which are closely related to the instincts, the instinctual. The boundary is really fluctuating. For however one may differentiate the mind from the body, differentiate mental functioning from biological functioning, in these, too, forces operate which are essentially related to the instincts. They are closely related, as is evidenced by the fact that the word instinct belonged to biology before it did to psychology, and therefore cannot be used in psychology undisputedly and without terminological difficulty.

From the other route we come upon a more defined border. The individual endowed by its ancestors with general mental qualities, special tendencies and ways of behaviour, lives in a world; his instincts have no other intention than to become effective in this world. According to our view the tendency of the instincts toward the world can be characterized briefly. One set—the R.-instincts—ensure the unwinding of the biological processes in the organism; they ensure, as Freud says, the individual road to death phylogenetically determined. The other—sexual instincts—seek stimulus-pleasure in similar phylogenetically determined ways. Both have a definite relation to the world. The one—R.-instincts—aims to annihilate the world: biologically, to devour it; mentally, not to take notice of it, or at least to ignore it as long as necessary, in order to overcome its disturbing quality. The other—the sexual instincts—aims to enjoy the world as a source of pleasure; they are prepared to change the world as far as is necessary in order to win from it the maximum pleasure. Both, however, come up against the resistance of the world and have to compromise with it in some way. This world is not biological and not mental. It is real. The world is given, and it evades all psychology and bio-psychology, too. This is a boundary that cannot be crossed, and we reach it when we speak of the perceptions of infants.

This is not the confession of an epistemological conviction; for this is irrelevant for modern psychology. For those particularly who do not consider the reality of the world worthy of thought will claim that it creates no problem for modern psychology. But even he who denies the reality of the world will be completely at a loss to understand the *quale* of perceptual objects from psychic determinants. Here a naïve viewpoint which is beyond all theoretical knowledge commends itself to us. Perceptions (their objects) are established by reality, they are the given, real world. They are not mental, but, on the contrary, the liberators, the aims, and governors of the mental unwindings. It is entirely unnecessary to remark that the act of perceiving, on the contrary, is entirely mental. It is important to remember this if one entertains the idea of imagining the infant's world from its reactions to the world—its instinctual reactions.

When we speak in this chapter of " world " and not—as heretofore—of stimuli, it is intended that one should think of a totality of stimuli, of a systematic, organized totality. This unification of stimuli into an organized whole has a meaning psychologically if it is related to an ego which is set over against this world. For going beyond this theory of knowledge one can think of the world of the ego as really given, but one cannot think of the world as really given. This implies a very precise standpoint relative to the theory of knowledge. In the title " The Infant and Its World," it is assumed that the child has an ego. I do not intend in this way to smuggle in an opinion of the much-disputed question of the origin of the ego. On the contrary, it will be discussed in detail, although we cannot come to any conclusion on this point; as the enduring, productive result of such a speculation we can only hope to formulate new questions for observation and experiment. The real world, which is given to me, contains parts which I experience in a definite relation to the ego as my body. It belongs to my ego; it does not belong to the world, which in this relationship I call *outer-world*. The proximity of the ego, the coalescence of the ego with my body can be seen only when analyzed, of course only phenomenally, by the fact that only the body is given to me in so many ways: optically, acoustically, tactually, etc., like the rest of the world; and by feeling data (pain, organic feelings, general feelings, and motor data). Ego and body are one for the unanalyzed experience. The experiences temporally and simultaneously organized with the ego relate to this my body and coalesce with it. The body has theoretically a middle position between the world and the ego since it belongs to both realms, but phenomenologically it is part (bearer, tool) of the ego. This fact is expressed by the term body-ego.

Schilder deserves the credit for having many times emphatically referred to this relationship. He underscores thereby, so it seems, some of Freud's casual observations. Developmental-psychology depends upon this concurrence. For, as far as I see, it calls attention to the necessity of giving heed to the reactions of the child, which has hitherto been neglected, as a factual field which certainly permit conclusions about the development of the ego. Preyer's observations,[1] which represent no more than a beginning, have not been systematically elaborated or extended since his time.

First of all, if we organize the scattered observations, one might then say: in the beginning the child behaves towards the parts of its own body exactly as it does toward foreign objects. Its eyes follow its own moving hand or foot exactly as they follow a candle flame; it observes its own grasping hand as attentively and with as much interest as it looks at any familiar foreign object; it observes and touches itself in the bath, especially its feet (39th week) (Preyer); it bites its finger, arm, toes, so that it cries out in pain (409th day), hits itself vigorously on its own head (41st week), presses one hand against the table with the other hand as it would a toy, etc. According to Preyer's observations, all such behaviour, especially that of attentive observations of itself, visibly stops only in the second year. It is as if the child now knows its own body and has no more interest in it.

The conclusion is obvious: the child has no knowledge of its own body at first, it must learn to distinguish it from the other things in the world. And, in so far as the ego coalesces with the body, its development must proceed in stages, which are co-ordinate with this recognition of the body. Since Preyer similar formulations have appeared from time to time in child-psychology. If we wish to attain a more precise realization of this rather vague conception it must be stated that the condition is essentially complicated by one factor; for at the same time that the child reacts to parts of its body as to foreign objects, it nevertheless knows these parts as its " own." The child who attentively observes its own grasping hand knows this hand by kinæsthetic data; the movement also occurs in the service of some " intention." What is here described as recognition of the body is an optical recognition, occasionally too a tactual and acoustic recognition. The child knows its body by simultaneous "motor-visceral data"

---

[1] Compairé's controversy with Preyer produces no new facts, and is directed only against Preyer's explanation, moreover confirming it in part.

exactly in the same way in which we, from the beginning, know our body as the one thing in the world. This should be stressed. Perhaps the child does not yet possess in the thought process the co-ordination of certain optical data with the motor data. It is still problematical how much of this co-ordination can be made except in order to experience a definite part of the body as a part of the body-ego. The mouth is certainly the seat of the most important and most impelling sensations of the infant, in it important and vivid experiences are enacted. But the mouth remains for life optically unperceived if we disregard the mirror. But in spite of this it is not treated like a foreign thing. Such behaviour is reported by Preyer, but it refers to a period after teething has begun, and therefore already involves very complicated reactions toward the body. The co-ordination of optical data with motor data, one may briefly say, is significant; but the body is from the beginning given one way which applies only to it: a motor way: and indeed it is here too given from the beginning in inextricable concurrence with actions, needs, gratifications, pleasure and ' pain.' Therefore in this co-ordination which certainly takes place, and which develops slowly in stages, it is a question not of the development of ego-feelings or ego-consciousness, but only of the co-ordination of optical experiences (*i.e.*, tactual, etc.) with the motor body-ego, and of its demarcation from the outer-world.

Since Preyer the pain sensations (*Schmerzempfindungen*) are made chiefly responsible for this process. This is very plausible and clear. We experience pain only on our own body. The child who originally treats part of its body as portions of the rest of the *outer-world* slowly makes the surprising and impressive discovery that there is a difference. If it bites its finger as it does its rattle it will feel differently, it feels pain. Although this is certain, and although painful experience is surely important in advancing the optical demarcation of the body-ego, nevertheless this factor should not be over-estimated. The infant reaction seems to indicate that its sensitivity to pain is very low. Dix, who estimates the significance of pain in the delimitation of the body rather highly, himself says elsewhere: " Bubi banged his own head while rocking himself on the *chaise longue* (tenth month). Instead of moving away he banged his head seven more times against the wall exactly as if it were a foreign object. At about the same time he grabbed his own belly and pulled at it vigorously. . . . Then he pinched himself, hit his head with his fist. . . ." In many instances the expected pain reaction does not appear in the infant. But even at a later age there are surprising forms of behaviour: Dix: " I was often and repeatedly surprised at how unconcernedly he responded to rather severe injuries. At one year and seven months he cut himself below the knee on a tin box, so that he had a wound 4 cm. long. He came to me quite cheerfully and only said: ' Papa, blood.' " From the first six to eight months the expressions of pain seem in general more intense and more frequent in reponse to stimuli from within the body (to stomach trouble, for example) than to those that take place on the skin surface. And for our discussion the latter are the decisive ones. In the last phase of infancy the reactions to pain become more frequent, more obvious, and unambiguous. But we have no basis for concluding that at this age biting the finger, banging the head, which produce pain, are undertaken because the child does not yet know its finger and head as its own. These actions may be of a very complicated nature. I assume that they really are complicated. The pain and its expressions are very uncertain tests of the co-ordination that took place. We have earlier renounced any claim to indicate incidentally a psychology of pain—which does not yet exist. But here it is necessary to recall two points: The expressions of pain are easily and durably influenced by the environment. It is as if even at this early stage, in response to impulsive expressions of pain, a motive plays a part like that found regularly in hyper-sensitive children or adults: the wish to obtain sympathy: it is as if the same motives are also effective in controlling the expressions of pain. What facts are covered by this analogy cannot be gone into here. Secondly, the observer easily gains the impression that the expressions of pain do not merely relate to the physical injury. Dix reports thus: " At one year and two months he jammed his little hand under a box-cover. Of course he felt pain when the cover closed on it, but it was absolutely out of proportion to the crying which followed it. I was perfectly sure at the time that it was not so much the pain as it was the inexplicable fact that he was held fast, that he was squeezed, without understanding how it happened. The sinister irritated him . . . at first I let him alone, expecting that he would free himself.

But after watching his false moves for a while, I liberated him. Because I laughed at the little booby's adventure, he looked at me quite bewildered, stopped crying, and held up the crushed paw for me to ' Blow.' I blew at it and—all, all was well again." This once more calls attention to the fact that there is a problem here. The rôle of pain in the delimitation of the body is not positively established. It is scarcely simple. But there are observations which predispose one to say, pain —in the adult sense—is the prerequisite of the development of the body-ego.

Accompanying and preceding the feelings of pain, a second factor has also since Preyer's day been explained. Preyer's often cited classical passage says: " Another important factor is the observation that by one's own activity alterations can be effected on familiar objects, and that the day in which the infant first experiences the relation of its movement with the sense impression that follows is psychogenetically the most remarkable—in any case, a most highly significant one in the infant's life." One sees here that the " ego-feeling," ego-consciousness as such, is referred to rather than the body-ego which interests us particularly. But Preyer's viewpoint can easily be applied. We have approached it closely before. I believe it is very plausible to say: the body-ego unfolds at the discovery of the submissiveness of the organs. At a definite time in development, the arms and fingers respond to the wish to bring a seen object into the mouth; at another time the legs follow the impulse to walk; from now on the arms, fingers, and legs belong to the body-ego. The co-ordination of optical and motor data is scarcely a process of especial difficulty and significance. For the child co-ordinates the data of the various fields of the senses very early—for example, optical-acoustic relationships in the third month. One may rightly detect a problem here, but it is not one specifically for the body-ego development. A schematic explanation of the above can be presented by an example: The motor data of arm movements and the optical data have no relation to each other before the third month; in the third month the motor data of the body are organized and thereupon the co-ordination of the motor with the optical is effected; they occur together. But it can casually be assumed that the motor-optical co-ordination existed before the organs were taken up into the body-ego. This is not relevant with relation to the process.

Before we follow up the idea of the "submissiveness" (*Folgsamkeit*) of the organs a difficulty *expressis verbis* must be recognized to which every consideration of the psychogenesis of the ego is subject. We are *a priori* inclined to value the ego as a highly complex phenomenon, and we would gladly see the appearance of ego-consciousness established late, as the crowning achievement of the mental development, so to speak. But conscientious observation and cautious interpretation show that it cannot be so; so that when one speaks of primitive co-ordination which has just occupied us, one must establish an hypothetical ego in it, in order to describe the origin of the ego itself. Preyer expresses this difficulty thus: " For what is meant by the following, ' to the child its feet, hand, teeth, appear like foreign toys ' ? and, ' the child bites its own arm as it used to bite unfamiliar objects ' ? To what part of the child does this appear ? What is it in the child that does the biting . . . ? Obviously the image in the mind is different from the actual part of the body." And Preyer considers it necessary to ascribe two egos to the child: " The brain-ego is different from the spinal-ego. The former speaks, sees, hears, tastes, smells, feels; the latter only feels; and both are from the beginning isolated from each other, so long as brain and spine are only loosely connected organic allies and functionally not at all connected. . . . One must, therefore, necessarily assume two egos in the child who has a brain and a spine and who imagines its arm as palatable or as something to be nibbled at. But if two, why not more ? At the beginning, when the seeing, hearing, smelling, and tasting centres in the brain are yet incompletely developed, each one of these perceives for itself. . . . Only through frequent simultaneous occurrence of disparate sense-impressions, as in tasting-touching, seeing-feeling, seeing-hearing, . . . could the various ideational centres, simultaneously the builders of the ego, lead, as in conception, to the formation of an homogeneous ego which is completely abstract."

Today one will readily attribute much value to Preyer's auxiliary idea (*Hilsvorstellung*); but some assumption must be made, for the ego is not of individual origin, but develops only in the course of ontogenesis. If one assumes a consciousness at the beginning of post-natal life, then one must have thought of an ego as accompanying it. It is difficult to think of consciousness, to think of perception, without thinking of a carrier, without reference to other earlier or simultaneous consciousness phenomena. From the beginning of conscious life the ego exists as a substratum. If one thinks of *consciousness* as originating at some point in the individual development, in any case at a very early one, then the ego arises simultaneously with it, and indeed in such a manner that a further analysis or derivation is not possible. Not only as a substratum nor as a relative system has the ego no psychogenesis, but from the beginning the ego is given as an institution, as an institution centrally organized for various discharges, heteronomous and heterogeneous in themselves. For the child is born as an individual. It manifests responses which treat the whole body as a unit, which organize certain " unwindings " (*Ablaüfe*), prerequisites for others, which harmonize the isolated processes with each other and which co-ordinate the body-parts to their functions. This is valid in principle also for the activities of the new-born, even if its beginning and the intensity of its organization may be hidden behind the physiological responses, and even though it is necessary to stress its lack of organization in certain relations. Sucking and crying are structuralized, organized " unwindings " from a certain centre. The mouth does not suck, the child sucks. The rest of its body participates; the rest of its psychic processes are brought into harmony with sucking. The structuralized centre which even if very undeveloped is still present in every activity, is the ego, regardless of how it is phenomenally given or represented in *consciousness*, or of whether it is given or represented in the infant's *consciousness*. Such general psychological discussions must seem uncertain and superficial, because we cannot apply any established terminology, any positive views of psychology to the study of child-psychology, especially when it is concerned with problems which are still in the making. And what important psychological problems are not in the making ? There is no doubt that some will accuse the author of eclecticism, others will charge him with being biassed; the latter will say that he has not clearly understood the various modern psychological viewpoints; the former will say, on the other hand, that he disregards them completely. But, as I see it, since a psychology of the infant would not otherwise be written, I must risk these reproaches and accept them now that I have made the attempt. This cannot be written any other way than as follows: Wherever decision of the method or of the merit of a general psychological question is to be made without much proof and discussion, the one which promises to be the most productive should be chosen. Of the definite views concerning the ego, it seems rather irrelevant that we assume—in order to formulate it without prejudice—that the ego of developmental psychology is not a developing object but a given object; to describe and understand its unfolding properly remains the task.

The body-ego, too, exists from the beginning, because from the beginning a number of organs respond to the needs of the body. A kernel of the body-ego exists from the beginning in the oral zone. Head, hands, arms, thighs, legs, and feet are added by stages to this kernel.[1] I should like to assume it thus. If we try to imagine this, we shall probably arrive at the following scheme for the infant's experience, which of course says nothing about the *quale* of the "phenomena of consciousness," no matter how intelligible a connection we can construct with our imagination. An object seen, awakes the impulse to oral mastery. The arms and fingers reach for it, grasp it, and lead it to the mouth. This situation can be compared with the one occurring simultaneously when the object is too far to be reached without moving the body. Here, too, the wish to master it occurs. The hand reaches for it, but the impulse neither leads the hand nor leads it toward the oral zone to fulfil the wish. The difference, which is certainly considerable in both situations, can perhaps be imagined thus: in both instances the infant experiences an impulse with all the appropriate sensations in the oral zone, and outside of it a whole series of motor-visceral data. These are not localized further. They are present, but there is no provocation for separating them from the longing. And we constantly experience situations in which we have a number of motor sensations, but these do not localize without particular provocation, and at times and in part cannot localize at all despite the provocation, but are experienced singly as excitement perhaps. In the first case, then, a series of such data arises from the profusion of other data—it enters into a definite

---

1 I here approach the idea of body-schema about which Schilder (2) comes to similar results. It is, however, a question of isolating the degree of imagination in the body-schema (*Körperschemas*) and of placing it in the foreground.

relation to the oral zone, it takes a direction, coalesces with the circumscribed zone: the arm and finger movements. From now on they occur simultaneously with the impulse. They belong to it and to its zone. In order to gain a point of contact with Bühler's idea of learning, one might say that success binds them to the ego. Whereas the unsuccessful leg movements in the second example remain in the coherent mass of motor impressions which belong to the wish, the desire, etc. Thus the body-ego would be grouped with the oral zone. If one wishes to extend the scheme to cover all the known facts fully, one should remember that the eyes belong to the oral zone. The first extension of this scheme would be that the cervical musculature and the ears would be added to the body-ego— of course only motorally, that is acoustically but not optically —in turning the head toward the source of the sound. Fingers and arms are added next; then the torso and legs, and ultimately the feet and the toes. These extensions must be connected with the relational experiences and experiences of direction, so that something results which we must express as "between mouth and leg." But since the body-ego has a continuity, indeed a localized spatial continuity, it indicates, first, that the whole surface of the body transmits sensations which do not belong to the principle of submissiveness to the body-ego as tools, but which play a considerable rôle as the goal of wishes and strivings. The skin as a whole is erotogenic, its erotogenicity is experienced during a bath for example, in connection with activities, and this skin zone is interspersed with more sensitive erotogenic zones. It seems as if skin were in general the usual and primitive projective surface for "inner" sensations. Throughout life we localize certain inner stimuli towards the outside; we feel the pain of the tooth in the gums, we feel the stimulus of the bronchia as a cough stimulus in the larynx, the headache on the forehead, we hold the stomach during a stomach-ache, etc., and where projection does not occur quite on the surface, we are inclined nevertheless to transfer the painful stimulus to the surface, to treat it as a foreign body (Federn). But if there is such a mechanism—although it may be completely unintelligible— it makes easier for us the understanding of the co-ordination of the optical and motor experiences which occur early. But perhaps, too, this projection-tendency is reversed, to a certain point optically conditioned. In general it should be formu-

lated that the erotogenic zones are especially " submissive ";
for they create pleasure as soon as adequate contact occurs.

An observation which can be easily made will serve as
illustration: we are inclined to exclude an unresponsive organ
from the body-ego. The biblical proverb says: " If thine eye
offend thee, pluck it out." And when a painful organ which
appears like a foreign body rages within us we sympathize with
it—*e.g.*, we experience a leg which has fallen asleep as if it did
not belong to us, or we are estranged from the hand which
has upset a glass of water, and for a moment considered it
reproachfully. This behaviour may on occasion be of some
significance for the psychology of the infant—for example, in
those transformations which we, so to speak, placed in the
mouth of the teething child.

The relation of toes to the body-ego mentioned above is
indeed only a simple and unimportant detail, but it fits in
so well with our view that it deserves a few words. Even
much later the child reacts to the toes as if they were a
foreign toy. Thus Preyer, for example, reports: " The same
child who gladly offers the *Zwieback* to the mouth of the relative whom it likes, offers this cake of its own accord to its
own toes; in the same way while sitting on the floor it holds
the cake expectantly to its toes; and this remarkable instance
occurred in the twenty-third month many times. The child
entertained itself in that way."

At this age one must, of course, already assume a rather
complicated psychic situation, so that here perhaps something
quite different from a mere interchange of *outer-world* and its
own bodily parts must be implied. In any case the toes seem
to be further from the body-ego than the legs, for example.
From our view one might conjecture that this is because
the toes are not " responsive." They are not used for any
" purpose-activities." In walking and standing they are
scarcely separated from the feet, they have no special function
in kicking. They are not experienced in connection with
" submissiveness"; they can therefore remain foreign to the
body-ego until other factors are conducive to their delimitation and to finer structuralization. I think it is wrong to
conclude that a part of the body does not belong to the
body-ego because the infant behaves as if it allowed itself to be
separated from the body. The inability to separate (without
pain) may be an experience which is achieved rather late. This

assumption is obvious, because the child's clothing, although removable, is nevertheless very near to the primitive ego, even if perhaps it does not belong directly to the body-ego.

A conclusion from what has been said is imperative, but if it is not carefully weighed it may easily become an objection. The infant must find things which do not belong to its own body, just as submissive as definite parts of its own body. When the child cries and the mother's breast appears, is it not essentially the same process as when it wants the rattle and it grasps it ? I believe one must say it is. This means that the outer-world is a part of the body-ego. One must assume something of the kind for a part of the outer-world; and indeed in essentials that part of the outer-world which is called mother. She, parts of her body, breasts, mouth, eyes, hands, a whole series of her actions, may very easily not be distinguished from the body-ego, may belong to it. Perhaps, too, some portions of the child's habitual environment may belong to the body-ego. We here approach a very important range of ideas which Ferenczi (1) follows up more closely in elaborating Freud's (4) ideas. More will be said about the idea later. Perhaps the conviction that there are at least two different mental processes which are decisive for the development of the body-ego suffices here. One arises from the patterns = (*Gestalten*) of the world developing in stages around a nucleus, the oral zone and its unlocalized motor dependents which correspond to the body-ego. It forms the body-ego from the world. The other refines this process by simultaneous and additional correctives, it separates the body-ego definitely from the outer-world. Thus it operates in two directions. One time it finds the body-ego too big, the mother must be pushed out; another time it finds it too small—for example, when the toes are added to the body-ego, to return to a previously mentioned instance. One is also tempted to state what the motive power of this refined delimitation is, the *disappointment*. When the child learns that a part of its own body-ego refuses to be submissive, it exiles this part from its body-ego. Such a disappointment, to link up once more with the foregoing, is the central point of weaning. Here, then, the decisive casting out of the mother from the body-ego ought to follow the biblical proverb. She becomes the outer-world. Now one can treat her affectionately, an act which had no

18

meaning before. Yet this statement leads to further reflections which link up with earlier ones.

In conclusion, it should not be forgotten that these developments are of a libidinal nature. They play no part, or only an unimportant part, in the sphere of the intellectual and rational. They are instinctual processes, they occur by libidinal displacement. Even at this point, this suggestive allusion must suffice.

THE AFFECTIVE ATTITUDES

Those who have observed the infant in the fourth quarter of the first year cannot describe its behaviour in any other way than by using the various affective designations. They will find anger, pride, fear, and vexation. Of course, this impression is by no means proof of the actual existence of this complex of affective attitudes and not always proof in the ordinary case; but it shows that in the first period of life the beginning of a rather uniform mode of behaviour has been broken up into a number of easily distinguishable states. Very little has been done to date systematically in order to attain to an understanding of these states. We are still very far from giving an explanation of the psychogenesis of these affective attitudes. Their beginnings and their differentiations are still very obscure. This is the more lamentable, since one might hope to draw plausible conclusions for the development of the ego from the development of the affective attitudes. Every new attitude, every differentiation, every intensification, must accompany, call forth, or have as a prerequisite, an expansion, a refinement and strengthening, respectively, of the ego. For the attitudes are total reactions of the individual; we understand them as reactions having a definite relation to the ego. And we speak of affective attitudes and attitudes in general in the infant, only when we are of the impression—or conviction—that it is a question of concise, organized, homogeneous reactions. We admit that the boundary is very flexible; and that the impression from both sides may be very deceptive. But if we compare two ways of behaviour from the first days of life with those of the sixth month, we can understand what is meant. Let us compare, for example, a simple action of Reaction Type I—closing the eyes in response to a dazzling light appearing suddenly as described by Scupin: " Now he sighs impatiently; he stretches his body stubbornly forward, throws himself suddenly forward and, stiffening himself, repeats this backwards; these movements give the impression that he is incredibly capricious. Since we did not react to this, he suddenly uttered a prolonged screech ' i '; there our son sat with flushed face and clinched fists, the contracted eyes directed against us with a furious expression, and, making a strenuous effort, he screeched his prolonged hoarse ' i ' again." In the first instance only the eyes, so to speak, take part; in the second the whole body. In the first it is a question of a simple inherited mechanism with a simple feeling of displeasure; in the second a large number of inherited mechanism and a goodly portion of the acquired, rich store of knowledge are operative together; it is accompanied by a gamut and a variety of different, mixed affects and emotions. The conduct in the second example is highly organized in comparison with that of the first example.

In accordance with Reaction Types I and II the attitudes can be divided into defence attitudes and desire attitudes. They are fundamental and primitive modes of behaviour, the primal attitudes which can be directed toward the world. They are—irrespective of any relation to the ego and therefore purely objective—the properties of all that is organic. We have spoken in detail in various places of desires, of the aims of desire, of the methods of gratification, and of the instinctual basis. Thence the elaborations which now become necessary will be appended when we speak about defence.

The affective attitude, defence, has not obtruded itself conspicuously upon the observer. Although the simple defensive actions are so frequent and general from the beginning, the affective attitude, defence, cannot easily be sharply distinguished. We, therefore, look for a striking example. The two following quotations from Scupin serve as such an example: " Seventh month. Weaning . . . a special kind of milk . . . the child had to take it from the bottle through a nipple. Already after the second draught the young one energetically pushed this substitute away, struck the bottle, kicked its arms and legs about, wrinkled its forehead, eyes and brows, looked indignantly and complainingly at its mother, and began to scold vigorously: ' awa-wa-wa-ba-mam-mam,' etc., and between these cries at every approach of the nipple, he refused it by turning his head sideways, and pleaded:

'want, want !' The instant the child opened its mouth the nipple was quickly thrust into it, and the restless moving little head was held firmly. Bubi resisted furiously, clamped the nipple between his gums, and bit into it with his teeth. That amused him until a few drops of milk got into his throat; making a wry face as if it tasted abominable, he pushed the hand and bottle away." " Seventh month. The child became furious if an attempt was made to put him into a carriage when he wished to be carried. His face became flushed, he screeched hoarsely, and stubbornly stiffened his body so that it became almost impossible to sit him down."

An evident and superficial analysis of such complicated defence-activities shows us the obviously intelligible—banal —efforts to keep the *outer-world* at a distance from the body, to remove it from the body, toward which end all the already acquired motor capacities are bent: turning the head away, moving the body away, awkward and successful attempts at flight by crawling, running, walking; pushing the disturbing object away with hands, feet, head, and body. The repeated " pushing away " becomes pushing and hitting. On the other hand, biting, scratching, holding fast to the arm of the enemy, etc., are not primal modes of behaviour, but are taken over from the desire-activities to the defence-activities, after an insight has been gained into the effect of 'pain' in response to refused objects or into the conditions of an action to be warded off. The opportunity for such defence is given most usually by persons who wish to force upon the child a position, an article of clothing, a contact which it refuses; or by an attempt to put something into a body opening which is unpleasant to it, such as an enema; or cleaning its nose, ears; or changing its favourite food and dishes. But the child applies the same action in removing an insect or an uncomfortable article of clothing (blanket). This defence presupposes, of course, a certain development of the motor apparatus, but its principle is already established in the first days of life when the satiated child actively ejects the breast from its mouth. The complexity of this defence action increases with the growing means to power and insight, but the principle is the same: ejecting the hostile object out and away from the body.

Next to (and instead of) the ejection and pushing away is the less obvious resisting. The mouth is firmly closed when the rejected rubber nipple is to be put into it; the anus is vigorously contracted when it wants to prevent the irrigation. Perhaps the stiffening of the limbs should be added to this kind of reaction. Otherwise a separate grouping must be assigned to it. Resisting is used more exclusively than rejection against the intervention of the attending person. It plays an important rôle in " house-breaking " the infant (and small child). For a long time it can be seen how well the child controls the anal muscles, and how well it understands, too, that it is expected to direct the defæcation into the pot, and how for a long time it occasionally refuses to do this, but releases the pressing mass as soon as the pot is removed. And when an object is wrested from the child's mouth one becomes acquainted with its very energetic resisting-defence (*Absperr-Abwehr*).

Finally, crying belongs to the defence actions. This crying is different from the universal activity, crying, and is soon recognized and understood by observant attendants as a specific expression. But any possibility of formulating its characteristics scientifically is at present still lacking. When one formulates one's impressions of defensive crying as a short, vigorous percussion with noticeable pauses, accompanied by a mouth position representing the sounds m, n, p, b, t, d, it is characteristically described. One must renounce the prospects for the genesis of speech which perhaps follow hypothetically; not only because they threaten to lead to speculation, but also and above all because the development of speech can explain retrospectively only the manifestations of the infant age from the psychology of early childhood.

The most radical defence against the disturbing or disagreeable outer-world is the suspension of perception, the breaking off of relations with the outer-world: falling asleep, fainting, somnolent states and similar manifestations. For many obvious reasons, a primal mode of behaviour can be seen in this radical one; but nothing feasible can be said about it because no observations of any sort exist—that is, nothing is contained in the literature which was available to me—which approximate such an interpretation. Of course the states of apathy and sleep—which have already been spoken about in this sense—are to be included here. But we are not able to distinguish the various causes for falling asleep. The so-called natural fatigue after a certain period of waking is not to be marked off from the special " fatigue " which is due to disappointment or due to warding-off stimuli. And therefore nothing definite can be reported of the infant period about the process—unquestionably existing later—of surrender of psychic apparatus to katergic force, as an active ego process, as an activity of the libido. But lest it be forgotten completely, our attention should be called to the fact that *a priori* it was obvious to assume that the defence-activities would show a certain nearer affinity to the katergic process. For the most radical defence is certainly the withdrawal of the libido from the objects, drawing it back into the ego. And the ego-libido is very close to "organ-libido," to katergy; narcissistic states in their completed evelopment in general stand theoretically the border line of the psychical.

The discussion of defence attitudes shows us two other affective states in close relationship which could not be so plausibly organized without this analysis. Defiance (obstinacy) is, at least in its forms of expression during infancy, nothing else than an energetic defence of the "resisting" type. I do not wish to maintain that expressions of defiance and obstinacy which contain other elements do not occur even at so early a time, but it cannot be a matter of indifference for the psychogenesis of these affects that the genetic analysis of the manifold attitudes, so important later, have their roots in defence and firstly in "resistance" (*Absperrung*). Nevertheless, this will occupy us in more detail in the presentation of early childhood. A direct line of development extends from the defence of the ejection type to a number of affective ways of behaviour, which are inaccurately studied in the adult; in the child they have not been organized and therefore are summarized roughly as: attack, combat, destruction, to punish. Bearing in mind the further development of defence we shall see that very soon the defence-actions will appear in the service of desire, and that we shall be faced with very involved conditions in the psychology of early childhood. Having said this we must reserve a more exact presentation for another place, assuring ourselves that our present knowledge even where it is not as scanty as in the psychology of infancy will leave difficulties and tasks enough for a coherent penetration of the subject-matter.

The analysis of desire-actions has occupied us in detail in the earlier chapters. If supplementations are necessary they will fit in well later. And we can maintain that desire, in itself a very varied affective attitude already in early life, contains the possibility of circumscribing other states—namely, when the desire-action leads to no result. Desire consists of the relatively simple conditions of the infancy period in its effort, its wish to bring an object close to the body. It is exactly the reverse defence which always wants to hold things off from the body. As far as I can observe, there is but one exception to this formulation preceding the throwing away of objects: wanting to see, which does not always demand the bodily proximity of the object seen, but is satisfied with the emotion it causes. This should be noted; but it should also be remembered that being satisfied may be secondary, and never excludes attempts at and intentions of mastery. Originally desire is certainly the impulsion toward mastery. But already in later infancy a certain moderation has taken place which is tied up with one differentiation. Obstructing this desire for mastery, interference with it, creates a definite affective state which develops into attitudes: anger, rage.

The passage cited above from Scupin (p. 275) gives a graphic picture of anger. It in any case has traits which are closely related to aggressive defence. Especially where the disturbance is produced by a real obstruction, anger will be nothing else than defence, increased aggressive defence. And a part of this remains characteristic for life in tantrums with their accompanying rampage. Anger could, therefore, be rightly added to aggressive defences. But I am of the opinion that it would be worth while to differentiate and characterize a state which is not an aggressive defence—at least not this alone. This is most clearly seen when the disturbance is not a bodily interference, and is less obviously seen when the disturbance is one which cannot be mastered. The infant who calls vainly for his mother, as in the instance cited, does not feel hindered by anything, and is yet not in any position to attain his aim. He cannot bring the mother's image within the proximity of his body. He cries louder and louder until he gets into paroxysms and finally weeps complainingly, during which his hands and his body are in vigorous but unorganized motion. This represents a picture of powerless rage, which authors, who have perhaps in vain written down their reminiscences of infancy, have described as a fundamental life situation. (I shall later treat such records.) This state is directed not only at the outer-world, but has an intention against the whole ego. What gives powerless rage its character is that in it a definite relation of the ego to the outer-world is given, namely powerlessness—an extremely unpleasant state which phenomenally has a very special aspect. In it rage, anger, vexation, resignation, and sorrow are united, irrespective of their differences and of the distinctly unified attitude of both these groups to the ego. We do not know how all this happens in the infant, but there is no reason for not assuming the nucleus of this state in the infant also. The differentiation is, of course, not sufficiently developed. It therefore seems high-handed to include anger among the frustrated desires. It could be placed equally well under the defence attitudes, but this classification stresses the element of powerlessness. It would be better to create a more exact nomenclature, but this would, of course, presuppose a more defined phenomenological line of demarcation of the attitudes. We, therefore, keep the ambiguous designations. And anger is a sort of counterpart of defiance, quite obvious when it develops into resigned powerlessness and apathetic submissiveness. But in any case, from one aspect anger is a reaction to an ego-powerlessness, defiance is an ego-victory. There are many varied differentiations within the wider range of the disturbances of desires; they cannot yet be formulated, however, for infancy. Here a survey in place of such differentiations may show, without any desire on my part to prejudice the results, what to expect from future investigations.

Overcoming an obstruction to desire results in joy. We have already spoken of this, but we must also classify this affective state and without hesitation place it opposite anger. Laughing is the same loud unorganized agitation except that it is highly pleasurable whereas crying is unpleasant. Joy is also an experience related to the ego and the outer-world, and indeed a victory of the ego over the outer-world. The chart gives us a basis for separating joy from defiance. This basis cannot be formulated in technical terms from the material of infant psychology. Joy, too, is only a marked representative of a whole group: self-regard—triumph.

All these attitudes have a decisive relation to the ego: they are conceivable in their complete development and differentiation only as attitudes of the ego. If we notice their slow development from a completely undifferentiated state in the course of the further months of life, if we see that their motor

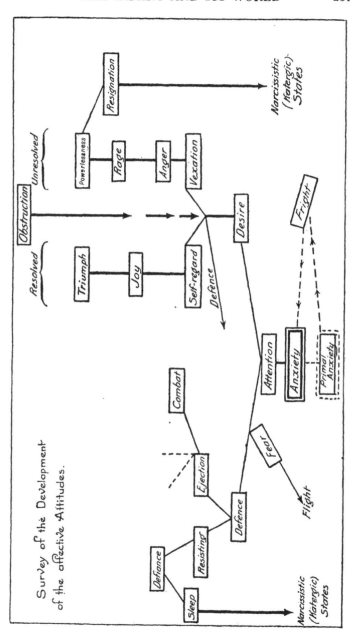

Survey of the Development of the affective Attitudes.

or bodily part, linked, with the inherent primitive reactions of Type I to III, becomes continuously more manifold and precise, if we see further that, from a definite time, the parts of the body become continually less important, less precise, less characteristic in comparison with the composite picture, then the assumption will force us rightly to recognize that in the development of the affective attitudes we have an index of the precision, and differentiations of the ego.

The affective attitudes are achievements of the ego. They are presumably at the same time the creators of the ego. Since the environment forces certain attitudes—releases instincts—and simultaneously resists the consummation (maintenance) of these attitudes—produce disturbances and obstructions—it forces the unfolding of the ego, creates possibilities of comparison, creates reality and ego as antithetical: reality as the occasion of desire and defence, reality as that " something " resistant to desire and defence. If we could say that the expansion of the body-ego starts from the fact of the submissiveness of the organs, then we could say that the antithesis, world and ego, is connected with the situation of the unsubmissiveness of objects. As long as a cry of the infant, an out-stretching of its hand, a push of the body, a shove of the foot, magically produces or removes things necessary for gratification, no distinction between the ego and reality exists. The child possesses an omnipotent ego. Or better still, there is only one ego in which the means for the needs and their gratification are given side by side; the means for gratification are determined, are given by the needs. Life is very agreeable, " im Besitz von solchen Flubissen und Golchen," as the profound Morgenstern says. The world responds to the magic of the simple body movement, and to the intense sounds, one might say, agreeing with Freud (4) and Ferenczi (1) who have formulated this train of thought.[1] Only when, and in so far as this magic fails, is the ego placed into opposition to the world. At these points on the chart: combat, obstruction, vexation, anger, this cleft begins; it is experienced in rage and powerlessness; in joy and triumph the ego conquers the hostile world; by powerlessness and resignation the ego is conquered. By defiance the ego maintains itself by negating the cleft.

[1] Reference: The technique of magicians actually consists in rhythmic movements and spoken formulæ.

PERCEPTION AND INSTINCT

Up to this point we have dealt with the affective side of life; for its psychological significance, certainly not in sufficient detail but perhaps even in more detail than our knowledge should permit. It is time to deal with the sensory side. This is certainly not less important, and psychology has concerned itself incomparably more with it than with the affective side, but not infant psychology. We know even less about the sensory life of the infant than of its affective life. I must, therefore, be satisfied with a few remarks about it, which will be no more than aphoristic because of their limited factual content as well as their perceptible incompleteness.

First I must make a terminological comment: I speak of perception and mean the process: perceiving, turning toward. The content, the object of perception, should be designated as such. I use the word perception as it is customarily applied to the sensory process. But it should not be forgotten that a perceptual element belongs also to the affective processes, that the localized sensations in the inner part of the body are perceptions as well as data coming through the eye, etc. All that is generally said about perception may apply to the affective process and certainly to the one important fact—namely, these perceptions also involve *Gestalten* and *Struckturen*. There are in life as few kinæsthetic sensations as there are visual ones. The former, too, are structuralized—are given, *e.g.*, " movement-melodies."

All indications point to the fact, as was already discussed in both the first sections of the book, that the infant's *consciousness*, from the beginning, is built on structures, and that only these patterns attain perception (in the precise meaning of the term). The theory of an initial chaos of sensation is untenable. It may apparently answer our purposes to think of the beginning as far removed from the developed state, to imagine the complicated as a result of the simple. But logical simplicity is not psychological simplicity here. Another possibility suggests itself, that of satisfying in this complex of phenomena also our ideal of scientific knowledge in developmental-psychology. Since the structure of objects belongs to primitive perception too, it must not, of course, be concluded that it is of the same kind as in the adult or older child. Volkelt,

proceeding in this line of thought, has investigated the images
of animals. He shows that the chaos (mosaic) theory cannot
apply to them either. He comes to the conclusion that perceptions are in a certain sense " disconnected " in animal
consciousness, that complexity predominates, but that the
same thing " outside " of a limited range of situations is not
represented by a similar thing-picture as when it is within
this range. There is " an inconsistency in the modification
of animal consciousness by objects which to us appear
the same."

To make these findings and the consequences resulting
from them fruitful for child-psychology, there must first be
in them a stimulation to experimental investigation and
systematic observation. Only then can we come to any conclusion. At this stage only an arbitrary impression based on
the previous observations can be expressed. And this shows
that it must be quite different in infants than in the animals
mentioned by Volkelt. As far as I see the infant completely
lacks the manifestations which Volkelt describes as complete
inadaptability. The infant may be put into a position where
it cannot overcome a situation, and it is very often in such an
embarrassing situation, but it is not a question of whether the
infant has the means (inclusive of sensory experience) to
conquer the situation and does not apply them merely because
it misjudges the sensory conditions. Volkelt's spider found
itself in this situation: the spider daily destroyed a gnat, if it
was caught on a definite place in the web; but when the gnat
was on a different part of the web, not only did he not seize
it but he became frightened and withdrew. Thus the gnat is
recognized not as a harmless or savoury morsel, as gnat, but
by means of a group of other given data which we do not consider as belonging to the object gnat. Such an example of
complete inadaptability does not seem to occur in the infant.
The infant does not adapt to a number of categories of situations only because it has no control over its arms, fingers,
etc. But it does not break down, so it seems, in a special
situation within a category to which it has adapted itself.

Whereas only a combination of a whole series of conditions
release in the spider the impulse to seize, which means that a
very complex object is conceived as a structure; and whereas,
arising from an omission of what to our perception would be
a very trivial element, the spider perceives a fundamentally

different structure, with which no impulse, or the opposite impulse, is associated; in the infant a few attributes of a situation are sufficient to call forth a response. Perception in the infant, differing from that in the spider, may be represented somewhat as follows: moving objects—near enough—small enough—snatch it ! I will not dispute that in this situation also Volkelt's formulation can perhaps be applied. But it seems to me more important to refer to the difference. The infant has structures which are built up of a few elements. And these structures are centralized mostly around colours, kinds of emotions, and geometric relations—that is, the infant has, as one of its properties, the abstract faculty for building structures. This is one step from its perceptions to intuitive concepts and to general imagination—which expresses the idea intelligibly without using terminology which will prejudice.

Alongside of these general structures very complicated ones are soon built. The mother is one of them. The general attributes of the person are not enough to call forth a definite attitude, but perception has advanced to the recognition of the elements of the individual. What the example of the spider taught applies, therefore, only in a certain sense: an apparently trivial detail makes the well-known person an unfamiliar one (see p. 135 with reference to the change of hat and its result). We are not attempting to deduce the latter structure from the general one, nor are we undertaking any specific speculation. Let us be content with noting the facts and summarizing them: this special structure applies at first only to the persons of the child's immediate environment; perhaps only to its mother.

In the third quarter at the latest, perhaps even earlier, the constructed world of the child—so the facts seem to indicate— has become essentially more varied. It behaves as if it has essentially the same configuration of a fairly good number of things as we ourselves have. Although the assumption is near at hand, I question our right to assume here development due to experience, for one will wish to make certain determinants responsible for this development. This has already been spoken about. It must be stressed that things important to the life-situation are not given to the infant. Expressed in our psychological terminology, it reads: perception is not first and foremost in the service of the R.-instincts. This biological relationship, considered as primal, is divided in the infant.

It sees, hears, touches quite independently of the R.-instinctual impulses. Its senses are in great part under the supremacy of the sexual instinct. Perception is in great part a libidinal process. This means, that the structures do not develop solely according to the relations and elements essential to life. Perception extends only as far as consumption requires; it not only reports on the quality of the disturbance which should be removed, but it extends beyond this to a wider field; it becomes embedded within the object itself and as such offers pleasure.

I have already often indicated that the concept, "important or essential to life," cannot be used without great care in relation to the development of the human infant. It is important to be clear on this point. This idea can refer only to the future. That the infant should recognize its mother is not at all essential for the maintenance of life, but this ability may become necessary for the older child. And the fact that this occurs in the perceptual structure with the clearness which is the final consequence of development, is necessary (important for life) only because the child is brought up in a very definitely constructed society which imposes definite demands. It may, therefore, be that these capacities once had a biological relation when they were phylogenetically acquired. In the infant (child) of today they are inherently delineated, or are the result of society's influence: the reaction to them. That means that it is superfluous and confusing to seek the biological relation in child-psychology.

It is really contained in the inherited modes of response; it is of a social-psychic, but not of a biological, nature. The life of an organism is not dependent upon specific human modes of perception; other organisms have their perceptions and they safeguard their life equally well. We, therefore, gain nothing by showing that the infant maintains its life by living as the results of its ancestral heritage and its spontaneous reaction. A psychological understanding does not result from this last harmony between organism and environment; but we must uncover the course for this harmony, and our problem, therefore, cannot be the relationship of these courses to the result, and surely not the teleological relationship.

The requirements of developmental psychology are not satisfied by explaining the complicated phenomena as derivatives of the simple ones. We find perceptions, from those beginnings which can be explained at all, equal to adult perception in essential tendencies. And we must be content with the quantitative difference. If we add that the affective components obviously predominate in the earliest perceptions, that the sensations which emanate from within the body presumably receive more attention than is usual for the mature function, and if we add that perhaps the significance of the data of various sense organs is to a certain degree different because perhaps the olfactory organ plays a bigger rôle for the perceptions of infants, or that the ear plays a different rôle than in the adult, then we have constantly before us a number of very plausible deviations, even if none of them can be designated as essential.

One must set a term to one's speculations about it. We must agree that in discussing perceptions we speak of *consciousness*. And if we establish the fact that the primitive perceptions are already structuralized and are indeed presumably similar in essentials to adult perceptions, then nothing else is meant but that consciousness—we are not speaking of objects here— is provided from its very beginning with the same or intrinsically similar *quale*, which is attributed to it all through life. Our consciousness is a quality which is not experienced as such, but which runs its course on or with definite structuralized phenomena. One can try to assume and construct the development of consciousness in various ways, but in this one direction it is hardly possible—namely, to assume that consciousness means to maintain the occurrence of definite structures and relations. And human consciousness will surely have in its most primitive form human world structures and ego-relationships. The latter seems directly evident. The former seems no less evident if one bears in mind that perceptions—it is immaterial what one's theory of knowledge is— have object-intention for the subjective experience and that these are certainly the established relations for human consciousness. According to naïve realism which we here hold to solely in order to simplify psychological phenomena, we could also say that perceptions are in some way the result of outer psychic stimuli, influences of a world. They are constant; so is the ego-relation; the world of consciousness is, therefore, identical from two angles in the infant and adult. Thus we cannot expect anything else than an intrinsic similarity. Of course, empiricism always forsakes us to a certain degree when it comes to making a decision upon this question. We will, therefore, for the present assume the intrinsic similarity and therefore do not need to prove it: the contrary, however, must be proven to us indisputably, if we are to recognize it conclusively.

We have spoken of perception up to this point without clearly separating " concept " from it, and for good reasons. In the first place, we know even less about concepts than about perceptions. In the second place, there are certain important points of contact close at hand which enable us to assume very different relationships for the psychology of the infant than for that of the psychology of the adult. Psychoanalysis and *eidetic* research meet in the same interpretation. The boundary between perception and conception is very indefinite in early childhood; both worlds, perception and conception, differentiate themselves out of a common " fore-stage." In visual perception this indefinite differentiation gives rise to an experience which Jaensch calls palpable image (*Anschaungsbild= A.-B.*).[1] It is clear that we are speaking of hallucinatory reproduction. One may assume that the difference between reproduction and perception in the beginning does not lie in the vividness of its sense qualities; indeed, one cannot really believe that the relation of perception to an *outer-ego-world*, to reality, already exists at the earliest age. But it is convenient to assume that we have states very similar to the infant's perceptions, in dreams, in palpable images, in hallucinations and visional states. Plasticity is common to all these states. Jaensch shows that it is obviously so in his visual palpable image (*A.-B.*). In them spatial-field changes, optical shifts, changes in size relationships, and in some types very extensive changes of different kinds, are presented. These alterations exist not in the conditions of the real world but in mental states, in mental functions. The *A.-B.* follows the psychic trend, whereas the completed perceptions resist the psychic trend. Perception has a constancy which is lacking in the *A.-B.* Jaensch develops the genetic point of view showing that the *A.-B.* represents the original type out of which perception evolves. One might say that with perception a tendency comes into being, whose aim of pure receptivity is never attained. A more exact analysis of these changes is lacking in the studies published by Jaensch and his collaborators; the

[1] (*A.-B.*) will be used to designate *Anschaungsbild.—Translator.*

motives, too, have not been specifically investigated. Nevertheless, the significance of the affective factors, interest and attention, is indicated. From the presented material one gains the impression that in the *A.-B.* the object seen is treated like an instinctual object; it is pulled toward one, it is pushed away, made larger, placed in the centre, held firmly, treated quite as if it were a real thing on which instinctual modifications were undertaken with the hands.[1] Jaensch does not speak explicitly of the infant's perceptions; yet there is no doubt that what he says generally of early childhood certainly applies to infancy. Freiling, a collaborator of Jaensch, mentions an observation from Stern: " In fun a doll's bottle, which was one-fifteenth the usual size, was held before Stern's eight-months-old son when he was expecting his own bottle. He became very much excited and snatched at the bottle as if it were the real one. Stern concludes from this that a constant of magnitude (*Grössenkonstanz*) is lacking;" and interprets it from the point of view of *eidetic*: " We would not deduce from Stern's assumption of uncertainty in judging magnitude that the association in the child between impressions of distance and size, which, according to him, condition the correct judgment of size, is sufficiently determined. We tend much more to the explanation that here also the affective factors bring about a subjective enlargement of the object."

If we link up Freud's proofs with Jaensch's views, in part combining what has already been said, we arrive at the following conception. Reproduction and perception are intrinsically and primarily similar to each other. The infant's visual phenomena are of the same kind whether they are responses to visual stimuli or to stimuli from inner needs (instincts or associations). The instinctual activities adapt themselves to these visual phenomena which are themselves transformed to a certain extent by the instincts. On the other hand, the appearance of the visual phenomena is occasionally itself, in a certain sense, an instinctual activity. For the wished-for phenomena are attained by motor activity—namely, by crying (till mother comes), by offence-movements[2], etc., or by reproduction. This phase might be called magic hallucination. It

[1] This is not formulated by Jaensch; but he approaches it when he says: " Here the possibility of connecting the perceptual theory to the theory of instincts is indicated." By no means an indifferent moment for the development of psychology.

[2] *Zuwendungsbewegungen.*

carries with it intense 'pain' experiences, connected mostly, perhaps, with the nutritional instinct. This must soon bring about the realization that there is a difference between the hallucinated breast and the real one, and will converge into clear concepts of reality, differentiated from other visual phenomena. Towards this end an impulse for development will more surely emanate from the instinct of mastery as it expresses itself in the delimitation of the ego-body, which, indeed, tends to the co-ordination of perceptions of various sense spheres. It can now be assumed from this that a kind of repression of the $A.-B.$ sets in, that it becomes impoverished, less vital. But the findings of Jaensch would not agree with this. Furthermore, the world of reproduction remains more accommodating instinctually than the world of perceptions. It will, therefore, give pleasure, and this opposes repression; and accordingly the $A.-B.$ of adults and adolescents is more brilliant than reality. In spite of this it is difficult to conclude that perception is impoverished in energy. There will, therefore, be complicated processes which we as yet cannot clearly conceive, but which in some way effects a differentiation within the world of reproduction during the "period of magic"; in certain fields some $A.-B.$ remains intact, others—obviously those which are closely tied up with the manifestation of mastery—are delimited by a closer understanding. In agreement with the earlier discussion it could be presumed that the disappointing, and the unsubmissive visual phenomena, are loosely related to the ego; they become somehow non-ego: objective. But some of the visual phenomena enter into an especially close union with the ego; they become, so to speak, subjective, reproductions, parts of the ego. The greater number, however, have no expressed relation to the ego. Those phenomena which are made alien to the ego are the beginnings of perception, of *world*; those brought close to the ego are the beginnings of imagination, of phantasy; those neutral to the ego are a kind of reservoir from which both these worlds receive their contribution. With these distinctions, processes set in which will lead to production as opposed to reproduction (and perception). We then deal here with the phase of the first limitation of magic hallucination. It synchronizes (temporally and dynamically) with the phase of the delimitation of the body-ego; it supplements this by adding to it the intellectual-ego, which similarly to the body-ego is set off from the non-ego by excluding disappointing phenomena (*i.e.*, the world), and by supplementing it from the neutral-ego.

All this is directly valid only for the sphere of vision. We must think of the development of the other sense spheres in some intrinsically similar way. Nevertheless, it would not surprise us to find very different relationships in some cases if the empirical material would permit a more detailed discussion. The psychology of space suggests problems, which can at present scarcely be adequately formulated. No wonder that the Psychology of the Infant has to offer so little to this theme. Nevertheless, we are very well informed upon some points. Stern (2) has given very conscientious study to the development of space perception in early childhood. He differentiates, into original space (*Urraum*), near space (*Nahraum*) and distant space (*Fernraum*). The original space is " the region of the mouth." " In the second week the child can already follow bright objects which are brought within its range of vision and slowly . . . shifted. With this accomplishment the child goes from the ' original ' space into the ' near ' space to the control of which space it remains limited for about one-quarter of year. It is an approximate hemisphere which, with the child's head as the centre, extends in front for a radius of about one-third of a meter." " In the course of the second quarter of the first year the visual ' distant ' space begins."

One sees that space, its growth and precision, is closely related to the development of the body-ego, of the ego and of the world. Stern (2) interprets this as follows: "Just as the conquest of ' near ' space was very incomplete so long as the child only passively surrendered itself to the visual and tactual impressions and could not actively grasp them, so the capture of ' distant ' space is extremely incomplete so long as the child must passively wait till the distant impressions meet its eye (or ear). The development of ' distant ' space is completed only by the child's active control of it. Its own locomotion helps to serve this end." The emergence of space first completes the delimitation of ego and world. For the processes of delimitation, elimination and omission, of which we have spoken up to this point, may have no relation to space. For every conscious perception—even in the infant—some "space" must be assumed, just as perceptions cannot be thought of without any ego-relation, just as an ego cannot be thought of purely as substratum, as subject, and just as perception without memory could scarcely have any meaning; but these spaces are not space *per se*. Conscious perception is the central focus of all these spaces, and has first of all a fixed relation to the ego (body-ego). But space *per se* is outer space, outside the body, removed from the ego (in *Ich-Ferne*). Internal space is thereby established, even if it is hardly psychically given simultaneously. In this interior space which is bounded by the body surface, everything which is or will become near-ego (*Ich-nah*) is localized. If this space is established, then the phenomena alien to the ego, or thought of as alien to the ego, are pushed out of it. Those phenomena near to the ego coincide with the interior space. In this way the ego comes into the body; everything in the world that is non-ego goes into the outer space. We must assuredly assume that this is a process of long duration. The boundaries are flexible. A phenomenon does not have to belong to the one space for any length of time; it can oscillate from one to the other. And there may be a large group of things which are spaceless for a long time, just as they are also ego-neutral. We have before us the beginnings of the neutral mechanism of projection (Freud). It is throughout analogous to the activity of pushing away, of ejecting. It is this kind of an act; only it is not executed motorially. But the reversed process, unmistakably evident from the observational records, ought to be considered: the analogy to the activity of incorporation, mental incorporation. We are dealing with the beginning of that mental mechanism, identification, which should be discussed in detail in the psycho logy of early childhood.

That all these developments in the order given run their course along hereditary conditioned paths cannot be doubted. But in spite of this we are, in the Psychology of the Infant, justified in inquiring into those motives which appear, to the individual, as causes, demands, inhibitions of the conditioned unwinding. We know them, on the one hand, as libidinal pleasure, on the other hand as disappointments. The problem which occurs here is easily stated: the psychogenesis of the ego and the infant's world can be proven comprehensively by including both instinct groups; it is then to be classified under the theory of energy. But this problem, although easily stated, is very difficult to solve, even if one can allow what was set down merely as tentative, speculative suggestion, mere statements not sufficiently well-founded to be considered as a solution. But I must leave this problem to be dealt with later. What will later be said will be more valuable when it is connected with material of the ego development of later childhood. Conclusions about the ego of the infant are perhaps a little more acceptable—where they touch the most disputable material—when they are based on the expressions of the two to five-year-old children, than when they are put into the mouth of the dumb infant.

THE SIGNIFICANCE OF WEANING

If now after building up a temporary conception of the infant's relation to the world, of its perceptual and " phantasy " life, we try to construct a view of the significance of weaning, we are not so inclined to doubt as we were after the study of the actual weaning process. An important coincidence will lead us to express an hypothesis which allows us to adhere to all that heretofore has been established and conjectured about libido development, and to add new facts and suppositions to it. We saw, on the one hand, that the mother's breast loses its value as a libido object for the child soon after weaning. On the other hand, we saw how almost at the same time the outer-world is set up by ejection against the ego, as the sum-total of " unsubmissive " objects. Both are modifications of libidinal cathexis; both are similarly regulated. The diminution which the libido quantum experiences when the breast becomes a more indifferent object, and the removal from the ego experienced by all those objects which are projected into the outer-world, are both processes which are to be interpreted as reactions which were produced by deprivation and disappointment. It can be easily assumed that the kernel about which the outer-world projection forms is the disappointing breast which is excluded from the body-ego because of the withdrawal of libido from it. The other objects are, figuratively speaking, torn with the banished mother's breast and projected into the outer space. The fact that at this age the mother's breast has not for a long time been an isolated object for the child, but has been a part of the mother, speaks in favour of this extension of projection to other objects which are not so very " unsubmissive "; the mother's image as a whole, therefore, must share the fate that the breast experiences, which was originally intended for the breast.

This assumption is intended merely as an hypothesis. Should it, however, attain its purpose of inducing new observations, it will still be necessary to make it more attractive by further support. One objection is already at hand. How does the matter stand among those people who wean late? Where are the results corresponding to their *world-image* (*Weltbild*) to be seen? We know nothing about this as yet, and, therefore, this objection has little weight; it must first produce evidence. But even our limited information extends far enough to gain an argument for the view presented. Actually the cultured European and American civilized races, who wean early, are in contrast to all others unique in this respect. No other nations have so well-defined a sense of reality, an external world so sharply distinguished from the ego as have those nations under the present-day capitalistic régime. The test of reality, as Freud says, the close distinction between actuality and phantasy, is one of civilization's most imperious demands; deficiency in the " test of reality " indicates a neurotic person; he is thus, by this word neurotic, considered as being not completely adjusted to the demands of his time. And the trend of this civilization inclines toward rationalization and the elimination of magic animistic thinking and acting. Although the Laplanders and the Chinese are such different races and have such different cultures, nevertheless, compared with the Europeans and Americans, their *world-image* contains rationalizations essentially not as advanced as those of the Europeans and Americans, their sense of reality is less sharply outlined. The probability, it seems to me, cannot be rejected off-hand, that the early date of weaning and the sudden method of weaning are the starting-points, the first impetus to development which finally leads to the already named characteristics of the *world-image*, by the fact that marking off body-ego from *outer-world* among these peoples takes place early, energetically, definitely and severely. Of course this one factor can determine only a portion of development; it can be perchance its impetus, but not more. I shall not pass over in silence the fact that the peoples listed with the Europeans in the weaning tabulation (p. 248) are exceptions to this discussion. Perhaps future investigations, among those peoples particularly, will uncover actual facts corresponding to our problematical assumptions.

The fact that no one, as far as I know, remembers the time when he still imbibed at the mother's breast is very surprising, and at first sight a weighty argument against the after effects of weaning. Authors such as Spitteler, Stifter, Tolstoy (*Ossipou*), and Jean Paul (2) who have recorded reminiscences from the first year, do not mention taking nourishment preceding weaning. Tolstoy thinks this is very remarkable in his own case: " It is singular and shocking to think that no matter how I search my memory I can find not one single impression besides . . . (two recollections) . . . for the period from my birth to the age of three years in which I suckled the breast, in which I was weaned, began to crawl, walk, and began to speak. When did I begin ? . . . Was I not alive then . . . as I slept, suckled, kissed the breast, and laughed and delighted my mother ? I lived and lived happily (*Ossipov*).

But this hiatus in memory is by no means an objection, for we know that earliest childhood as a whole and also the moments most significant for its later development and its experience of this time sink almost completely into amnesia. And thus this frustration at the breast as an instinctual aim is very soon forgotten. This forgetting makes the " overcoming " of the frustration and applying the libido to other aims easier. But, according to our conception, this is not a question of ordinary forgetting. The nutritional instinct from the beginning learned to desire the breast as the means of its gratification. Similarly from the first weeks of life the libidinal strivings of the oral zone have been bound in no small measure to this object. The breast was desired and enjoyed for months. A very strong tie must have been formed between the wishes which originated at the oral zone and the breast which gratified them. And the hallucinatory, reproductive image of the breast must have become equipped to react to the oral wish. This bond must be resolved, if the frustrating, disappointing object is to cease to be the instinctual aim, is to cease continually to evoke unfulfilled and unrealizable longing. This bond is broken up by the withdrawal of all attention, of cathexis; it is made easier by distinguishing it from the original visual phenomena in the *outer-world*: real breast and imaginary one: memory of the gratifying situation. Memory becomes impossible; it can be reproduced neither by the oral needs and hunger, nor by the sight of the real object. This means that recalling the breast as an instinctual aim, imagining the breast as an instinctual aim, is not merely forgotten but repressed. Of course, the term repression which is borrowed from the developed state of the adult ego is not precisely applicable here. Nevertheless, its essential properties exist in these processes which concern us, and the detailed study of repression must be reserved for another connection.

That a process which we must call repression takes place during weaning is concluded from the fact that the psychoanalysis of healthy and sick people can prove in numerous cases that the forgotten situation is retained in the unconscious, that it impels toward consciousness and passes through the process of becoming conscious, passes through memory in various distorted forms, in dreams, phantasies, activities and symptoms, which of course, without analysis are unknown to the ego. Freud (15) has made this very plausible in the example of the famous reminiscences of Leonarda da Vinci. It reads: " It comes to my mind as a very early memory when I was still in the cradle, a vulture came down to me, opened my mouth with his tail and struck many times with his tail against my lips." The deepest level of this memory or phantasy is certainly a distorted return of repressed suckling experiences. Perhaps this is similarly valid for Jean Paul's only early memory: "I am able to my great ioy to draw out of my twelfth month—at most my fourteenth month—a little, faint memory which is at the same time the first spiritual flowering of the snowdrop from the dark earth of childhood. I also recall that a poor scholar liked me very much and I him, and that he held me in his arms—which is pleasanter than to be held in the lap as one is later—and that this resident pupil gave me milk to drink in a big black room. His distant, dark image and his love hovered over me in later years" (Jean Paul, 2).

A glimmer of a recollection of the weaning period is perhaps to be found in Stifter's lines. Stifter's recollections are little known, but they coincide in important points with the opinion presented here, and I quote them in detail as far as they relate to the earliest period. They are certainly no more direct than are all the other earlier memories or documents, but they show that the emphatic poet, creating on the residue of actual memory and the "return of the repressed," attains results similar to those of developmental psychology. He cites the following as a primal memory: " Far back in the empty ' nothingness ' is something like bliss and ecstasy, that penetrated into my being, holding me powerfully, almost destroying me, and which can compare with nothing in my later life. The features which were retained are: it was brilliancy, it was tumult, it was below. This must have happened very early, for it seems to me that a high, wide darkness of *Nothingness* encircles the *thing*. Then there was something else that gently and lingeringly permeated my inner being. And the sign of it is that there were chimes. Then I swam in something flat, I swam back and forth, it was softer in me; then I was as if drunk, then there was nothing more." The following points were ever more distinct, ringing of bells, a broad sheen, a red dawn. Something which was being repeated was very clear. A voice that spoke to me, eyes that looked at me, arms that eased everything. I cry for these things. Then came wretchedness, the insufferable, then sweetness and tranquillity. I remember efforts which attained nothing, and the ceasing of the horrible and destructive. I recall a brightness and colours which were in my eyes; I remember tones in my ears, graciousness in my being. I felt the eyes that gazed on me and the tones that assuaged everything evermore. I remember that I called it ' Mam.' I felt these arms carry me once. There were dark spots in me. My memory later tells me that they were woods which were outside of me. Then there was a sensation like the very first one of my life, bliss and ecstasy, then nothing more. After this sensation there is again a large gap. States that were must have been forgotten. Thereupon the outer-world arose before me, which hitherto must have been perceived only as sensations. Even ' Mam,' eyes, voice, and arms were merely sensations in me, indeed the woods too, as I have just said above. . . . ' Mam,' whom I now call Mother, stood as a form before me and I here distinguish movements, then father, grandfather, grandmother, and aunt. I call them by name, receive love from them, but can recall no difference in their forms."

Perhaps we can justly substitute weaning in that " large gap."

What happens to the bottle-fed baby ? The question deserves, in view of the deficiency of conclusive observational material, at least short consideration. It is freely admitted that in the various relations between feeding by breast and by bottle considerable differences may exist—as far as weaning is concerned there is scarcely any essential difference. For the infant who from birth or from the first weeks of life gets a bottle instead of the breast must be weaned, that is, in place of the loved bottle-nourishment it receives food, which must be chewed, the solidity and method of feeding of which do not correspond to its erstwhile instinctual aims. To the infant the milk bottle becomes a part of the mother; when the milk bottle disappointed it the mother disappointed it, just as the breast and the mother disappointing the breast-child. It is compelled to change its instinctual aim, and this is made possible by repression and projection. In those children who receive their nourishment from a bottle given to them by so many different people that they do not learn to recognize the mother (nurse) and source of milk, bottle, as a coherent whole loved object, the process is essentially changed. Infants who are brought up in institutions can be cited as instances. We may expect that a study of these institution infants will teach us interesting facts about which we as yet know nothing specifically. It is well known that the name institutionalism generally implies that children so brought up are usually not desirable, that they develop differently from others.

Accordingly, weaning is to be considered as a very significant frustration which applies to the oral group of the sexual instincts, and to which the child reacts, after a short rebellion of rage and defiance by withdrawing the libido from the disappointing object through projection and repression. The frustration is mitigated by the beginning of the desexualization of the oral zone during dentition—connected with the beginning of the processes of repression and projection. The libido withdrawn from the old object is obviously given in part to the new method of feeding, and the new kind of food, but another part is directed as aggression and tenderness toward the mother, who has become an object in the *outer-world*. This is a process which I should like to indicate here, but the understanding of which will perhaps better link up with the consideration of early childhood.

The process of " overcoming " the frustration is for all that, however, not concluded. The disappointment which the child experiences because of the frustration is an injury to, and a weakening of, its ego, a blow to, and a very considerable curtailment of, its narcissistic omnipotence. After weaning, however, we see the child's ego considerably grown, not only because it stands over against the *outer-world* more sharply delineated, but also because the ego has gained supremacy over the whole body; the legs have become submissive, the child can move about in space in the service of the strivings for mastery as an entity; it has finally, by overcoming the anxiety of walking along, of walking without a breast-stomach-support, undertaken a decided release from the mother's body, from the proximity to the mother; has freed itself from the fœtal situation during its waking period as completely as an adult has, and thus to a considerable degree consummated an adaptation to the post-fœtal biosphere. This development, setting in toward the end of the first year, has become to some extent intelligible to us from the impulse toward mastery, from the desexualization of the legs, from the supplying of freed libido to the ego and its great increase in power. The transformation of that anxiety into pleasure-in-walking and pride, its binding into spontaneous rhythmical articulation in walking, the transference of libido which belonged to mother to " space," has clarified some details.

But we can consider the same process from the point of view of weaning, and then perhaps we may attain an understanding for the first time of another phase of it. A part of the libido, drawn from the object, breast-mother, seems to be used for identification. Disappointment follows sorrow; it may be short, and, as the first sorrow that befalls man, not yet deep and still obscure, may be free of all prolonged and painful complications which are acquired later. But in principle this, too, will have the same work of sorrow to do as all sorrows that follow (Freud, 7). Sorrow changes the outer deprivation into an inner gain, the lost object is irrevocably erected in its own ego by identification with it. The child treats its mother and the many objects of its interest— its toys, for example—as it itself is treated; the loss, the deprivation which it passively experienced through an outer force it now disperses by turning away, walking away, throwing away, and, indeed, by actively using force to a certain degree. What it once experienced as a prolonged privation (*Entzug*), it now practises in numerous repetitions. Here, too, we can see indications of this repetition in the game of throwing things away, perhaps prepared for some months by teething and perhaps also by the steady rhythm of the mother's coming and going, hunger and satisfaction, yearning and gratification.

Until more conscientious investigation is undertaken, it cannot be decided what is the relation between the following developmental directions: the strengthening of the ego, which is indicated by walking, and the strengthening of the ego which is the result of the first sorrow mechanism. Both of these coincide approximately in time in the forms of child-rearing dominant at present in cultured European and American circles. If a definite answer is to be hazarded, weaning might be called the releasing factor; nevertheless, it seems as if it need not be so under all circumstances, but as if the relations under other forms of rearing were reversed. The coincidence will lead to a reinforcement of the results; from that unyielding delimitation of reality a stronger ego will also result. The early, sudden frustration at the important time, and the end of the first year of life, prepared in many ways for such an ingress, would offer the possibility, so it seems, for the unfolding of an energetic ego. On the other hand, this energetic form of frustration often has traumatic effects: the overcoming is not successful and leaves behind a disposition for various faulty developments. To discuss these in this book is not my task. It must suffice to indicate the fixation points and to stress the fact that from these faulty developments which are rightly so called emanate not only striking deviations of the further development from the normal, and what we call normal, but also those many numerous nuances which are within the realm of the normal and are spoken of as individual differences. One can, therefore, speak metaphorically of the trauma of weaning. By this, however, nothing more is meant than a frustration, which includes injuries of all kinds as possible dangers. Weaning is not a trauma in the sense that the defence mechanisms have been broken through and that the psychic apparatus has been flooded with energy from the *outer-world*, as we understand it in the expression, " Trauma of Birth." The latter is a term applied to the theory of " psychic energy "; the former would be a term stressing the frustration-character, and thus is a term applied to the theory of instincts.

But, bearing this difference in mind, the expression, "Trauma of Weaning " (Stärke), serves to call our attention to two relations which unite birth and weaning. First: the mechanisms which overcome the trauma and the frustration are the same; the former, however, is enacted on a quantity of psychic energy, the latter on instincts and *faculties*: the fractional, rhythmic repetition, transformed from passivity into activity, running its course on a portion of psychic energy instead of on a considerable quantum (*i.e.*, on isolated instinctual impulses rather than on the instinct as a whole). Secondly: birth and weaning are the crises of the biological, psychical, and social development of the individual, determined from without, which assign to the individual definite tasks, the fulfilment of which means approaching the development of one's self, and approaching the adult state to a considerable extent. Hence, the period of development which the infant has come through can be formally designated as: "*from the trauma of birth to the trauma of weaning.*"

BIBLIOGRAPHY

ABRAHAM, K., *Versuch einer Entwicklungsgeschichte der Libido*, 1924.

ALLERS, R.,." Psychologie des Geschlechtslebens," G. Kafka, *Handbuch d. vergl. Psychol.*, 1922.

BALDWIN, J. M., *Mental Development in the Child and Race.*

BLEULER, E., *Naturgeschichte der Seele und ihres Bewusstwerdens*, 1921.

BERNFELD, S., " Die Psychoanalyse in der Jugendforschung," Bernfeld, *Vom Gemeinschaftsleben der Jugend*, 1922.

BIEDERT, Ph., *Die Kinderernährung im Säuglingsalter*, 1900.

BREHMS, *Tierleben*, Bd. i, 1893.

BÜCHNER, M., *Die Entwicklung der Gemütsbewegungen im ersten Lebensjahr*, 1909.

BÜHLER, K., *Die geistige Entwicklung des Kindes*, 1921.

CANESTRINI, S., *Über das Sinnesleben des Neugeborenen*, 1913.

CLAPARÈDE, E., (1) " Esquisse d'une Théorie biologique du Sommeil," *Archives de Psychologie*, iv, 1905.
(2) *Psychologie de l'Enfant*, 1922.

CLARETIE, L., *Les Jouets* (Maison Quantin, Paris).

COMPAIRÉ, G., *Die Entwicklung der Kindesseele*, 1900.

CRAMAUSSEL, E., " Le Sommeil d'un petit Enfant," *Archives de Psychologie*, x-xii, 1910-12.

D'ALLEMAGNE, H. R., *Histoire des Jouets* (Chez l'Auteur, Paris).

DARWIN, Ch., (1) *The Expression of Emotions in Man and Animal*, 1872.
(2) " A Biographical Sketch of an Infant," *Mind*, ii, 1877.

DEKKER, H., *Naturgeschichte des Kindes*, Frankh. Stuttgart, 21 Aufl.

DEUTSCH, F., " Die Psychoanalyse am Krankenbett," Kongressbericht, *Intern. Zeitschr. f. Psychoanalyse*, x, 1924.

DIX, K. W., *Körperliche und geistige Entwicklung eines Kindes*, 4 Hefte, 1911-13.

DYROFF, A., *Über das Seelenleben des Kindes*, 1911.

EISLER, M. J., " Über Schlaflust und gestörte Schlaffähigkeit," *Intern. Zeitschr. f. Psychoanalyse*, vii, 1921.

FELDMAN, W. M., *The Jewish Child*, London, 1917.

FERENCZI, S., (1) " Entwicklungsstufen des Wirklichkeitssines," *Intern. Zeitschr. f. ärztl. Psychoanalyse*, i, 1913.
(2) *Versuch einer Genitaltheorie*, 1924.

FRANKE, E., *Die geistige Entwicklung der Negerkinder*, 1915.

FREILING, H., " Über die räumlichen Wahrnehmungen der Jugendlichen," *Zeitschr. f. Sinnesphysiol.*, Bd. 55.

FREUD, S., (1) *Interpretation of Dreams*, 1913.
(2) *Three Contributions to Sexual Theory*, 1924.
(3) " On the Transformation of Instincts with Special Reference to Anal Erotism," *Collected Papers*, vol. ii.

(4) " Formulations Regarding the Two Principles in Mental
    Functioning," *Collected Papers*, vol. iv.
(5) " A Note on the Unconscious in Psycho-Analysis," *Collected
    Papers*, vol. iv.
(6) " The Unconscious," *Collected Papers*, vol. iv.
(7) " Mourning and Melancholia," *Collected Papers*, vol. iv.
(8) " Narcissism: An Introduction," *Collected Papers*, vol. iv.
(9) *Beyond the Pleasure Principle*, 1922.
(10) *The Ego and the Id.*, 1927.
(11) *A General Introduction to Psycho-Analysis*, 1920.
(12) *Totem and Taboo*.
(13) *Wit and the Unconscious*, 1917.
(14) " Notes upon a Case of Obsessional Neuroses," *Collected
    Papers*, vol. iii.
(15) *Leonardo da Vinci—A Psychosexual Study of an Infantile
    Reminiscence*.

FRIEDENTHAL, H., *Allgemeine und spezielle Physiologie des Menschen-
    wachtstums*, 1914.

FRIEDJUNG, J. K., (1) *Erlebte Kinderheilkunde*, 1919.
    (2) " Beobachtungen über kindliche Onanie," *Zeitschr. f.
    Kinderheilk.*, iv, 1912.
    (3) *Die kindliche Sexualität*, 1923.

GALANTH, " Das Lutscherli," *Neurol. Zentralbl.*, 1919.

GARLEY, D., " Der Schock des Geborenwerdens," *Intern. Zeitschr. f.
    Psychoanalyse*, x, 1924.

GAUPP, *Psychologie des Kindes* (Aus Natur und Geisteswelt, nr. 213).

GENZMER, *Untersuchungen über die Sinneswahrnehmungen der neuge-
    borenen Menschen*, 1873.

GOERGES, Th., *Das Kind im ersten Lebensjahr*, Ullstein, Berlin.

GROOS, K., (1) *The Play of Man*.
    (2) *Das Seelenleben des Kindes*, 1913.

HEILIG, G., *Die sinnlichen Gefühle des Menschen*, 1919.

HERZ, " Einige Bemerkungen über das Saugen des Kindes," *Jahrb. f.
    Kinderheilk.*, vii, 1865.

HOCHSINGER, " Über Ernährungsneurosen im frühen Kindesalter,"
    Berl. klin. Wochenschr., 1910.

HOVORKA, O., und KRONFELD, A., *Vergleichende Volksmedizin*, 2 Bde.,
    1908-9.

HUFELAND, Ch. W., *Guter Rath an Mutter über die wichtigsten Punkte
    der physischen Erziehung des Kindes*, 1903.

HUG-HELLMUTH, H., *Aus dem Seelenleben des Kindes*, 1921.

ISCHIKAWA, T., *Beobachtungen über die geistige Entwicklung eines
    Kindes in seinem ersten Lebensjahr*, 1910.

JAENSCH, E. R., *Über den Aufbau der Wahrnehmungswelt*, 1923.

JUNGKEN, J. H., *Wohlunterrichtender sorgfältiger Medicus*, 1729.

KEMPF, E. J., *Psychopathology*, New York and London, 1921.

KEY, A., *Schulhygienische Untersuchungen*, 1889.

KIRKPATRICNK, E. A., *Fundamentals of Child Study*, 1916.

KOFFKA, KURT, *The Growth of the Mind : An Introduction to Child-
    Psychology* (International Library of Psychology).

KÖHLER, W., *The Mentality of Apes*, 1927 (International Library of
    Psychology).

KRAUSS, F. S., " Folkloristisches von der Mutterschaft," Schreiber, *Mutterschaft.*

KROH, O., *Subjektive Anschauungsbilder bei Jugendlichen,* 1922.

KRUEGER, F., *Über Entwicklungspyschologie,* 1915.

KUSSMAUL, *Untersuchungen über das Seelenleben des neugeborenen Menschen,* 1859.

LEHMANN, *Hauptgesetze des menschlichen Gefühlsleben,* 1892.

LINDNER, S., " Uber das Saugen an den Fingern, Lippen, usw., bei den Kindern (Ludeln)," *Jahrb. f. Kinderheilk.,* xiv, 1879.

MITCHELL, Chalmers, *The Childhood of Animals,* 1912.

MOLL, A., *The Sexual Life of the Child,* 1924.

MORO, E., " Das erste Trimenon," *Münch. med. Wochenschr.,* 1918.

MÜLLERHEIM, R., *Die Wochenstube in der Kunst,* 1904.

OFFNER, M., *Das Gedächtnis,* 1913.

OSSIPOW, N., *Tolstois Kindheitserinnerungen,* 1923.

PAUL, Jean, (1) *Levana; or, The Doctrine of Education,* Boston, 1863.
(2) *Meine Kindheit,* 1921.

PEREZ, B., *Die Anfänge des kindlichen Seelenlebens,* 1902.

PLOSS, H., (1) — Bartels, *Das Weib in der Natur- und Volkerkunde,* 2 Bde., 1895.
(2) Renz, *Das Kind in Brauch und Sitte der Völker,* 2 Bde., 1911-12.

POPPER, E., " Studien über Saugphänomene," *Archiv f. Psychiatrie,* Bd. 63, 1921.

PREYER, W., *The Mind of the Child,* 1884.

QUECK-WILKER, H., *Ein erstes Lebensjahr.,* 1912.

RANK, O., *The Trauma of Birth,* 1929 (International Library of Psychology).

REIK, Th., *Probleme der Religionspsychologie,* 1919.

REUSS, A. v., " Über transitorisches Fieber bei Neugeborenen," *Zeitschr. f. Kinderheilk.,* iv, 1912.

RÜHLE, O., *Das proletarische Kind.,* 1922.

SADGER, J., " Haut-, Schleimhaut- und Muskelerotik," *Jahrb. f. psychoanalytische Forschungen,* iii, 1912.

SANCTIS, S. de, *Psychologie des Traums,* Kafka, " Handbuch d. vergl. Psychol.," III Bd., 1922.

SCHILDER, P., (1) " Über den Wirkungswert psychischer Erlebnisse," *Archiv f. Psychiatrie u. Nervenkrankh.,* Bd. 70, 1923.
(2) *Das Körperschema,* 1923.
(3) *Medizinische Psychologie,* 1924.

SCUPIN, G. u. E., *Bubis' erste Kindheit,* 1907.

SHINN, M. W., *Notes on the Development of a Child,* 2 vols., 1907, 1909.

SIGISMUND, B., *Kind und Welt,* Ausgewählt Schriften, 1900.

SIKORSKY, J. A., *Die seelische Entwicklung des Kindes,* 1908.

SPITTELER, C., *Meine frühesten Erlebnisse,* 1914.

SPRANGER, E., *Psychologie des Jugendalters,* 1924.

STÄRKE, A., " Der Kastrationskomplex," *Intern. Zeitschr. f. Psychoanalyse,* vii, 1921.

STERN, L. William, (1) *Psychology of Early Childhood up to Sixth Year of Age,* 1924.

20

(2) " Die Entwicklung der Raumwahrnehmung in der ersten
     Kindheit.," *Zeitschr. f. angew. Psychologie*, Bd. 2, 1909.
(3) " Die Anwendung der Psychoanalyse auf Kinder und Jugend-
     liche," *Zeitschr. f. angew. Psychologie*, Bd. 8, 1913.

STIFTER, A., *Selbstbiographie, Betrachtungen und Bilder* (Amalthea-Verlag,
     Leipzig).

SULLY, J., (1) " Extract from a Father's Diary," *Studies of Childhood*,
          1896.
     (2) " The Psychology of Tickling," IV Congrès Intern. de Psycho-
          logie, 1901.

TRACY, F., *The Psychology of Childhood*, Boston, 1894.

TRÖMNER, " Zur Biologie und Psychologie des Schlafes, "*Klin. Wochen-
     schrift*, 1910.

VIERORDT, K., " Physiologie des Kindesalters," Gerhardt, *Handbuch
     d. Kinderkrankheiten*, I Bd., 1877.

VOLKELT, J., *Uber die Vorstellungen der Tiere*, 1914.

WATSON, J. B., *Psychology from the Standpoint of a Behaviorist*, 1911.

WEBER, M., *Grundriss der Sozialokonomik*, III Teil, 1922.

INDEX

ACTIVITIES:
defence, 58, 93, 276, 278
desire 275
offence, 58, 93, 64
tenderness, 205, 206, 241
warding off. *See* Defence,
resisting
Altruism, 204
Ambivalence, 209
Anal zone, 36, 146, 194, 276
Anger, 242, 274
Anxiety, 113, 134, 141, 142, 172,
· 206
primal, 216
state, 13, 215
Appetite, 188
Attention, 41, 48, 84, 85, 90, 92

Birth, 1, 17, 22, 24, 34, 40, 59,
111, 134, 211, 301
Biting, 240, 276
Body-ego, 261
Breathing, 1, 13, 20, 35, 40, 64,
113, 215

Cathexis:
counter, 92
energy, 92, 115, 131, 140,
173, 219, 226
Chewing, 240
Climbing, 154
Complexity, 284
Compulsion, repetition, 72, 102,
175, 218
Concept, 288
Consciousness, 16, 29, 32, 187,
268, 269, 283, 287
Couvade, 8
Creeping, 154, 167, 170
Crying, 19, 34, 51, 69, 103, 238,
246, 279

Death instinct, 98, 242
Defence:
actions, 278
See Activities
attitude, 275
resisting, 277
Defiance, 280

Dentition, 171, 178, 228
Desexualization, 173, 239
Differences:
consequences, 214
individual, 74, 75
vicissitudes, 225
Disappointment, 131, 239, 273, 290
Discharge:
See Movements
phenomena, 67, 68, 69, 92,
162, 149, 159, 172, 219
Dresseur, 7, 166, 170

Ego, 69, 177, 192, 239, 263, 273,
274
I, 137
body. *See* Body-ego
intellectual-ego, 290
instincts, 100
omnipotence of, 282
Egotism, 204
Energy:
cathectic. *See* Cathexis
katergic. *See* Katergy
psychic, 33, 52, 62, 71, 115,
144, 172, 244
Expressive:
-gesture, 19, 22, 50, 51, 52, 91,
216
-movements, 51, 52
External. *See* World

Fatigue, 277
Fear, 135, 274
Feeling:
of familiarity, 132, 135
of self-regard, 191, 280
Fever, 240
Fœtus, fœtal situation, 1, 20, 28,
46, 61, 137, 145, 150, 161, 222
Fright, 42, 45, 83, 91, 102, 136
Fusion. *See* Instincts

Gain:
mental, 67
psychic, 163
Genital zone, 35, 194
Gestalt psychology, 59, 121, 123,
146, 168

Gorging instinct. *See* Nutritional instinct
Grasping, 151, 168, 170, 178, 181, 205
-reflex, 152, 180

Habit, 75, 245
Hallucination, 129, 136, 288
Hate, 240
Hearing, 1, 40, 46, 83, 179, 180, 205
Hunger, 11, 19, 20, 21, 22, 25, 34, 73, 130, 135, 188, 238

Identification, 257, 259, 299
Image, palpable, 288
Infant:
   feeding, 6, 247
   mortality, 7, 8, 9
   protection, 8
   rearing, racial superstitions of, 2, 18, 80, 148, 155, 158, 230, 247, 248
Initiation rites, 8, 236
Instinct:
   death. *See* Death
   ego. *See* Ego
   fusion of, 208
   mastery. *See* Mastery
   nutritional, 27, 28, 34, 38, 58, 62, 77, 94, 130, 186, 290, 295
   pleasure, 38
   R =instincts, 101, 136, 140, 162, 175, 192, 238, 285
   reproductive, 27
   self-preservative, 26, 27, 96
   sexual. *See* Sexual.
Intellectual. *See* Ego
Interest, 70, 135, 183

Joy, 65, 68, 160, 190, 282

Katergy, 143, 209, 242

Laughing, 51, 68, 102
Libido, 90, 121, 136, 137, 139, 172, 193, 242
   object, 202, 208
   organ, 144, 221
Locomotion, 149, 165
Longing, 257, 259
Love, 203

Magic, 282
Masochism, 243
Mastery, 95, 137, 149, 240
Masturbation, 194

Memory, 38, 64, 128, 130
Movement:
   discharge, 48, 67
   impulsive, 48, 149
   -melody, 173
   -towards, 64

Narcissism, 139, 141, 202, 278
Neurosis, nutritional, 258
New-born, 1, 68, 77, 118, 138, 150
Nutrition. *See* Nutritional instinct

Object. *See* Libido
Offence. *See* Activity
Olfaction. *See* Smell, sense of
Oral zone, 37, 47, 72, 140, 184, 230, 239
Organ. *See* Libido

Pain, 36, 92, 114, 117, 238, 243, 265
Perception, 121, 283
Play, 119, 193, 260
   -toys, 147
Pleasure:
   kinæsthetic, 151, 153
   " pain," 35, 97, 166, 172, 217
   tactual pleasure, 77, 89
Possession, 137
   See Mastery instinct
Pride, 190
Privation. *See* Disappointment
Projection, 242, 244, 292, 293
Psychology:
   gestalt. *See* Gestalt
   theoretical, 117
Pushing, 276

Reaction type, Rt., 1, 11, 53, 66, 85, 86, 111, 275
Reality, test of, 294
Reflexes, 48, 55
Repetition. *See* Compulsion
Repression, 77, 130, 244, 259
Resisting, defence, 277
Rhythm, 87, 118, 152, 226, 260

Sadism, 242
Seeing, 2, 42, 63, 187, 188
Sense of hearing. *See* Hearing
   sight. *See* Seeing
   smell, 1, 39, 45, 180
   taste, 38
   touch, 2, 35, 89
   See Pleasure, tactual
Sexual instincts, 27, 79, 98, 137, 139, 151, 169, 186, 192, 201, 239, 262, 286

Shock-reaction, 41, 83, 174
Sitting, 154, 170
Sleep, 11, 27, 28, 34, 74, 100, 135, 206, 277
Society, 60, 108, 147, 286
Sorrow, 257, 259, 280
Space, 223, 292
Speaking, 227, 239, 243, 255
Spontaneity, 175, 226, 260
Standing, 159, 167
Sucking, 24, 34, 37, 47, 66, 72, 133, 178, 227, 245
Suffering, 104

Tactual. *See* Pleasure
Talking. *See* Speaking

Teething, 171, 178, 228
Tickling, 120, 194
Touch. *See* Sense of

Value, 52, 177, 206, 208
Vernix caseosa, 2
Vexation, 274, 280, 281

Walking, 137, 159, 222, 227, 255
Weaning, 171, 178, 225, 226, 245, 293
Weeping, 102
Work, 156
    effort, 191
World, outer, 125, 130, 201, 238, 261